P9-AGT-112

THE NEW WORLD OF
HEALTH PROMOTION

New Program Development, Implementation, and Evaluation

EDITED BY

Bernard J. Healey, PhD
Professor, Health Care Administration
King's College
Wilkes-Barre, PA

Robert S. Zimmerman Jr., MPH
Former Pennsylvania Secretary of Health
Adjunct Professor, Health Care Administration
King's College
Wilkes-Barre, PA

JONES AND BARTLETT PUBLISHERS
Sudbury, Massachusetts
BOSTON   TORONTO   LONDON   SINGAPORE

World Headquarters

Jones and Bartlett Publishers
40 Tall Pine Drive
Sudbury, MA 01776
978-443-5000
info@jbpub.com
www.jbpub.com

Jones and Bartlett Publishers Canada
6339 Ormindale Way
Mississauga, Ontario L5V 1J2
Canada

Jones and Bartlett Publishers International
Barb House, Barb Mews
London W6 7PA
United Kingdom

Jones and Bartlett's books and products are available through most bookstores and online booksellers. To contact Jones and Bartlett Publishers directly, call 800-832-0034, fax 978-443-8000, or visit our website www.jbpub.com.

Substantial discounts on bulk quantities of Jones and Bartlett's publications are available to corporations, professional associations, and other qualified organizations. For details and specific discount information, contact the special sales department at Jones and Bartlett via the above contact information or send an email to specialsales@jbpub.com.

This publication is designed to provide accurate and authoritative information in regard to the Subject Matter covered. It is sold with the understanding that the publisher is not engaged in rendering legal, accounting, or other professional service. If legal advice or other expert assistance is required, the service of a competent professional person should be sought.

Production Credits

Acquisitions Editor: Shoshanna Goldberg
Senior Associate Editor: Amy L. Bloom
Editorial Assistant: Kyle Hoover
Production Assistant: Jill Morton
Associate Marketing Manager: Jody Sullivan
V.P., Manufacturing and Inventory Control: Therese Connell

Composition: Arlene Apone
Cover Design: Kristin E. Parker
Cover and Title Page Images: © Katarzyna Malecka/ShutterStock, Inc.
Printing and Binding: Malloy Incorporated
Cover Printing: Malloy Incorporated

Library of Congress Cataloging-in-Publication Data

Healey, Bernard J., 1947-
  The new world of health promotion: new program development, implementation, and evaluation / by Bernard J. Healey and Robert S. Zimmerman Jr.
      p. ; cm.
  Includes bibliographical references and index.
  ISBN-13: 978-0-7637-5377-1
  ISBN-10: 0-7637-5377-7
  1. Health promotion. I. Zimmerman, Robert S. II. Title.
  [DNLM: 1. Health Promotion—organization & administration—United States. 2. Epidemiologic Methods—United States. 3. Health Education—methods—United States. 4. Health Planning—methods—United States. 5. Program Development—United States. 6. Program Evaluation—United States. WA 525 H4336n 2010]
  RA427.8.H427 2010
  362.1068—dc22
                        2009014464

6048

Printed in the United States of America
13 12 11 10 09   10 9 8 7 6 5 4 3 2 1

Dedication

To Kathy, my wife of 37 years, my two wonderful children, Alison and Bryan, and my new grandson, John.

Bernard Healey

To Jean, my lovely wife of 39 years, our dear children, Wendy and Steven, their spouses, Steve and Brooke, and our precious granddaughters, Tyler Rose and Bradley Grace.

Bob Zimmerman

Contents

Chapter 2: Epidemiology as the Catalyst in the Development of Health Promotion Programs   23

Bernard J. Healey, PhD
Robert S. Zimmerman Jr., MPH

Chapter 3: Needs Assessment   41

Bernard J. Healey, PhD
Robert S. Zimmerman Jr., MPH

Chapter 4: Program Development   57

Bernard J. Healey, PhD
Robert S. Zimmerman Jr., MPH

Chapter 5: Health Promotion Program Marketing Techniques   73

Bernard J. Healey, PhD
Robert S. Zimmerman Jr., MPH

Chapter 6: Program Evaluation   89

■ PART II: EMERGING PRIORITIES IN HEALTH PROMOTION PROGRAMS

Chapter 7: Health Promotion in People with Disabilities   107

Chapter 8: Health Promotion Programs in the Workplace   **139**

Chapter 9: Toward Health Equity: A Prevention Framework for Reducing Health and Safety Disparities   **163**

Chapter 10: The truth® Campaign: Using Countermarketing to Reduce Youth Smoking   195

Jane A. Allen, MA
Donna Vallone, PhD, MPH
Ellen Vargyas, JD
Cheryl G. Healton, DrPH
American Legacy Foundation

Chapter 11: Case Study of a Data Informed Response to Youth Gun Violence: Pennsylvania Injury Reporting and Intervention System (PIRIS)   217

Michelle R. Henry, BA
Robert D. Ketterlinus, PhD

Chapter 15: Partnerships and Collaboration: Critical Components to Promoting Health   283

Chapter 16: Economic Evaluation of Health Promotion Programs   313

Chapter 17: MAPP: A Strategic Approach to Community Health Improvement   329

Julia Joh Elligers, MPH

Appendix A: Health Promotion and Health Education Resources for Health Educators and Health Promotion Specialists   359

Appendix B: Case Studies of Successful Workplace Wellness Programs   367

Appendix C: Partnership Steps Checklists   373

Appendix D: MAPP Case Studies   379

Foreword

As the wealthiest nation on earth, it is a travesty that we are also not the healthiest. We spend far more on health care than all other countries, yet we consistently underperform on such key health indicators as healthy life expectancy, infant mortality, and many others. The rising costs of health care delivery, the tens of millions of uninsured or underinsured Americans, the widespread high-risk health behaviors, and the epidemic of chronic diseases in this country are symptomatic of our wrong-headed approach to achieving health.

As an emergency physician, I came to understand the problem of failing to invest in prevention. Later, as a local and then state health official, I have had the privilege of learning that many of these disease states are preventable and some can be mitigated; quality of life can be improved; health disparities are not inevitable; and wellness can be achieved. We have the evidence for improved outcomes, but far too often we have the way but not the will. Far too often, the focus on individual health obscures the benefits of a more comprehensive approach to health and wellness.

Achieving a healthier nation is within our reach. But we have been going about it the wrong way. We need a more holistic approach; one that puts more emphasis on wellness and prevention rather than focusing primarily on cure.

This book provides many of the answers. It offers a very different approach. It lifts up health promotion activities as a solution to some of the major problems faced by our current health delivery system in this country. Community interventions such as cancer screenings, tobacco cessation programs, and childhood vaccinations are proven to reduce premature death and disability. Workplace wellness programs improve worker health and productivity. Programs for those with disabilities can improve outcomes for those living with specific conditions. This book also provides tools for planning, implementing, and evaluating health promotion programs. Community partnerships, for instance, are often essential in reaching goals.

The authors are well established in the field of public health, having practiced in academic, management, and program settings. They are well trained and experienced and have approached the problem of improving health in a focused way. This text reminds us that the value of health promotion goes beyond improving the health of the individual. It promotes and protects the health of the community as well. It is my hope that this book will stimulate wider use and acceptance of population-based programs. It should be read by those in both practice and academic settings and will be a valuable tool for many practitioners working in the trenches to improve the health of the public.

Georges C. Benjamin, MD, FACP, FACEP (E)
Executive Director, American Public Health Association

Preface

This book was written with one overriding theme. Comprehensive, evidence-based, and cost-effective health promotion strategies, policies, and programs offer the best hope of continuing to increase the longevity, quality of life, and positive contributions of all Americans while reducing health care costs for all Americans, their employers, and governments. The best way to prevent illness, disease, and injuries is to consider all of the influences on health as health promotion initiatives are developed and implemented in future years. The new world of health promotion requires bringing high-risk health behaviors to center stage in our effort to reduce health care costs and to increase access to health care services for all Americans. Health promotion programs work.

It is interesting to note that life expectancy in 1900 was only 49 years of age while life expectancy has now increased by almost 30 years. This increase in life expectancy is not due to better medical care but is due in large part to a better understanding of how disease occurs and how to prevent these diseases. By learning the real causes of disease, health care is starting to change from the concept of cure to the idea of primary care, focusing on prevention of health problems before they occur.

This book is devoted to the development and implementation of health promotion programs that work. This text begins with chapters that discuss the necessary prerequisites of the development of a new health promotion initiative. The focus then shifts to several chapters that explore some of the emerging priorities in health promotion programs. The third part of the text looks at many of the competencies that can help health promotion programs achieve their goals and increase their funding stream.

Throughout this book, the authors looked for health promotion programs that were successful in order to share these success stories with others. We found many examples of success in promoting good health and several concepts that were repeated in each successful initiative. We were very pleased to have attracted several coauthors who have been successful in national efforts to promote a healthy lifestyle. We were also successful in receiving permission from the National Association of County and City Health Officials (NACCHO) to utilize several of their case studies and other resources as part of the text.

This book is unique in that it has chapters devoted to program leadership, continuous quality improvement, developing partnerships, evidence-based programs, and economic evaluation of health promotion programs. These are skills that will be required of the individuals responsible for the success of health promotion programs in this century.

The vision of a healthy America can only become reality if leadership and collaboration by all sectors becomes a reality. Strong community partnerships will ensure that health promotion initiatives are developed, implemented, evaluated, and continuously improved in order to achieve all of the objectives outlined in *Healthy People 2010*. This is the vision offered by this book.

Acknowledgments

We begin by acknowledging the dedicated people who strive to advance the public's health and to accomplish so much despite limited resources. Our combined 70-plus years of public health and health promotion experience has been a privilege because of *those we serve* and *those with whom we serve*. To our readers, we wish you the same life-long privilege and satisfaction.

This health promotion text was a labor of love for both of us in so many ways.

We have had the opportunity to collaborate with talented and caring coauthors and other partners—old and new—to share our collective knowledge, experiences, and ideas. We were also blessed with a wonderful book publisher enabling us to offer a comprehensive addition to the discipline of health promotion.

During the process of writing this book, we have benefited from the work and assistance of many dedicated professionals. We thank our contributors whose excellent work has enriched this text as they have done throughout their distinguished professional lives.

Rose Cheney, Amy Liao, and Douglas J. Wiebe of the University of Pennsylvania

Larry Cohen, Rachel A. Davis, and Lisa Fujie Parks of the Prevention Institute

Julia Joh Elligers of the National Association of County and City Health Officials

Michelle R. Henry and Robert D. Ketterlinus of the Public Health Management Corporation

Andrew Lanza and Sarah Olson of the Centers for Disease Control and Prevention

Donna Vallone of the American Legacy Foundation

We would also like to thank the following individuals and organizations for sharing their ideas and time with us.

Karen Baker, National Sexual Violence Resource Center
Tamar Bauer, Nurse Family Partnership
Ronald David, National Commission on Infant Mortality, Joint Center
    for Political and Economic Studies
Brian Ebersole, Pennsylvania Department of Health
Cheryl Healton, American Legacy Foundation
Secretary Calvin B. Johnson of the Pennsylvania Department of Health
David Olds, University of Colorado School of Medicine
Michele Ridge, Former First Lady of Pennsylvania
Delilah Rumberg, Pennsylvania Coalition Against Rape
Stephen Thomas, University of Pittsburgh Center for Minority Health

Lastly, thank you to the reviewers of this text. Their voices, criticism, and support have truly made this a better text:

John Janowiak, PhD, Professor, Health Education, Appalachian
    State University
Corinne Kyriacou, PhD, MPH, Hofstra University
Jennifer Dearden, EdD, Morehead State University
Tetsuji Yamada, PhD, Rutgers University

The only way to reduce the costs associated with the delivery of health care services in this country is to keep people healthy. We also need to keep those of us with chronic diseases away from the high-risk health behaviors that lead to the many complications that can occur as a result of these diseases. The collective chapters in this book offer the reader the opportunity to gain from the experiences of many individuals who have developed and implemented successful health promotion programs.

About the Authors

Bernard J. Healey, PhD, is a professor of health care administration at King's College in Wilkes-Barre, Pennsylvania. He began his career in 1971 as an epidemiologist for the Pennsylvania Department of Health, retiring from that position in 1995. During his tenure with the government, he completed advanced degrees in business administration and public administration. In 1990, he finished his doctoral work at the University of Pennsylvania. Dr. Healey has been teaching undergraduate and graduate courses in business, public health, and health care administration at several colleges for more than 30 years. He is currently the director of the graduate program in health care administration at King's College in Wilkes-Barre, Pennsylvania.

Dr. Healey has published more than 100 articles about public health, health policy, leadership, marketing, and health care partnerships. He has also written and published two books about leadership in health care and children's high-risk health behaviors.

Dr. Healey is a member of the American Association of Public Health and the Association of University Programs in Health Care Administration. He is a part-time consultant in epidemiology for the Wilkes-Barre city health department and a consultant for numerous public health projects in Pennsylvania.

Robert S. Zimmerman Jr., MPH, is an accomplished leader and public executive in health and human services at the state and national levels, including service as regional director of the U.S. Department of Health and Human Services (DHHS), Pennsylvania's Secretary of Health in the cabinets of both Governors Tom Ridge and Mark S. Schweiker, and as Pennsylvania's deputy secretary of medical assistance programs. He is now an adjunct professor of health care administration at King's College in Wilkes-Barre Pennsylvania, and a consultant in health and human services. He was recently president of Public Health Works, LLC, and also CEO of a nonprofit consulting firm.

At DHHS, Mr. Zimmerman was the secretary's principal representative for DHHS Region 3. He worked on initiatives on Medicare, Medicaid, health disparities, public health preparedness, global health, and diabetes (for which he received the Secretary's Award for Distinguished Service for National Public Health Leadership).

As Pennsylvania's Secretary of Health, Mr. Zimmerman played a key role in developing Pennsylvania's tobacco settlement spending plan—later responsible for implementing a broad health research program and comprehensive tobacco use prevention and cessation programs. His tenure included development of Pennsylvania's first bioterrorism–public health preparedness plan, statewide electronic disease reporting and surveillance systems, and the first rural and minority health plans. Mr. Zimmerman led a major expansion of community health partnerships and improved quality of care oversight and major regulatory reform for health care services–facilities, disease reporting, managed care, and patient safety. He received the First Annual Minority Health Leadership Award from the Center for Minority Health, University of Pittsburgh, and the Exemplary Service Award from the MCP Hahnemann University School of Public Health (now Drexel School of Public Health).

As deputy secretary for medical assistance programs, Mr. Zimmerman led implementation of the Medicaid HealthChoices managed care program, expanded access, improved special needs services, and directed major initiatives in clinical quality management and long-term care.

His earlier career included senior positions in health planning, disease prevention, health promotion, and maternal and child health.

Mr. Zimmerman has a sociology degree from King's College, a masters of public health from the University of Tennessee, and attended Harvard University's Executive Leadership Program for State Health Officials. He was a captain, USAR Medical Service Corps, and before that a sergeant, USAR.

About the Contributors

Jill D. Morrow-Gorton, MD, is a developmental pediatrician serving as the medical director for the Office of Developmental Programs, Department of Public Welfare, Commonwealth of Pennsylvania. She graduated from the University of Pennsylvania School of Medicine and did her pediatric internship and residency at Tufts New England Medical Center at the Boston Floating Hospital. She completed a developmental pediatric fellowship at the St. Louis University at the Knights of Columbus Developmental Center at Cardinal Glennon Children's Hospital. She is board certified in both pediatrics and developmental and behavioral pediatrics. In 2004, she completed a masters of business administration at Lebanon Valley College in Annville, Pennsylvania.

Dr. Morrow provides consultation for children with developmental disorders at Wyoming Valley Children's Association in Wilkes-Barre, Pennsylvania, and is the chair of the Early Childhood Committee for the Pennsylvania chapter of the American Academy of Pediatrics. She also sits on the Health Advisory Committee for the Capital Area Headstart. She previously directed the Child Development Clinic at Polyclinic Hospital in Harrisburg, Pennsylvania, and was on the faculty of Pennsylvania State University Hershey Medical Center as the director of pediatric rehabilitation. She continues to teach child psychiatry residents. In the past, Dr. Morrow has taught pediatric and family practice residents at the Pennsylvania State University Hershey Medical Center and at Polyclinic Hospital and has lectured for medical students at the University of Pennsylvania School of Medicine. She has also provided consultation for Dauphin County Case Management Early Intervention Program. She is the author and coauthor of numerous articles and chapters related to children and adults with developmental disabilities.

Rachel A. Davis, MSW, is managing director at the Prevention Institute, a nonprofit national center dedicated to improving community health and well-being by building momentum for effective primary prevention. Ms. Davis oversees the Institute's work in the areas of health disparities, community health, health care reform, violence prevention, and mental health. She develops tools for advancing primary prevention and provides consulting and training for various community and government organizations. With funding from the Federal Office of Minority Health, Ms. Davis developed and piloted THRIVE, a community resilience assessment tool that helps communities bolster factors that will improve health outcomes and reduce disparities experienced by racial and ethnic minorities. Other projects include coauthoring *Health for All: California's Strategic Approach to Eliminating Racial and Ethnic Health Disparities*, facilitating a statewide interagency violence prevention partnership in California's state government, writing state and county violence plans, and conducting training for federal violence prevention grantees. In addition, Ms. Davis coauthored a report for the California Endowment called *Good Health Counts: A 21st Century*

Approach to Health and Community for California and is the project director of UNITY (Urban Networks to Increase Thriving Youth through Violence Prevention), a national initiative to ensure long-term sustainability of youth violence prevention efforts. With a background in mental health, Ms. Davis has documented the effectiveness of prevention and early intervention approaches for the Center for Mental Health Services, Substance Abuse, and Mental Health Services Administration and conducted training and technical assistance to mental health program staff. She has authored several published articles on health disparities and community health. She worked previously as a school social worker and counselor.

Larry Cohen, MSW, is the founder and executive director of the Prevention Institute, a nonprofit national center dedicated to improving community health and well-being by building momentum for effective primary prevention. He has been an advocate for public health and prevention since 1972. Mr. Cohen's work focuses on local policies that support health and wellness and spur legislation at the state and federal levels. He formed the first coalition in the nation to change tobacco policy; helped catalyze the nation's food labeling law; and helped shape strategy to secure passage of bicycle and motorcycle helmet laws, strengthen child and adult passenger restraint laws, and establish fluoridation requirements in California. Mr. Cohen is the coeditor for *Prevention is Primary: Strategies for Community Well-Being*, an academic text that defines best practices of quality prevention.

Mr. Cohen has authored numerous publications on primary prevention, including a report outlining promising approaches and next steps for reducing health disparities, *The Imperative of Reducing Health Disparities through Prevention*, and *Health for All: California's Strategic Approach to Eliminating Racial and Ethnic Health Disparities*, a report produced with the California Campaign to eliminate racial and ethnic disparities in health on the statewide public–private sector initiative to advance systemic change to improve health outcomes. He was also a major contributor to *Good Health Counts: A 21st Century Approach to Health and Community for California*, which synthesizes findings from nearly 100 community report cards and indicator reports from throughout the country and broadens the understanding of all the elements that contribute to community health.

Mr. Cohen is the recipient of numerous awards, including the American Public Health Association Injury Control, the Emergency Health Services Section Public Service Award, and the Secretary's Award for Health Promotion from the U.S. Department of Health and Human Services, and he has received recognition from the American Cancer Society and the Society for Public Health Educators.

Sharon Rodriguez, BA, works at the Prevention Institute, a nonprofit national center dedicated to improving community health and well-being by building momentum for effective primary prevention. Ms. Rodriguez focuses her efforts on developing training tools and strategies that aim to eliminate health disparities and promote health equity and community health. She has been instrumental in designing and delivering a health disparities training series for grantees of the California Endowment. She also works on Advancing Public Health Advocacy to Eliminate Health Disparities, a national effort to strengthen public health capacity through policy. A key component of this effort is to develop, pilot, and disseminate a web-based tool to provide policy and prevention training to assist public health professionals and local elected and appointed officials in eliminating health disparities and improving health outcomes within their communities.

Prior to joining the Prevention Institute, Ms. Rodriguez worked as a project manager in the Department of Future Initiatives for Planned Parenthood Federation of America where she managed efforts to develop and promote the organization's long-term vision and goals. She graduated from Brown University with a BA in semiotics. While at Brown, she was awarded the Isabelle Scott Bollard Scholarship, a Literary Forum Grant, and a Creative Arts Council Grant. She is also a certified yoga instructor with the Yoga Alliance, a national nonprofit organization that recognizes teachers meeting specified training standards.

Jane A. Allen, MA, is a senior research associate at American Legacy Foundation.

She has been a member of Legacy's Research and Evaluation Department and the truth® Campaign evaluation team since 2000.

Ms. Allen holds a master's degree from the Annenberg School for Communication at the University of Pennsylvania, where her focus was health communication. She has published 11 peer-reviewed articles and numerous reports, the majority of which are related to countermarketing and tobacco use.

Donna Vallone, PhD, MPH, is the senior vice president of Research and Evaluation at the American Legacy Foundation. She oversees Legacy's portfolio of internal, contract, and grant-funded research and evaluation studies. Major studies include the ongoing evaluation of the national truth® Campaign and evaluation of EX, Legacy's cessation program for adult smokers. Dr. Vallone is also leading efforts to establish the National Institute for Tobacco Research and Policy Studies being formed by Legacy in affiliation with Johns Hopkins University School of Public Health.

Some of Dr. Vallone's recent peer-reviewed publications include "How Reliable and Valid is the Brief Sensation Seeking Scale (BSSS-4) for Youth of Various Racial–Ethnic Groups?" (*Addiction*, 2007); "A Closer Look at Smoking Among Young Adults: Where Should Tobacco Control Focus Its Attention?" (*American Journal of Public Health*, 2007); "Women's Knowledge of the Leading Causes of Cancer Death" (*Nicotine and Tobacco Research*, 2007); "Smoking, Obesity, and Their Co-occurrence in the United States: Cross Sectional Analysis" (*British Medical Journal*, 2006); and "Televised Movie Trailers: Undermining Restrictions on Advertising

Tobacco to Youth" (*Archives of Pediatric and Adolescent Medicine*, 2006). Dr. Vallone recently served as coeditor of a special issue of the *Journal of Epidemiology and Community Health*, which focused on tobacco control policy and women of low-socioeconomic status.

Dr. Vallone is a member of several research networks and expert panels that serve the tobacco control community. She is a member of the Tobacco-Related Health Disparities Research Network (TReND) and the Evaluation Task Force for the Tobacco Control Section of the California Department of Health. She serves on the expert panel that guides the evaluation of the Health and Human Services National Network of Tobacco Cessation Quitlines Initiative. Dr. Vallone received her doctoral degree in sociomedical sciences, an interdisciplinary degree combining public health and sociology, from Columbia University.

Ellen Vargyas, JD, is general counsel and corporate secretary for the American Legacy Foundation. Ms. Vargyas has long pursued a career dedicated to the practice of law in the public interest. Before joining the Foundation as general counsel, she served as legal counsel to the U.S. Equal Employment Opportunity Commission (EEOC). At EEOC, she directed the commission's regulatory and policy program under Title VII of the Civil Rights Act of 1964, the Equal Pay Act, the Age Discrimination in Employment Act, and the Americans with Disabilities Act. She was also the commission's in-house counsel.

Additionally, Ms. Vargyas has served as senior counsel for employment and education at the National Women's Law Center in Washington, DC, where she handled precedent-setting Title IX litigation that opened opportunities for women in athletics in educational institutions and developed the law prohibiting sexual harassment. She was actively involved in the passage of major legislation that redefined and expanded existing legal protections against discrimination in employment. Ms. Vargyas is published on legal issues of concern to women and has spoken widely on the topic. She directed the Access to Justice Project at the National Legal Aid and Defender Association. She began her career as an attorney with Community Legal Services in Philadelphia, where she provided legal representation to low-income clients. Ms. Vargyas is a graduate of Williams College and the University of Pennsylvania Law School.

Cheryl G. Healton, DrPH, is the president and chief executive officer of the American Legacy Foundation. Dr. Healton was selected for this post following a nationwide search and has worked to further the Foundation's ambitious mission: to build a world where young people reject tobacco and anyone can quit. During her tenure with the Foundation, Dr. Healton has guided the highly acclaimed, national youth tobacco prevention counter-marketing campaign, truth®, which has been credited in part with reducing youth smoking prevalence to its current 28-year low.

Dr. Healton holds a doctorate from Columbia University's School of Public Health and a master's degree in public administration at New York University for health policy and planning. She joined the American Legacy

Foundation from Columbia University's Joseph L. Mailman School of Public Health in New York, where she served as head of the Division of Sociomedical Sciences and associate dean for Program Development. She founded and directed the school's Center for Applied Public Health, conceptualizing and implementing applied research in emerging issues in public health, including AIDS care for women and children, staffing and burnout at AIDS care organizations, training and development for AIDS care professionals, and computer networking of medical records.

Michelle R. Henry, BA, is a research associate at Public Health Management Corporation (PHMC) in Philadelphia, Pennsylvania, where she works on numerous studies and is the current project manager for the quality improvement assessment of the Pennsylvania Injury Reporting and Intervention System (PIRIS) case management intervention.

Ms. Henry began her research career in 2001 at the University of Pennsylvania's Center for Bioethics before joining PHMC's Research and Evaluation group in 2004. She has worked on numerous qualitative and quantitative research and evaluation projects pertaining to at-risk youth and youth violence, including the Philadelphia Interdisciplinary Youth Fatality Review Team; an evaluation of the Norristown Truancy Abatement Initiative; and a Community and Youth Violence Prevention White Paper for Philadelphia's Behavioral Health System, which assessed opportunities for behavioral health involvement in youth violence initiatives.

Ms. Henry has published a number of articles and reports in the areas of bioethics and public health and has presented on both subjects at local and national conferences.

Robert D. Ketterlinus, PhD, is the founder of Robert D. Ketterlinus, PhD & Associates, where he provides program evaluation, program development, grantsmanship, and other consulting services to nonprofits. He is a developmental psychologist with expertise in early childhood and adolescent development and the prevention and treatment of substance abuse, violence, and other high-risk behaviors. Dr. Ketterlinus is adjunct assistant professor of psychology at St. Joseph's University.

Dr. Ketterlinus has 21 years of experience conducting human services and public health research and program evaluations. He graduated summa cum laude from Pennsylvania State University, where he earned a bachelor's degree in social sciences, and he graduated with honors from Catholic University of America, where he received his doctorate in human development. He served as a staff fellow at the National Institute of Child Health and Human Development at NIH and was a senior research associate at Public Health Management Corporation, Public–Private Ventures, Treatment Research Institute, and CSR, Incorporated.

Dr. Ketterlinus has published in peer-review journals and books, is editor–author of two books on adolescent development, and has presented his work at numerous professional conferences.

Andrew Lanza, MSW, was a commissioned officer in the U.S. Public Health Service since 1976, after receiving his masters of social work from Marywood University in Scranton, Pennsylvania. During his public health career, he has had numerous progressively challenging managerial, administrative, and programmatic assignments. Mr. Lanza has received a masters of public health with a concentration in health administration from Columbia University in 1988. Since then, he has focused on health promotion and disease prevention particularly in the workplace and community settings, while holding leadership positions in Federal Occupational Health, Agency for Toxic Substance Disease Registry, and currently, with the Centers for Disease Control and Prevention. Mr. Lanza has been a member of the Commissioned Corps Readiness Force, attained the rank of captain (06), and retired his commission in the U.S. PHS in May 2006 after a 30-year career.

Through his role as program consultant and as the CDC's Diabetes Division's lead for working with businesses and health plans, Mr. Lanza focused on translating the well-defined and accepted standards of public health practices into the real world. He has published on this subject area; has presented at numerous national meetings, including national conferences sponsored by the National Business Coalitions on Health and the National Business Group on Health; and has coordinated the Business Consultation on Diabetes. He has also served as the CDC operational lead for the DHHS Secretary's Diabetes Detection Initiative, the National Diabetes Education Program's Business and Managed Care Workgroup, and is involved with the development of new and useful tools for businesses and health plans. He is currently a consultant with McKing Consulting Corporation, consulting with CDC's Division of Partnerships and Strategic Alliances, where he serves as a senior program consultant for the business sector. Through this role, Mr. Lanza provides technical and strategic support for CDC's partnerships with national business and health organizations, bridging the gap between evidence-based science and its practical applications in order to improve and protect health. His recent work includes serving as coeditor of and author in *A Purchaser's Guide to Clinical Preventive Services: Moving Science into Coverage*, which has been acclaimed as a comprehensive and useful tool to improve the purchasing and ultimately, the delivery, of evidence-based preventive services such as screenings, immunizations, counseling, and preventive medications.

Sarah J. Olson, MS, CHES, has more than 35 years of experience in health promotion and disease–injury prevention, training, management, and leadership. She earned her bachelor of science and master of science degrees from Tulane University and is a certified health education specialist. She was with the Texas Department of Health for almost 12 years as a health educator, including serving as the acting director of the Public Health Promotion Division, and the director of both the Health Education and Disease Management Divisions for a large HMO in Texas. In 1998, Ms. Olson joined the Injury Center, Centers for Disease Control and Prevention, in

Atlanta. In June 2005, she moved to the new Division of Partnerships and Strategic Alliances in the National Center for Health Marketing at CDC. She is the author of a number of health education and promotion materials and is a sought-after national speaker on a variety of topics, including building effective partnerships, older adult and childhood unintentional injury prevention, and cultural competency.

Julia Joh Elligers, MPH, is a senior analyst at the National Association of County and City Health Officials (NACCHO). She provides technical assistance and training to local communities, implementing a strategic planning process for community health improvement called Mobilizing for Action through Planning and Partnerships (MAPP). She also provides assistance to communities using the National Public Health Performance Standards (NPHPS); NPHPS helps local public health systems assess their capacities to deliver the ten essential public health services.

In addition to working at NACCHO, Ms. Elligers is pursuing her doctoral degree in American politics at the University of Maryland, College Park. Her academic work focuses on how politics affect governmental public health capacity. She received her bachelor of arts degree in biology and public policy from Cornell University and her master of public health degree in health policy and management from Columbia University Mailman School of Public Health.

PART

1

Developing a Health Promotion Program

Health Promotion in the New Century

Bernard J. Healey, PhD
Robert S. Zimmerman Jr., MPH

Bernard J. Healey, PhD
Robert S. Zimmerman Jr., MPH

OBJECTIVES

After reading this chapter, you should

- Understand the value of prevention efforts in medical care delivery
- Define and explain the components of our current health care system
- Become aware of the various problems found in our current medical delivery system
- Understand the problems associated with our health insurance system

KEY TERMS

Chronic diseases	Health promotion
Determinants of health	High-risk health behaviors
Epidemiology	Social insurance

Introduction

Throughout the twentieth century and into the first years of the twenty-first century, there have been dramatic changes in the health of individuals and populations. A complex array of factors has contributed to these changes and their pace, and complexity will no doubt increase and significantly shape health in the future.

The Centers for Disease Control and Prevention (CDC, 1999) reported that the average lifespan of individuals in the United States has lengthened by greater than 30 years since 1900. At least 25 of these years are directly attributable to advances in public health. The CDC listed ten great public health achievements for the period 1900–1999. The list is not ranked in any particular order and was chosen based on the opportunity for prevention and the impact on death, illness, and disability in the United States.

Ten Great Public Health Achievements—United States, 1900–1999

- Vaccination
- Motor-vehicle safety
- Safer workplaces
- Control of infectious diseases
- Decline in deaths from coronary heart disease and stroke
- Safer and healthier foods
- Healthier mothers and babies
- Family planning
- Fluoridation of drinking water
- Recognition of tobacco use as a health hazard

Source: Centers for Disease Control and Prevention. Ten great public health achievements—United States. 1900–1999. MMWR. 1999, 48:241-243.

These and other achievements of the twentieth century span what Breslow (2004) and others call the epidemiologic transition that occurred about mid-century as we moved from the first era, during which there was significant progress in addressing the presence and control of communicable diseases, to the second era marked by the prominence of noncommunicable or **chronic diseases**. Very significant public health progress was made against chronic disease (particularly in mortality) during the second half of the twentieth century.

This brings us to the twenty-first century to what Breslow (2006) refers to as *The Third Era in Health—The Pursuit of Health*. He believes that one indicator of this era is the tremendous increase in longevity—a roughly 50% increase in longevity in the last century. This has led to a different view and idea of health or what you might call a spectrum of health. Breslow (2004) points out that increasing numbers of people are not only living longer (into their 80s, 90s, and beyond) but living with less disability than in the past. He and others call this decreased disability in later decades "the compression of morbidity." He says this compression of morbidity can be advanced (as he and others have proven) by adherence to seven health practices: not smoking, drinking alcohol moderately or not at all, exercising regularly, getting regular sleep, maintaining moderate weight, eating regular meals, and eating breakfast. These may ring a bell (along with many others such as hand washing, eating more fruits and veggies, and so on) as the words of wisdom we have been hearing from our mothers (and wives, sisters) for generations. Think about it—a familiar, trusted, wise, and nurturing person with your best interests at heart with the authority and proximity to repeatedly reinforce the message. It does not get any better than the original and best health educators of all.

Stallworth and Lennon (2003) note the development of the Alameda Human Population Laboratory in 1965 and the follow-up health survey and studies establishing the benefit of these seven practices as perhaps Breslow's greatest public health achievement. He tells them that although the evidence points to the importance of individual initiative in health behavior change, people do have choices to make.

In *Health, United States, 2007* (National Center for Health Statistics, 2007), the National Center for Health Statistics (NCHS) points out that the progress made in life expectancy and longevity is accompanied by increased prevalence of chronic diseases. Unfortunately, progress in this area is slowing down or trending in the wrong direction. They note that the improvements that have been made are not shared equally depending on income, race, ethnicity, education, and geography. They express concern about the high prevalence, among all Americans, of unhealthy lifestyles and behaviors, such as insufficient exercise and being overweight, which are risk factors for many chronic diseases and disabilities including heart disease, diabetes, hypertension, and back pain. The obesity epidemic among our youth is very troubling. I remember learning about a wonderful prevention program that set out to address the childhood origins of the diseases of adulthood and realizing that we are now actually seeing adult diseases in childhood. The NCHS (2007) also notes the high prevalence of risky behaviors among children and young adults.

The State of Aging and Health in America 2007 (CDC/Merck, 2007) report makes several calls to action to encourage individuals, professionals, and communities to take specific steps to improve the health and well-being of older adults. They include the following recommendations:

- Address health disparities among older adults, particularly in racial and ethnic minority populations.
- Encourage people to communicate their wishes about end-of-life care.
- Improve the oral health of older adults.
- Increase physical activity among older adults by promoting environmental changes.
- Increase adult immunizations, particularly in racial and ethnic minority populations.
- Increase screening for colorectal cancer.
- Prevent falls, a leading cause of hospitalization and injury deaths among older adults.

The Future of the Public's Health in the 21st Century by the Institute of Medicine (IOM, 2002) also notes the great national achievements in health during the twentieth century but expresses concern about the government public health infrastructure's ability to meet future challenges without substantial changes. It reaffirms the vision of Healthy People 2010—healthy people in healthy communities (discussed more below)—and recommends six areas of action and change in the government, private, and nonprofit sectors to meet future challenges:

1. Adopting a population health approach that considers the multiple **determinants of health**.
2. Strengthening the governmental public health infrastructure, which forms the backbone of the public health system.

3. Building a new generation of intersectoral partnerships that also draw on the perspectives and resources of diverse communities and actively engage them in health action.
4. Developing systems of accountability to assure the quality and availability of public health services.
5. Making evidence the foundation of decision making and the measure of success.
6. Enhancing and facilitating communication within the public health system (e.g., among all levels of the governmental public health infrastructure and between public health professionals and community members).

The report also makes 34 detailed recommendations to what it sees as 6 public health system actors: governmental public health infrastructure, health care delivery system, community, businesses and employers, media, and academia (public health and health sciences).

A Look at Costs

The days of free health care and the waste of scarce resources on a health care delivery system that is destined to fail at keeping people healthy are also changing. The rising cost of health insurance premiums (including employer- and government-financed care), the escalation in self-induced chronic diseases, and the inability to provide health care services for millions of people in the richest country in the world, are clear signals that something is radically wrong with our current health care system.

According to Price Waterhouse Coopers Health Research Institute (2009), health care spending will reach $5.2 trillion dollars by 2020 and consume 21 percent of GDP. These increased costs for health insurance are forcing employers to ask their employees to pay more for their health insurance. There has been a 6% increase in the share of premiums paid by workers in recent years. Business owners contacted in the same survey indicated that there will probably be an increase in health care expenditures for employees every year into the future.

This same study revealed that 20% of these employers plan to hire fewer workers this year because of rising health insurance costs. As health care costs continue to rise above the inflation rate, everyone from state and federal legislators to the owners of businesses are struggling to reduce the costs associated with delivering health care services to their respective constituents.

On the government side, the Congressional Budget Office (2007) calculates that in 2006, Medicare benefit payments totaled $374 billion, accounting for 13% of federal spending, and they project net spending on Medicare to increase to $564 billion in 2012. The Kaiser Foundation (Kaiser Commission, 2007) cites many financing challenges to Medicare in the future due to the aging of the U.S. population, declining ratio of workers to beneficiaries, increasing health care costs, and other economic factors. The Kaiser

Commission Medicare Primer (2007) quotes the total federal and state spending on Medicaid in 2005 at $316.5 billion and that although federal government funds about 57% of those expenditures, the remaining 43% is funded by the states and amounts to about 18% of their general funds second only to education.

Breslow (2006) questions how we spend our money in relationship to its impact and influence on health. He says that many of the best studies show that access to medical care is seen to have about 10% of the influence on health status but 88% of the money goes to Medicare. Whereas health behaviors indicate about 50% of the influence but only 4% of the money is spent on health behaviors.

Changes in the Concept of Health Insurance

The health insurance industry is also changing in the early years of this new century. Feldstein (2003) argues that individuals buy health insurance to pass risk on to others because of the uncertainty of illness and the inability to pay the costs if long-term illness occurs.

More and more employers are asking whether they can afford health insurance for their employees and whether this health insurance is worth what it costs. The cost of the insurance does not seem to be as important as the fact that the current health care delivery system is plagued by failures in preventing the development of expensive chronic diseases in the insured population.

The health care system must face radical change in the next few years or the best health care delivery system in the world will go broke. This sounds very similar to the crisis we face in social security over the next several years. Trust for America (2009) argues that health insurance costs are rising at such a rapid rate that if not stopped, they will eliminate all profits for the average Fortune 500 company in the next several years. It seems like an opportune time for employee wellness programs to be considered by employers as a potential solution to the crisis.

Insurance is generally classified as casualty or **social insurance**. Casualty insurance is found in car or home insurance and has worked very well as long as most people practice safety measures concerning automobile and home use. Social insurance usually ignores risks and shares the costs equally among participants. Enthoven and Fuchs (2006) argue that a change from the concept of social insurance, where excess costs of high-risk behaviors are shared collectively, to health insurance based on actuarial principles, where the price for insurance is based on predictable risky behaviors undertaken by some individuals, is going to be the norm. In other words, you will be charged a higher premium for health insurance if you practice **high-risk health behaviors.**

Legislators are focusing on the tremendous number of Americans without access to the health care system. Barton (2003) states there must be incremental changes to health insurance plans if access to health insurance by the uninsured is ever going to happen.

The problems faced by the health care system in this country are not simply access issues. The ability to enter the health care system is not what is required to keep people healthy. It is the ability to avoid behaviors that cause illness that is the real problem for Americans. This ability to choose healthy behaviors is not currently provided by a collection of health care facilities. It is a question of access to information at an early age that can potentially shape the development of better health behaviors and carry them through the process of aging.

Busch, Barry, Vegso, Sindelar, and Cullen (2006) found one way of dealing with the escalation in the cost of health insurance entailed in an innovative approach by Alcoa. In order to reduce costs of health insurance, Alcoa increased employees' cost sharing. In January 2004, this company increased enrollees' cost sharing for many outpatient and hospital services while simultaneously eliminating all cost sharing for a large number of preventive services. This move by a large employer indicates their awareness of the value of preventive care as an investment in the future health of their employees.

These developments in the escalation of health care costs and the changing health insurance industry to provide incentives to practice healthy behaviors or to pay more for the insurance are providing an atmosphere of opportunity for well-developed **health promotion** programs for the school, the community, and the workplace.

State and federal governments are beginning to increase the use of incentive payments to providers of government sponsored care along with a variety of other initiatives designed to incorporate health promotion and disease prevention services and principles. The National Governors Association (2007) notes that states, impatient with lack of progress at the national level, are increasingly pursuing health care reform as a priority and seeking ways to achieve quality improvement in health care delivery by incorporating prevention and wellness into their health plans, and using information technology to further improve health care. The Healthy States Initiative, a partnership among the CDC, the Council of State Governments (CSG), the National Black Caucus of State Legislators, and the National Hispanic Caucus of State Legislators, has produced an excellent work titled *State Official's Guide to Wellness* (CSG, 2006) among other resources to help provide state leaders with information upon which to make sound public health decisions.

The Healthy People Concept

There has always been an interest in the prevention of health problems by many in this country. This interest is evident when we look at the strong support for the elimination of childhood diseases through the funding of vaccine development and distribution by public health departments. Unfortunately, there has been a reluctance to move past children and young adults with well-developed prevention programs.

The concept of healthy people began in 1979 as the result of a report by the Surgeon General of the United States titled *The Surgeon General's Report on Health Promotion and Disease Prevention*. This report was responsible for the start of a national discussion on the relationship of personal health behaviors in the development of many serious diseases and injuries. *Healthy People 2010* is a set of health goals and objectives for the nation to achieve by the year 2010. It includes 467 health improvement objectives in 28 focus areas. The focus areas established for *Healthy People 2010* are shown in Table 1-1 (U.S. Department of Health and Human Services [DHHS], 2000).

Table 1-1

Healthy People 2010

Source: U.S. Department of Health and Human Services. *Healthy People 2010* (2nd ed.). With Understanding and Improving Health and Objectives for Improving Health (2 vols.). Washington, DC: U.S. Government Printing Office.

Healthy People 2010 Objectives at a Glance

Healthy People 2010 consists of 467 target objectives organized into 28 broad focus areas, as follows:

- Access
- Arthritis, osteoporosis, chronic back
- Conditions
- Cancer
- Chronic kidney disease
- Diabetes
- Disability and secondary conditions
- Environmental health
- Educational and community-based programs
- Family planning
- Food safety
- Health communication
- Heart disease and stroke
- HIV–AIDS
- Immunization and infectious diseases
- Injury–violence prevention
- Maternal, infant, child health
- Medical product safety
- Mental health and mental disorders
- Nutrition and overweight
- Occupational safety and health
- Oral health
- Physical activity and fitness
- Respiratory diseases
- Public health infrastructure
- Sexually transmitted diseases
- Substance abuse (including alcohol)
- Tobacco use
- Vision and hearing

Determinants of Health

Improving the health of the population requires consideration and a better understanding of the various components that determine good or poor health. Although one of the major influences on health is the receipt of health services, it has become very clear to those in public health that there are other factors that determine good health that are of equal, or perhaps greater, importance than the health care system. Topics covered by the objectives in *Healthy People 2010* reflect the array of critical influences that determine the health of individuals and communities. For example, individual behaviors and environmental factors are responsible for about 70% of all premature deaths in the United States (DHHS, 2000). Developing and implementing policies and preventive interventions that effectively address these determinants of health can reduce the burden of illness, enhance quality of life, and increase longevity.

Major Determinants of Health
- Individual behaviors
- Environmental factors

Individual biology and behaviors influence health through their interaction with each other and with the individual's social and physical environments. In addition, policies and interventions can improve health by targeting factors related to individuals and their environments, including access to quality health care.

Biology refers to the individual's genetic makeup (those factors with which he or she is born), family history (which may suggest risk for disease), and physical and mental health problems acquired during life. Aging, diet, physical activity, smoking, stress, alcohol or illicit drug abuse, injury or violence, or an infectious or toxic agent may result in illness or disability and can produce a "new" biology for the individual.

Behaviors are individual responses or reactions to internal stimuli and external conditions. Behaviors can have a reciprocal relationship to biology; in other words, each can react to the other. For example, smoking (behavior) can alter the cells in the lung and result in shortness of breath, emphysema, or cancer (biology) that then may lead an individual to stop smoking (behavior). Similarly, a family history that includes heart disease (biology) may motivate an individual to develop good eating habits, to avoid tobacco, and to maintain an active lifestyle (behaviors), which may prevent his or her own development of heart disease (biology).

Personal choices and the social and physical environments surrounding individuals can shape behaviors. The social and physical environments include all factors that affect the life of individuals, positively or negatively — many of which may not be under their immediate or direct control.

Social environment includes interactions with family, friends, coworkers, and others in the community. It also encompasses social institutions, such as law enforcement, workplaces, places of worship, and schools. Housing, public transportation, and the presence or absence of violence in the community are among other components of the social environment. The social environment has a profound effect on individual health, as well as on the health of the larger community, and is unique because of cultural customs; language; and personal, religious, or spiritual beliefs. At the same time, individuals and their behaviors contribute to the quality of the social environment.

Physical environment can be thought of as that which can be seen, touched, heard, smelled, and tasted; however, the physical environment also contains less tangible elements, such as radiation and ozone. The physical environment can harm individual and community health, especially when individuals and communities are exposed to toxic substances; irritants; infectious agents; and physical hazards in homes, schools, and work sites. The physical environment also can promote good health, for example, by providing clean and safe places for people to work, exercise, and play.

Policies and interventions can have a powerful and positive effect on the health of individuals and the community. Examples include health promotion campaigns to prevent smoking; policies mandating child restraints and safety belt use in automobiles; disease prevention services, such as immunization of children, adolescents, and adults; and clinical services, such as enhanced mental health care. Policies and interventions that promote individual and community health may be implemented by a variety of agencies, such as transportation, education, energy, housing, labor, justice, and other venues, or through places of worship, community-based organizations, civic groups, and businesses.

The health of individuals and communities also depends greatly on access to quality health care. Expanding access to quality health care is important to eliminate health disparities and to increase the quality and years of healthy life for all people living in the United States. Health care in the broadest sense not only includes services received through health care providers but also health information and services received through other venues in the community (DHHS, 2000).

The determinants of health—individual biology and behavior, physical and social environments, policies and interventions, and access to quality health care—have a profound effect on the health of individuals, communities, and the nation. An evaluation of these determinants is an important part of developing any strategy to improve health.

Our understanding of these determinants and how they relate to one another, coupled with our understanding of how individual and community health affects the health of the nation, is perhaps the most important key to achieving our *Healthy People 2010* (DHHS, 2000) goals of increasing the quality and years of life and eliminating the nation's health disparities.

Value of *Healthy People 2010*

The healthy people process allows for continuous feedback regarding progress toward short-term and long-term goals and objectives toward better health for constituents. The determinants of health and the health status of the population allow communities to focus on the real cause of the health problems rather than wasting resources on the symptoms of the problems. The key to the healthy people concept is the premise that the personal habits and behaviors of individuals are the key determinants in whether or not that individual will remain well or become ill later in life.

Dever (2006) argues that support for using this framework to address health problems is based on the fact that the objectives must be supported by scientific evidence and also be prevention oriented. Therefore, the program is driven by sound epidemiological principles that can withstand criticism. It allows prevention to go beyond health systems and gate keepers, and into the community or workplace.

The healthy people approach utilizes expertise from many disciplines in dealing with diseases and their complications that are primarily the result of lifestyle behaviors. Dever (2006) also points out that because individual behaviors and environmental factors are responsible for about 70% of all premature deaths in this country, it stands to reason that the health care system will deal with these problems "downstream" after they have already occurred because that is where they see patients. In order to prevent these problems "upstream," there needs to be a concentrated effort of prevention supported by the community partnerships. In public health, the upstream approach looks for the cause of disease and disability and attempts to prevent the problem rather than treat it downstream. These prevention efforts over time can reduce the burden of illness and enhance the quality of life.

Three Levels of Prevention
- Primary
- Secondary
- Tertiary

High-Risk Health Behaviors

Turnock (2004) believes that a synonym for public health is prevention, which he defines as actions that are taken to reduce the possibility that something will happen.

Prevention can also minimize the damage if something bad does happen. The main problem with prevention activities is found in the fact that it is difficult to know if you were successful in your prevention activities. How do you measure something that did not happen?

One of the things that a public health system should be doing is promoting healthy behaviors. This activity includes behavioral risk factor monitoring, school and work site health promotion, community-wide risk reduction programs, health education, and media involvement. Public health departments attempt to do all of these things with a very limited budget, limited staff, and many other mandated programs to manage at the same time.

Satcher (2006) points out that the World Health Organization published a report in 2000 on the "health system efficiency," comparing the United States with 189 other countries. Despite spending more than any other country on health care, the United States was ranked seventh in overall health system efficiency. One of the major reasons for this poor performance was the fact that this spending lacked balance with population-based prevention. How ironic it is that a country that is so generous in sharing its public health expertise with third world countries does not practice the same public health knowledge in most of its own sectors.

The escalation of chronic diseases as America grows older is placing high-risk health behaviors in the forefront of any attempt to deal with the rapid costs found in our current health care delivery system. McGinnis (2006) argues that these costly chronic diseases require behavioral interventions involving public health incentives and education with strong reinforcement and constant monitoring by health care providers. This intervention ideally should begin very early in life, long before the behaviors begin.

McGinnis and Foege (1993) point out that daily habits like smoking, inactivity, diet, and alcohol use and their consequences contribute to the development of virtually all of morbidity and mortality in industrial nations. Adopting healthy behaviors such as eating nutritious foods, being physically active, and avoiding tobacco use can prevent or control the devastating effects of these diseases.

Leading Causes of Mortality

- Tobacco
- Physical inactivity
- Diet

Figure 1-1 offers a very good example of the use of **epidemiology** as a necessary adjunct to developing a better understanding of the need to separate the symptoms from the real problem when dealing with disease and disease causation. These figures also reveal the behavioral aspects of chronic disease development.

McGinnis, Russo, and Knickman (2002) point out that we know behavioral choices are responsible for at least 900,000 deaths annually. These deaths are

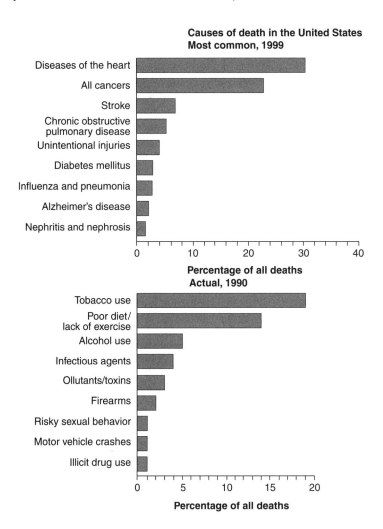

Figure 1-1
Comparison of Most
Common Causes of
Death and Actual
Causes of Death

Source: Centers for Disease
Control and Prevention,
National Center for Health
Statistics. (1997). National
Vital Statistics System and
unpublished data.

usually premature and preceded by loss of quality of life because of illness.
These daily choices of the practice of high-risk health behaviors account for the
vast majority of chronic diseases that are manifested in the individual later in life.
According to Turnock (2009), despite all the health improvements achieved
through prevention efforts, the country is still plagued by large numbers of
premature diseases, disabilities, and deaths that could have been prevented.

We have developed a health care delivery system in the United States that
is designed to respond to a medical emergency. The system is predisposed to
wait for an uninformed patient to enter the system after a medical event has
occurred. There should also be aggressive intervention even after the high-risk
behaviors have been practiced for many years. There is strong epidemiological
evidence that stopping high-risk behaviors can prevent or lessen the long-term
complications that usually result from practicing high-risk health behaviors.

Chronic Diseases

Chronic Diseases
- Long incubation period
- No cure
- Caused by high-risk health behaviors

The diseases facing Americans have changed dramatically since 1900. According to Brownson, Remington, and Davis (1998), the disease state in the United States has shifted from communicable diseases to chronic diseases that pose different threats to the public health. Although life expectancy has increased by over 40 years since 1900, the **chronic diseases** are capable of affecting the quality of life as one ages in this country.

Dever (2006) argues that the use of epidemiology has become very important among the methods of advancing the concept of risk in the causation of chronic diseases. He believes that in many cases high-risk health behaviors virtually guarantee the future development of expensive and deadly chronic diseases. These diseases are usually a result of one's lifestyle, which may include high-risk health behaviors.

Figure 1-2 shows the progression of the disease state for a communicable disease. Once you adjust for a longer incubation period for most chronic diseases,

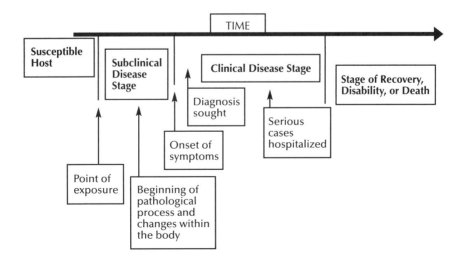

Figure 1-2 Natural Course of a Communicable Disease

Source: Merrill, R. M., & Timmreck, T. C. (2006). *Introduction to epidemiology* (4th ed.). Sudbury, MA: Jones Bartlett Publishers.

the same model can be used for studying a chronic disease. Following this model, a susceptible host would be anyone who practices high-risk health behaviors. In the case of tobacco use, it would also include anyone exposed to secondhand smoke from the tobacco user. The incubation period begins at first exposure and continues until the clinical disease stage. The last stage can include the same potential outcomes as a communicable disease—recovery, disability, or death.

Chronic diseases are noncontagious, have a long latency period, and are usually not curable. These diseases are usually caused by human behaviors, which, once developed, are very difficult to change. Tobacco use, poor nutrition, and physical inactivity are the main causes of chronic diseases. Once these diseases develop, they are virtually impossible to eliminate. They just continue to get worse as the individual ages and eventually become the catalyst in the individual's disability or death.

The CDC (2007) reports that today, chronic diseases, such as cardiovascular disease, cancer, and diabetes, are among the most prevalent, costly, and preventable of all health problems. Each year, 7 out of 10 Americans die from a chronic disease, and the costs associated with these diseases represent over 75% of our health care bill every year.

Because the incubation period of chronic diseases is usually years before onset of illness, it is very difficult to always determine the cause of these diseases. The best that can be done is to look at known risk factors and draw conclusions from the available data. It seems certain that most of these chronic diseases were acquired during the work years and could have been prevented in many cases at the workplace.

Brownson et al. (1998) argue that the concept of control has a different meaning when attributed to a chronic disease than it does for a communicable disease. A chronic disease interferes with good health long before this type of disease interferes with the length of life. Along with the direct costs associated with this type of disease, one must consider the indirect costs of pain, suffering, and disability that are also part of the chronic disease before it causes death.

Health Promotion

Health education is defined as the way that individuals and groups of people learn about good and bad health behaviors. Health promotion represents an enabling process to help people increase their control over their health by going beyond lifestyles to everything that can possibly affect one's health. There has always been a rising expectation concerning the value of health services, especially treatment for conditions that already exist. This belief has helped to shape our health care delivery system in this country into a provider of care after illness occurs. Because the individual has a primary role in determining his or her wellness before entering the health care system, the critical ingredient for good health in this country has become information.

McGinnis et al. (2002) argues that a major factor affecting investment in health promotion initiatives has been gaining consensus in decisions on what should be done to change high-risk health behaviors and how to measure the effectiveness of these new initiatives. Another reason for reluctance to embrace health promotion as a potential strategy to reduce both the incidence and complications of chronic diseases has been a misunderstanding, by even those in public health, of the real meaning of health promotion.

According to Timmreck (2003), the concept of health promotion was an outgrowth of several disciplines, including school health education, public health, medicine, and psychology. Timmreck (2003) defined health promotion as the "science and art of helping people change their lifestyle to move toward a state of optimal health." O'Donnell (1989), in his expanded definition, goes on to define optimal health as a balance of physical, emotional, social, spiritual, and intellectual health. The prevention of disease is the overriding concern in the evolving concept of health promotion as a discipline.

Laverack (2005) believes there is a great deal of disagreement among health educators as to the best definition of health promotion. It seems most authorities on the subject of health promotion believe it involves a structured effort to prevent disease and to promote good health rather than an attempt to fix health problems after they develop. Others focus on preventing the complications that usually arise from the disease once it occurs.

For example, type 2 diabetes is a chronic disease, but it is the complications from this disease that causes disability and premature death. The high-risk health behaviors that caused the disease are also responsible for causing the complications that ultimately result in disability and death from the disease.

Anspaugh, Dignan, and Anspaugh (2000) point out that health promotion programs usually spend a great deal of attention and focus on individual responsibility for their health. Easterling, Gallagher, and Lodwick (2003) argue that health promotion is a prevention strategy that needs to involve the community in the prevention effort.

Barton (2003) believes that the goal of health promotion is the achievement of optimal health, but that goal is not a very great concern to a health care system that spends the majority of its resources on curative medicine. In fact, the current system of health care services is not even trained in preventing things that have not happened. The system is educated to respond to crisis intervention when a patient is very ill.

Barton (2003) believes that two factors affect the success of health promotional activities. They are the individual's awareness of the danger associated with a poor lifestyle choice and the aggressiveness of the individual in seeking healthier behaviors.

According to McGinnis et al. (2002), about 95% of health care expenses go to direct medical services while only 5% goes to population-based health improvement. It seems that the major reason that our current health care system is not delivering high-quality good health is because the expenditures are being spent on individuals who are already ill and not on preventing that illness from occurring in the first place.

McGinnis (2002) argues that human behavior contributes to approximately 40% of premature mortality in this country. It seems obvious that more attention and resources need to be made available to the behavioral aspects of disease, disability, and premature death.

Laverack (2005) argues that there are five approaches to health promotion discussed in the literature: the medical approach, the behavioral–lifestyle approach, the educational approach, the client-centered approach, and the socioenvironmental approach. Anspaugh et al. (2000) describes health promotion in terms of purposeful activities that are designed to improve personal and public health. The focus in this definition is on individual responsibility after health information is provided. The individual workplace and community become empowered through the availability of accurate understandable information about how to maintain good health and to avoid disease. Health education requires individuals to be educated about their health. The health educator uses specific educational strategies to enlighten individuals and even communities about their health.

McKenzie, Neiger, and Smeltzer (2005) argue that health promotion is a larger concept than health education. Thus, health promotion includes many more concepts that are important to good health along with the educational piece of the puzzle. McKenzie et al. (2005) also points out the involvement of change, individual responsibility, and motivation in the assumption of a potentially successful health promotion program.

After review of arguments about whether individuals of society bear primary responsibility for individual health, Minkler (1999), like Breslow (2004), Stallworth, and Lennon (2003), strikes a balance between individual and social responsibility. The World Health Organization says that health promotion is the process of enabling people to increase control over, and to improve, their health. It goes on to state the following:

> Health promotion represents a comprehensive social and political process, it not only embraces actions directed at strengthening the skills and capabilities of individuals, but also action directed towards changing social, environmental and economic conditions so as to alleviate their impact on public and individual health. Health promotion is the process of enabling people to increase control over the determinants of health and thereby improve their health. Participation is essential to sustain health promotion action. The Ottawa Charter identifies three basic strategies for health promotion. These are advocacy for health to create the essential conditions for health indicated above; enabling all people to achieve their full health potential; and mediating between the different interests in society in the pursuit of health (WHO, 1998, p. 11–12).

The Institute of Medicine publication, *Promoting Health—Intervention Strategies from Social and Behavioral Research* (IOM, 2000), found the difficulty of any one intervention or set of interventions to address all behavioral and social influences and encouraged the use of multiple approaches.

Health promotion is therefore a mechanism to empower large numbers of people in the school, workplace, and community to remain healthy and to avoid illness and disease. This goal is accomplished through the sharing of accurate information about the long-term effects of high-risk health behaviors. Health promotion is not a panacea and will never change everyone, but in time, it can change the majority and that will postpone, if not end, the health care crisis in America. This helps to identify targets where the most effective intervention measures can be applied.

CONCLUDING REMARKS

The health care delivery system in the United States has reached the crisis stage. The escalating costs of health care insurance and the employer's desire to pass these costs on to employees have increased the incentives for action on this crisis. This crisis and the advancements in the art and science of health promotion make it imperative to reduce the escalation of resources being devoted to illness and disease and to increase attention and resources to wellness.

There is an increasing body of evidence of the real value of health promotion for individuals and society, and that without it society will be increasingly plagued with chronic diseases. These chronic diseases with their disability and loss of quality of life as we age have the ability to turn the newly acquired length of life for Americans into a nightmare of pain and suffering that is largely avoidable.

We have a responsibility to insist on, deliver, and support sound evidence-based health promotion strategies and programs and to affect public and private sector policies and decisions to improve on both longevity and quality of life for all Americans throughout the twenty-first century. The text that follows in this book provides both instructions on process and technique and substantive examples of how they are being put into practice.

DISCUSSION QUESTIONS

1. What is the difference between health education and health promotion programs?
2. Name and explain the three levels of prevention.
3. What are the major determinants of health in the United States?
4. What do we mean by upstream and downstream health care delivery?

REFERENCES

Anspaugh, D., Dignan, M., & Anspaugh, S. (2000). *Developing health promotion programs.* Long Grove, IL: Waveland Press Inc.

Barton, P. L. (2003). *Understanding the U.S. health services system* (2nd ed.). Chicago, IL: Health Administration Press.

Breslow, L. (2004). Perspectives: The third revolution in health. *Annual Review of Public Health, 25.*

Breslow, L. (2006). *The third era in health—The pursuit of health. University of Minnesota School of Public Health Public Lecture Series.* Available at http://blog.lib.umn.edu/sphpod/sphpod/2006/05/the_third_era_in_health_the_pu.html. Accessed August 20, 2007.

Brownson, R. C., Remington, P. L., & Davis, J. R. (1998). *Chronic disease epidemiology and control* (2nd ed.). Washington, DC: American Public Health Association.

Busch, S. H., Barry, C. L., Vegso, S. J., Sindelar, J. L., & Cullen, M. R. (2006). Effects of a cost-sharing exemption on use of preventive services at one large employer. *Journal of Health Affairs, 25*(6), 1529–1553.

Congressional Budget Office. (2007). *The budget and economic outlook fiscal years 2008 to 2017.* Washington, DC: The Congress of the United States, Congressional Budget Office.

Centers for Disease Control and Prevention. (1999). Ten great public health achievements—United States, 1900–1999. *MMWR, 48*(12), 241–243.

Centers for Disease Control and Prevention and the Merck Company Foundation. (2007). *The state of aging and health in America 2007.* Whitehouse Station, NJ: The Merck Company Foundation.

Council of State Governments. (2006). *State official's guide to wellness.* Lexington, KY: The Council of State Governments.

The Commonwealth Fund Commission on a High Performance Health System, The Path to a High Performance Health System: A 2020 Vision and the Policies to Pave the Way, The Commonwealth Fund, February 2009 http://www.commonwealthfund.org/Content/Publications/Fund-Reports/2009/Feb/The-Path-to-a-High-Performance-US-Health-System.aspx

Dever, G.E. (2006). *Managerial epidemiology: Practice, methods and concepts.* Sudbury, MA: Jones and Bartlett Publishers.

Easterling, D., Gallagher, K., & Lodwick, D. (2003). *Promoting health at the community level.* Thousand Oaks, CA: Sage Publications.

Enthoven, A., & Fuchs, V. (2006). Employment-based health insurance: Past, present, and future. *Journal of Health Affairs, 25*(6), 1538–1546.

Feldstein, P. J. (2003). *Health policy issues: An economic perspective* (3rd ed.). Chicago, IL: Health Administration Press.

Healthy People: The Surgeon General's report on health promotion and disease prevention (1979). Department of Health, Education, and Welfare, Washington, D.C.: U.S. Government Printing Office.

Institute of Medicine Committee on Capitalizing on Social Science and Behavioral Research to Improve the Public's Health. (2000). *Promoting health: Intervention strategies from social and behavioral research* (B. D. Smedley and S. L. Smyne, Eds). Washington, DC: National Academy Press.

Institute on Medicine Committee on Assuring the Health of the Public in the 21st Century. (2002). *The future of the public's health in the 21st century.* Washington, DC: National Academies Press.

Kaiser Commission on Medicaid and the Uninsured. (2007). *Medicaid a primer.* Washington, DC: The Henry J. Kaiser Family Foundation.

Kaiser Family Foundation. (2007). *Medicare a primer.* Washington, DC: The Henry J. Kaiser Family Foundation.

Laverack, G. (2005). *Health promotion practice power and empowerment.* Thousand Oaks, CA: Sage Publications.

McGinnis, J. M. (2006). Can public health and medicine partner in the public interest? *Journal of Health Affairs, 25*(4), 1044–1052.

McGinnis, J. M., Russo, P. W., & Knickman, J. R. (2002). The case for more active policy attention to health promotion. *Journal of Health Affairs, 21*(2), 78–93.

McGinnis, J., & Foege, W. (1993). Actual causes of death in the United States. *Journal of the American Medical Association, 270,* 2207–2212.

McKenzie J. F., Neiger B. L., & Smeltzer J. (2005). *Planning, implementing and evaluating health promotion programs: A primer.* (4th ed.). San Francisco, CA: Pearson Benjamin Cummings.

McKenzie J., Neiger B., & Thackeray R. (2009) *Planning, implementing and evaluating health promotion programs: A primer.* New York: Pearson Benjamin Cummings.

Minkler, M. (1999). Personal responsibility for health? A review of the arguments and the evidence at century's end. *Health Education & Behavior, 26,* 121–141.

National Center for Health Statistics. (2007). *Health, United States, 2007 with chartbook on trends in the health of Americans.* Hyattsville, MD: U.S. Government Printing Office.

National Governors Association Center for Best Practices. (2007, July 11). *Leading the way: State health reform initiatives* (Issue brief). Washington, DC: National Governors Association Center for Best Practices.

O'Donnell, M. P. (1989). Definition of health promotion: Part III: Expanding the definition. *American Journal of Health Promotion, 3*(5).

Price Waterhouse Coopers. (2008). *The factors fueling rising health care costs.* Available at www.pwc.com/extweb/pwcpublications. Accessed February 3, 2009.

Satcher, D. (2006). The prevention challenge and opportunity. *Journal of Health Affairs, 25*(4), 1009–1011.

Stallworth, J., & Lennon, J. L. (2003). Faces of public health–An interview with Dr. Lester Breslow. *American Journal of Public Health, 93*(11), 1803–1805.

Timmreck, T. C. (2003). *Planning, program development, and evaluation: A handbook for health promotion, aging, and health services* (2nd ed.). Sudbury, MA: Jones and Bartlett Publishers.

Turnock, B. J. (2004). *Public health: What it is and how it works* (3rd ed.). Sudbury, MA: Jones and Bartlett Publishers.

Turnock, B.J. (2009). *Public health: What it is and how it works* (4th ed.). Sudbury, MA: Jones and Bartlett Publishers.

U.S. Department of Health and Human Services. (2000, November). *Healthy people 2010* (2nd ed.). With understanding and improving health and objectives for improving health. 2 vols. Washington, DC: U.S. Government Printing Office.

Trust for America's Health (2009). Blueprint for a Healthier America. Available at http://healthyamericans.org/report/55/blueprint-for-healthier-america. Accessed February 23, 2009.

World Health Organization. (1998). *Health promotion glossary.* Geneva, Switzerland: World Health Organization (WHO), Division of Health Promotion, Education and Communications (HPR), and Health Education and Health Promotion Unit (HEP), *98*(1).

Epidemiology as the Catalyst in the Development of Health Promotion Programs

Bernard J. Healey, PhD

Robert S. Zimmerman Jr., MPH

OBJECTIVES

After reading this chapter, you should

- Be capable of understanding the need for an understanding of the principles of epidemiology when developing health promotion programs
- Become aware of the cause of many of the leading contributors to morbidity and mortality in the United States
- Understand the role of high-risk health behaviors as the cause of chronic diseases
- Become aware of the need for a multidiscipline approach in the development of health promotion programs

KEY TERMS

Analytical epidemiology
Chain of infection
Descriptive epidemiology

Morbidity and mortality weekly report
Rate

Introduction to Epidemiology

In order to develop health promotion programs that have the best chance of success, there needs to be a very clear definition of the real health problem. The key to this definition is the use of epidemiology in defining the real health problems. In fact, those given the task of developing health promotion programs need to have a firm grasp of the principles of epidemiology in order to separate symptoms from the problem that is causing a given disease.

The most important tool used in public health is epidemiology, which has been a part of medicine as well as public health departments since the very beginning of the first outbreak of illness and disease. The purpose of epidemiology is to discover what people do that cause disease. Turnock (2004) believes that the ultimate goal of epidemiology is to find the cause of disease and to apply this knowledge to the development of prevention and health promotion programs. It seems that epidemiology is a necessary adjunct to the development of a successful health promotion program.

Leading Causes of Mortality
- Tobacco
- Physical inactivity
- Poor diet

The major reason for the advances in longevity for most Americans over the last several years has been the discovery of the real causes of illness by epidemiologists, and public health used this information to establish prevention programs. The epidemiologist acts like a disease detective, examining clues and determining the ultimate cause of health problems. Epidemiology examines the health of the population, not the health of the individual, and is often referred to as population-based medicine. An epidemiologist studies a problem or health event, gathers required data, analyzes the data, and attempts to offer an unbiased interpretation of what the data means.

This tool has served us well over the years by solving many of the mysteries surrounding the causation of illness and disease. This public health science has now expanded into occupational injuries and chronic diseases. This science can also be utilized to solve managerial and marketing problems using the approach of looking for cause and effect. Epidemiology has matured over the years and has been accepted as a very important discipline in the medical sciences.

There are those who believe that epidemiology is nothing more than a different way to use medical statistics to solve a disease outbreak. This perception has developed and been reinforced by the media attention that has been focused on large outbreaks of disease that gained national attention. The media portrays the epidemiologist as nothing more than a government employee gathering data about illness. This allows the perception by many that epidemiology ranges from a very complex science to believing that it is nothing more than common sense.

In order to make epidemiology a useful tool to be utilized by health promotion specialists, there needs to be a demystification of the topic. This can only be accomplished by explaining the development of the science through its historical evolution and the reader achieving a better understanding of the most important tools utilized by the epidemiologist in the solution of complex public health problems.

Epidemiology is the study of the determinants, distribution, and frequency of disease. The epidemiologist utilizes a concept called the **chain of infection** to explain how disease is transmitted from an infected individual to someone who is not infected. It is a time-tested method that is used to solve medical problems of unknown etiology. Epidemiology can also be the starting point for the planning process in the control and prevention of many health problems. This science can also be very helpful in the development and evaluation of health promotion efforts for schools, workplaces, and communities.

The Evolving Discipline of Epidemiology

There are many who believe that epidemiology is a recently discovered science. The fact is that individuals have been using the principles of epidemiology to solve health problems for centuries. Since the beginning of civilization, people have wondered why sickness occurred and why some people became ill and others did not.

According to Merrill and Timmreck (2006), epidemiology is a very sound method of investigation that utilizes statistical techniques to evaluate a hypothesis about the causation of any disease. If you gather enough good data about something and use sound statistical analysis, you can usually understand why it happened. For example, epidemiology of chronic diseases, injuries, environmental and occupational exposures, and personal behaviors is now used on a frequent basis.

Epidemiology can be as difficult or as easy as you want it to be. It consists of semantics, statistics, and a great deal of common sense. In order to get a good understanding of the value of the science of epidemiology, it is helpful to understand the evolution of the discipline of epidemiology.

Hippocrates Epidemiologists frequently classify large numbers of cases of disease as an epidemic. According to Merrill and Timmreck (2006) this medical meaning of the term was first developed by Hippocrates. The term epidemic came from the Greek words *epi* (on) and *demos* (people). In the fifth century, Hippocrates was instrumental in authoring *Corpus Hippocraticum* containing seven books titled *Epidemics*. There is also substantial evidence that Hippocrates used epidemiology for recording outbreaks of communicable diseases like the plague, cholera, and dysentery. As the science and art of epidemiology grew in stature and understanding, its many possibilities in the scientific field also expanded.

John Graunt According to Merrill and Timmreck (2006) in 1662, a London councilman, John Graunt, was responsible for the first publication of a comprehensive analysis of mortality data. His publication offered data concerning birth, death, and disease occurrence, and he was able to evaluate differences in vital statistics by location. This was the first utilization of a surveillance system, which is useful in reporting demographic data.

William Farr   This concept of data collection was further developed by William Farr, who is considered the father of vital statistics and surveillance. He developed the concepts used today in vital statistics and the classification of diseases. He was able to build on Graunt's work by collecting the data, evaluating the data, and reporting that data to the responsible authorities and the general public.

John Snow   Merrill and Timmreck (2006) point out that one of the more famous case studies of communicable disease solved by the use of epidemiology occurred in 1849 in London during a cholera epidemic. A physician, John Snow, used epidemiology to find the cause of the spread of cholera through the water supply on Broad Street in London. Based on his prior years of studying the transmission of cholera through contaminated water, Snow surveyed households of cholera victims and traced their water supply to one of the three wells being used by the town. Once the suspect well was closed at his urging, the illness in the town ended. This is one of many instances of the successful use of the principles of epidemiology to solve an outbreak of an unknown communicable disease.

Epidemiology at the Centers for Disease Control and Prevention

According to the CDC (2009), epidemiology began at the CDC with Dr. Alexander Langmuir in 1949. He served as first chief epidemiologist and remained at the CDC until 1970. He convened the first Conference of State and Territorial Epidemiologists, which represents over 2,500 epidemiologists working today in all states. He defined disease surveillance and was responsible for the development of the *Morbidity and Mortality Weekly Report* (MMWR), which communicates weekly reports on disease prevalence and outbreaks of disease.

Doll and Hill Study   CDC (2009) reports that another epidemiologic study was conducted by Doll and Hill in the 1950s, implicating the use of tobacco with a rare form of cancer at that time—lung cancer. This landmark study paved the way for additional chronic disease studies that linked secondhand smoke to the same deadly form of cancer. Tobacco became identified as the leading cause of death for 430,000 Americans every year. Secondhand smoke was also identified in 1966 as the cause of lung cancer in over 80,000 nonsmokers every year (CDC, 2009).

Framingham Study   After Doll and Hill's study, it seemed like a natural follow-up to start using epidemiology to evaluate high-risk health behaviors as a potential cause of other chronic diseases. The Framingham study, beginning in 1948, in the town of Framingham, Massachusetts, did just that. It followed residents of this town for 50 years in order to discover how people develop the leading cause of mortality, heart disease. Turnock (2004) refers to the 28,000 residents of Framingham who volunteered for this first longitudinal study of heart disease as having given a gift to this country.

This was an analytical study that revealed that by changing a few health behaviors like not smoking, following a better diet, lowering weight, and increasing physical activity, one can reduce their chances of developing heart disease. The success of this study signaled that epidemiology was moving rapidly into the very important area of chronic disease causation even though chronic diseases were usually caused by multiple factors. Epidemiology was now ready to deal with diseases involving very long incubation periods that had no visible starting point. Epidemiology is the starting point for a movement from secondary prevention to primary prevention.

Levels of Prevention

Primary prevention
Activities taken to prevent disease in the future

Secondary prevention
Early detection and treatment of disease

Tertiary prevention
Rehabilitation therapies to prevent complications or further illness

---

Acquired Immune Deficiency Syndrome

The Acquired Immune Deficiency Syndrome (AIDS) epidemic began in the United States in 1981. Through case investigations, it was discovered in 1983 that this deadly disease was caused by the Human Immunodeficiency Virus (HIV). There is now better treatment for individuals once the virus is detected, but there is no vaccine to prevent infection and no complete cure to prevent premature death from this virus.

Descriptive epidemiology is used to characterize the extent and the distribution of disease involved in the investigation. The use of descriptive epidemiology in the beginning of this epidemic helped us to better understand how the virus is spread but caused some confusion by utilizing the high-risk group labeling of those infected. It is not belonging to a high-risk group that causes infection with HIV; it is the practice of high-risk behaviors that causes infection. This disease is now characterized as both a communicable disease because it is spread person to person and a chronic disease because of the long incubation period and the long time from infection to death.

Injury Control

Injuries, both unintentional and intentional, are a major threat to disability and death in this country. According to Christoffel and Gallagher (2006), they are preventable. They also are capable of being better understood and prevented through epidemiology and health promotion.

Figure 2-1 demonstrates the use of a surveillance system to help with learning more about how to prevent injuries.

Behavioral Health Problems

In recent years, behavioral health problems have become the target of intense research by public health agencies. The CDC has begun the use of new intervention strategies for HIV that is behaviorally and socially oriented. Public health departments have developed Behavioral Risk Factor Surveillance Systems that have concentrated on gathering information about high-risk health behaviors. Because chronic diseases are the new disease epidemic facing Americans, this new interest in behavioral health problems is entirely appropriate.

Epidemiology in the Future

The CDC (2006) predicts that epidemiologists will continue to respond to communicable disease emergencies, natural disasters or bioterrorism, and other public health problems. The future will also include providing information for health promotion specialists concerning cardiovascular diseases, obesity, tobacco use, and injuries. The epidemiologists will work with other disciplines concerning the prevention of high-risk health behaviors. They will

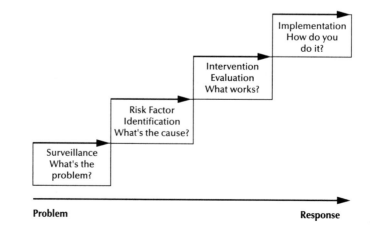

Figure 2-1
Public Health Approach
Source: Christoffel, T., & Gallagher, S. S. (2006). *Injury prevention and public health practical knowledge, skills and strategies* (2nd ed.). Sudbury, MA: Jones Bartlett Publishers.

utilize new technology and be instrumental in fostering collaborative partnerships to increase disease prevention activities in the schools, workplaces, and communities.

Descriptive Epidemiology

It is virtually impossible to work on health promotion programs without understanding the value and the limits of epidemiology. It is useful to define epidemiology as descriptive or analytical depending on the stage of the investigation. Those involved in all aspects of health promotion programs will be using descriptive and analytical epidemiology in their work.

There are several different types of studies utilized in epidemiology. For our purposes, they range in design from descriptive to analytical types of studies. Merrill and Timmreck (2006) define **descriptive epidemiology** as that part of epidemiology that involves the description of health events in terms of time, place, and person. This allows the epidemiologist the opportunity to start looking for clues as to the cause of the event. Several questions require answers before more time-consuming and expensive studies can begin: What do cases of the event in question have in common? Why do some people become ill and others do not? What is the time period and location of the diseases of concern?

Epidemiologists are then able to describe the health event by gathering and interpreting data in some meaningful way. The time of the occurrence, where the event took place, and who was affected by the event are the major components of descriptive epidemiology.

Szklo and Nieto (2000) point out that descriptive epidemiology allows the use of available data to determine how rates of health events differ based on time, place, and person. It is from these rates that high-risk groups can be revealed in order for prevention efforts to be developed and implemented for the groups affected by the disease.

Analytical Epidemiology

Merrill and Timmreck (2006) define **analytical epidemiology** as an attempt by investigators to identify the cause of an event and to test their developing hypothesis. These studies are better able to prove that high-risk behaviors are the cause of illness and disease because they utilize a comparison or control group in the study.

Szklo and Nieto (2007) argue that analytical epidemiology allows the evaluation of a hypothesis, to the association of various risk factors, with the health event being observed. Figure 2-2 demonstrates the basic analytical approach used in a cohort study.

A *cohort study* involves a group of healthy people followed over time to determine the occurrence of health events. This figure looks at those exposed to a factor and those not exposed to the same factor. It then compares illness

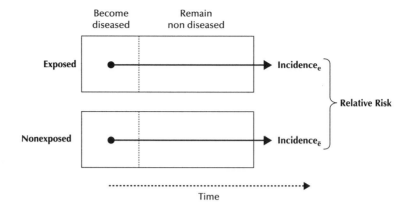

Figure 2-2
Basic Analytical
Approach in a
Cohort Study

Source: Szklo, M., &
Nieto, F. J. (2007).
*Epidemiology beyond the
basics* (2nd ed.). Sudbury,
MA: Jones and Bartlett
Publishers.

with wellness in the study group. There are advantages and disadvantages to this type of study, but it is usually one of the first methods utilized to indicate potential disease causation.

Epidemiologist Tool Kit

Merrill and Timmreck (2006) describes epidemiology as the distribution and determinants of health in a certain population with the goal being to use the information gathered about people for the control of health problems. Merrill and Timmreck (2006) support this definition of epidemiology as the study of the occurrence of a health event and the application of the study results to the prevention or the control of the event. Both of these definitions of epidemiology consist of the use of information to prevent disease. This is very similar to the goal of health promotion programs.

The starting point for an epidemiological investigation is the report of an abnormal occurrence or clustering of illness or disease, like a detective methodically solving a crime by determining the causative factors and then determining the best way to prevent future occurrence of disease. Detectives work with motives, circumstances, and profiles of the victim and the criminal; epidemiologists analyze the disease–injury–illness and profile the victims and circumstances of environments, habits, and motivations for healthy or unhealthy lifestyles. Epidemiologists evaluate ill and well individuals in an attempt to find the reasons some people become ill and others do not become ill.

The usual starting point for this type of investigation is the use of a survey to gather information from ill and well individuals exposed to a potential cause of disease. Then, an attempt is made to uncover the determinants of the disease and to document locations and numbers of old and new cases. The data gathered from potentially exposed ill and well individuals allows the opportunity to develop a rough hypothesis that may explain the cause of disease.

Figure 2-3 illustrates the chain of infection of how injury, disease, and many other health events occur. It is considered to be a step-by-step process

Figure 2-3
The Chain of Infection

PATHOGEN — RESERVOIR — MODE OF TRANSMISSION — HOST

that results in the health event. The starting point in the chain of infection is the introduction of a pathogen, which is the cause of the illness or disease. This pathogen can be a bacterium, virus, parasite, or anything capable of causing illness or disease in humans.

The reservoir is where the pathogen lives. Humans often serve both as a reservoir and a host. The mode of transmission is the way that the pathogen gets from the reservoir to the new host. It can be direct contact, which involves person-to-person transmission, or indirect transmission involving person to object to the new host. In order to prevent illness or disease, the chain of infection must be broken.

Table 2-1 illustrates the various forms of information required to affect public health policy and individual health decisions. This information can be found through the use of epidemiology and can also be interpreted by the same epidemiological process. The table demonstrates the assessment, cause of the problem, completion of the clinical picture, and program evaluation. These components are also very necessary to develop and evaluate a health promotion program.

Table 2-1
Types of Epidemiologic Information Useful for Influencing Public Health Policy and Planning and Individual Health Decisions

Source: Merrill, R. M., & Timmreck, T. C. (2006). *Introduction to epidemiology* (4th ed.). Sudbury, MA: Jones Bartlett Publishers.

1. Public health assessment
   - Surveillance
     - Identifying individuals and populations at greatest risk for disease
     - Identifying where the public health problem is greatest
     - Monitoring diseases and other health-related events over time

2. Finding causes of disease
   - Identifying the primary agents associated with disease, disorders, or conditions
   - Identifying the mode of transmission
   - Combining laboratory evidence with epidemiologic findings

3. Completing the clinical picture
   - Identifying who is susceptible to disease
   - Identifying the types of exposures capable of causing disease
   - Describing the pathologic changes that occur, the stage of subclinical disease, and the expected length of this subclinical phase of the disease
   - Identifying the types of symptoms that characterize the disease
   - Identifying probable outcomes (recovery, disability, or death) associated with different levels of the disease

4. Evaluating the program
   - Identifying the efficacy of the public health program
   - Measuring the effectiveness of the public health program

The corner stone of public health practice is the ability to gather accurate and useful surveillance data. There is an enormous amount of health data available; in fact, there is so much available data that those charged with gathering the data have difficulty in determining what data is most valuable for the problem under consideration.

The primary consideration needs to be finding the cause of the illness or disease. This step requires defining the real problem and not concentrating on the symptoms of the problem. Luck, Chang, Brown, and Lumpkin (2006) argue that local health information can be an invaluable component in the discovery of health problems and a potential source of the solution to these health problems. This local data can be a very strong tool to open up opportunities for collaboration among businesses, government, and communities in the improvement of health. Therefore, the right data can help us better define the real problem and develop collaborative prevention efforts. This represents the real starting point in the development of health promotion programs.

Table 2-1 also illustrates the importance of completing the clinic picture of diseases. This is an important contribution of epidemiology because it can identify those who are most susceptible to disease. When evaluating chronic diseases, the science of epidemiology is very capable of uncovering the high-risk health behaviors that place individuals at risk for disease and, more importantly, cause the long-term complications from having the chronic disease.

Table 2-1 also demonstrates the important role for epidemiology in program evaluation. Prevention programs must be evaluated in terms of efficacy and effectiveness. In order to obtain resources from the government or foundations, the prevention effort must survive evaluation that demonstrates success in reducing the disease burden at a cost that is acceptable to the funding agency. Health promotion programs are being subjected to cost-effectiveness evaluation just like clinical services and drug therapy regimens.

The key components in Table 2-1 include surveillance, disease causation, completion of the clinical picture, and evaluation. These are the same components that are a prerequisite to a successful health promotion program. Merrill and Timmreck (2006) argue that this model is the very foundation of all epidemiological models. Although it is primarily used for communicable diseases, its components are applicable to other health events.

This model better explains the role of behavior and lifestyle in the causation of the current epidemic of expensive chronic diseases in this country. The model uses causative factors rather than agents in explaining the etiology of these diseases.

This is more reflective of the new wave of diseases with long incubation periods and with more than one cause. It places primary prevention as the only defense against infection. This model also considers behavior over time and the culture of the group practicing unsafe behavior as factors to consider in disease prevention programs. Therefore, health promotion programs will gain new stature as the best intervention against infection.

Case Definition and Surveillance Systems

The epidemiologist now begins building a case definition. Turnock (2004) argues that a case definition includes standardized criteria for determining whether a person has a disease or health-related condition. This case definition includes clinical and personal qualities of the health event under investigation. A case definition is like a well-developed problem statement. The old adage that a problem well defined is half solved can be true in illness and disease prevention programs. This case definition is the major component of a well-developed surveillance system.

> **Surveillance Systems**
> - Active system
> - Passive system

A surveillance system is the use of gathered data to observe health events in order to better understand the event and, more importantly, to prevent or control the event. Although surveillance systems are usually used for communicable diseases, they can be used to gather data on chronic diseases or injuries. In fact, these systems can be used to gather data on anything that we are interested in better understanding.

Health data usually comes from people, the environment, and health providers of care and health facilities. Some data reporting is mandatory, and other data is requested for different purposes. Surveillance systems can be active, requiring mandatory reporting, and passive surveillance systems can be requested by government. These systems are one of the most important tools found in the tool kit of the epidemiologist.

A survey instrument is the mechanism utilized to gather data for the surveillance system to operate efficiently and effectively. These surveys are developed in order to obtain very specific information about a representative population and then generalized for the entire population.

Rates Used in Epidemiology

Figure 2-4 demonstrates how to obtain a rate for use in epidemiology. A **rate** is a measure of some event, condition, disease, injury, or illness in relation to a unit of population during some specific time period. It makes it much easier to compare health events if the population exposed and infected is taken into consideration. The rate of illness, disease, or injury makes more sense if evaluated in terms of some type of morbidity rate. The cause of death makes more sense in comparison of causes of death if the health event is evaluated in terms of mortality rates.

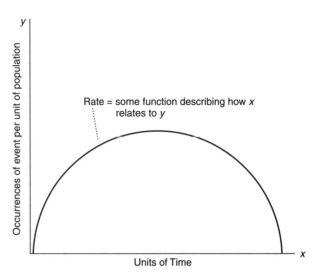

Figure 2-4
Determination of a Rate

There are many other rates that are used in epidemiology and are very useful for making comparisons of disease in the community. The incidence rate is quite useful in a short-term evaluation or a developing epidemic of some type of community hazard or illness that is being evaluated. This rate looks at new cases of something over a short period of time

Another useful rate for the community is the prevalence rate. This rate looks at disease over a longer period of time, like a year. It is very useful in looking at long-term exposure to community hazards and changes in the reporting of chronic diseases in individuals over the long run. The attack rate is utilized when there is a rapid increase in new cases of disease over a short period of time. It is usually expressed as a percentage, and some consider it a cumulative incidence rate.

The more important rates to an epidemiologist would certainly be incidence rate, prevalence rate, and attack rate. In order to have reliable rates, one must be using good data gathered from an established surveillance system. One of the most important tools utilized by the epidemiologist in an investigation is a rate. In fact, it is noted by those in public health that what separates an epidemiologist from other scientists is the development and comparison of rates in order to form a hypothesis.

Epidemics

One of the most feared words in the epidemiologist's dictionary is epidemic. This much-abused term simply means more cases of disease or "Event A" than one would normally expect. The word *epidemic* can be used with communicable and chronic diseases, injuries, and environmental and occupational health problems. Rowitz (2006) argues that the definition includes small facts or events that have large and long-lasting consequences, and how to prevent additional cases.

There are examples of epidemics are all around us on a daily basis. The city of New York is experiencing an epidemic of diabetes, the nation is preparing for a possible pandemic of Avian Influenza, women are experiencing an epidemic of heart disease, and some occupations are experiencing an epidemic of homicides. It is interesting to note that all four of these epidemics can be prevented with the help of good epidemiological data and a well-developed prevention program.

Behavioral Epidemiology

The CDC (2006) believes that there is a very important role to be played by the behavioral and social sciences in the mission of their agency. Although this is a recent belief, it is becoming very evident that the value of behavioral and social science is increasing at the CDC, as demonstrated by the creation of new organizational units and the recent emphasis on unhealthy behavior as the cause of many diseases.

High-Risk Health Behaviors
- Begin early in life
- Are learned behaviors
- Are responsible for causing many of the chronic diseases

The addition of these disciplines to the epidemiology tool kit brings new approaches to the major goal of public health, the prevention of disease. Including sciences like sociology, anthropology, psychology, and economics can increase the emphasis on the development of better disease intervention programs.

Behavioral research has already been utilized with diabetes, HIV, and obesity programs with great success. These positive intervention approaches need to be combined with epidemiology to improve prevention efforts, program evaluation, and policy analysis.

Epidemiologic studies conducted over the last several years have consistently implicated certain high-risk behaviors as the cause of many of the chronic diseases. These high-risk health behaviors usually begin early in life and increase in intensity as people grow older. Because these behaviors involve human behavior, the epidemiologist cannot tell us why they happen, only that they do increase susceptibility to disease.

> **Cause of Obesity Epidemic**
> - Poor diet
> - Lack of physical activity

Value of the Use of Epidemiology in Health Promotion

Epidemiology is a prerequisite for the development, implementation, and evaluation of a successful health promotion program. For example, public health disease control programs start with a very pessimistic reason for existence. Is the best that we can hope for to control the occurrence of disease? Why can we not utilize the scarce resources to prevent rather than to control disease? Why do we always use the word *control* when we address public health problems in this country? For example, when discussing communicable disease control programs, chronic disease and injury control programs, should we not start using the word *prevention* instead of control?

Turnock (2009) takes this concept a step further by questioning the responsibility for health promotion, health protection, and disease prevention. Where is the responsibility for these functions? Does the responsibility rest with the patient, the health care system, or does responsibility rest with society? Epidemiology offers no questions about responsibility. Instead of assuming that responsibility lies somewhere else, the science of epidemiology gives us the data and attempts to help us to work together to prevent health problems at the earliest stage of development.

When developing prevention programs, it must be realized that there are three levels of prevention that must be considered when attempting to improve the health of Americans: primary, secondary, and tertiary. All of these levels require the need for good information about the cause of disease and how to prevent disease from occurring.

The most important area of prevention is found at the primary level. This level entails the use of health promotion techniques in order to prevent high-risk behaviors from ever developing in the first place. Epidemiology can be utilized at any of these levels to help develop, implement, and evaluate disease and disease complication promotion efforts or moving to the next stage.

There is a need for a different thought process when dealing with the concept of health prevention programs. Christensen, Baumann, Ruggles, and Sadtler (2006) point out that this country spends more money per capita on health care than any other nation but falls behind other nations on basic health indicators like infant mortality. They claim that these results occurred because of misdirected investments that use money to maintain the old way of delivering health care to consumers.

Ecological Component of Disease

Ecological studies involve comparisons of groups on exposure and disease.

The Institute of Medicine (IOM, 2003) argues that the public health model using the epidemiological triad (agent, host, and environment) is able to understand the ecological component of disease prevention. This model allows the use of many disciplines along with public health skills in solving a disease problem.

The IOM (2003) recommends extensive use of research in the development, implementation, and evaluation of health promotion efforts. The agency also recommends that those involved in the evaluation of health promotion programs utilize cost-effective analysis in the evaluation of new and old promotion efforts. These recommendations strongly support the need for those assigned health promotion responsibilities to have extensive training in epidemiology.

Table 2-2 reveals the eight leading causes of death in this country. This table also presents the risk factors associated with the development of these often fatal chronic diseases. The same behaviorally related risk factors are also responsible for the health complications that come forth from these diseases once they are fully manifested in the individual.

The discovery of the association of the risk factors with disease and justification for prevention programs is the responsibility of those trained in epidemiology. Those charged in the development of behavioral change programs are trained in other equally important disciplines. It becomes clear that understanding and appreciating both the discipline of epidemiology and behavioral health are required prerequisites for the development of a successful preventive health effort.

McKenzie, Neiger, and Smeltzer (2005) argue that the major problem with health promotion programs is that everyone knows that they make economic sense, but these worthwhile programs are either not funded for political reasons or are underfunded and fail because of a lack of resources. There is a major role for epidemiological data in the support for the rationale of health promotion programs.

Epidemiological data can link the health problem to behaviors that can be changed or prevented. It then becomes easier to attract much needed support for the health promotion program. For these reasons, health promotion specialists need to understand and use epidemiology in the development of their programs. According to Green and Kreuter (2005), the health promotion planner requires the ability to offer description and quantification to a health problem in order to get others to prioritize intervention efforts required to prevent the health problem.

Risk Factors	Heart Disease	Cancer	Stroke	Accidents	Diabetes	Cirrhosis	Suicide	Homicide
Behaviorally Related								
Smoking/tobacco use	X	X		X				
Alcohol use/abuse	X	X		X		X	X	X
Nutrition/diet	X	X	X		X	X		
Lack of exercise/fitness	X	X	X		X			
High blood pressure	X		X					
Cholesterol levels	X		X					
Overweight/obesity	X	X			X			
Stress	X			X			X	X
Drug use/abuse	X		X	X			X	X
Lack of seat belt use				X				
Environmentally Related								
Worksite risks/exposures		X		X				
Environmental hazards		X		X				
Vehicular hazards				X				
Household hazards				X				
Medical care risks	X	X	X	X	X	X	X	
Radiation exposures		X		X				
Infectious pathogens	X	X						
Engineering/design hazards				X				
Biological/Genetic Related								
Chromosome/genetic defects	X	X	X		X	X	X	
Congenital anomalies	X	X	X		X	X	X	
Developmental defects	X	X	X		X	X	X	
Socially Related								
Poverty	X	X	X	X	X	X	X	X
Low educational level	X	X	X	X	X	X	X	X
Lack of work skills	X	X	X	X	X	X	X	X
Disrupted families	X	X	X	X	X	X	X	X

Table 2-2

Top Eight Leading Causes of Death in the United States According to Selected Risk Factors

Source: Merrill, R. M., & Timmreck, T. C. (2006). *Introduction to epidemiology* (4th ed.). Sudbury, MA: Jones and Bartlett Publishers.

Kaplan, Everson, and Lynch (2000) argue for a multilevel approach when attempting to understand disease determinants. There needs to be a focus on upstream determinants of health and disease with no one discipline claiming supremacy. Rather, an effort needs to be made to build bridges between the levels. An honest evaluation of disease determinants requires at least a limited understanding of each discipline with something to add to the understanding of the disease upstream before it manifests itself.

CONCLUDING REMARKS

A very good understanding of the principles of epidemiology is a necessary prerequisite in the development of successful health promotion programs. The science of epidemiology has to be demystified to the point where those assigned with health promotion responsibilities not only understand how it works but begin to embrace the logic of the process.

On the other hand, epidemiologists need to realize the limits of their science when it comes to human behavior. It is one thing to understand the fact that many chronic diseases are caused by human behavior, but it is an important expansion of causation to understand why people deliberately practice these dangerous behaviors.

Perhaps the reason why health promotion programs have not achieved even greater success in preventing chronic diseases and their complications has been the poor understanding and utilization of the principles of epidemiology in their mission.

In order to develop a good health promotion program, a great deal of planning needs to be done before the effort even begins. This planning requires a better understanding of the real problem for which the prevention effort is being developed. Understanding the problem requires the use of tools that have been developed and perfected over the years by epidemiologists.

Those controlling resources can become more interested and supportive of the health promotion program being developed if they have a better understanding of the problems and the impact on their school, business, or community.

Epidemiology becomes one of the more important areas of concern for the health promotion specialist. It can be an exciting and formidable tool to develop and use in the efforts to develop, prioritize, and receive funding for the health promotion effort. Epidemiology can truly become the catalyst for the development of health promotion programs.

DISCUSSION QUESTIONS

1. What role should the principles of epidemiology play in the development of a health promotion program?
2. Why can we not utilize the scarce resources to prevent rather than to control disease?
3. What are the major differences between descriptive and analytical epidemiological methods?
4. Can the principles of epidemiology be utilized to provide answers to the epidemic of chronic diseases in the United States?

REFERENCES

Christensen, C. M., Baumann, H., Ruggles, R., & Sadtler, T. M. (2006). Disruptive innovation for social change. *Harvard Business Review, 84*(12), 94–101.

Christoffel, T., & Gallagher, S. S. (2006). *Injury prevention and public health practical knowledge, skills and strategies* (2nd ed.). Sudbury, MA: Jones and Bartlett Publishers.

Green, L. W., & Kreuter, M. W. (2005). *Health program planning: An educational and ecological approach* (4th ed.). New York, NY: McGraw Hill Publishers.

Institute of Medicine. (2003) The Future of Public's Health in the 21st Century. Washington DC: The National Academies Press.

Kaplan, G. A., Everson, S., & Lynch, J. W. (2000). *The contribution of social and behavioral research to an understanding of the distribution of disease: A multilevel approach*. Washington DC: Institute of Medicine.

Luck, J., Chang, C., Brown, E. R., & Lumpkin, J. (2006). Using local health information to promote public health. *Journal of Health Affairs, 25*(4), 979–991.

McKenzie, J. F., Neiger, B. L., & Smeltzer, J. L. (2005). *Planning, implementing and evaluating health promotion programs: A primer* (4th ed.). San Francisco, CA: Pearson Benjamin Cummings.

Merrill, R. M., & Timmreck, T. C. (2006). *Introduction to epidemiology* (4th ed.). Sudbury, MA: Jones and Bartlett Publishers.

Rowitz, L. (2006). *Public health for the 21st century: The prepared leader* (1st ed.). Sudbury, MA: Jones and Bartlett Publishers.

Skolt, M., & Nieto, F. J. (2000). *Epidemiology beyond the Basics.* Gaithersburg, MD: Aspen Publications.

Szklo, M., & Nieto, F. J. (2007). *Epidemiology beyond the Basics* (2nd ed.). Sudbury, MA: Jones and Bartlett Publishers.

Turnock. B.J. (2004). *Public Health What It Is and How It Works* (3rd ed.). Sudbury, MA: Jones and Bartlett Publishers.

Turnock. B. J. (2009). *Public Health What It Is and How It Works* (4th ed.). Sudbury, MA: Jones and Bartlett Publishers.

U.S. Centers for Disease Control and Prevention. (2009). www.cdc.gov

3

Needs Assessment

Bernard J. Healey, PhD
Robert S. Zimmerman Jr., MPH

OBJECTIVES

After reading this chapter, you should

- Understand the major data that is required for a community health promotion program
- Become aware of the value of a needs assessment in the development of a new health promotion program
- Understand the value of primary and secondary data in completing a needs assessment
- Become aware of all of the data required to complete a comprehensive needs assessment
- Be capable of explaining the use of a focus group in the completion of a needs assessment

KEY TERMS

Community health problems
Focus group
Needs assessment

Observation
Probes
Problem assessment

An Introduction to Needs Assessment

The IOM developed a very important report on promoting health a few years ago that consisted of a series of recommendations concerning health promotion intervention strategies using input from social and behavioral research (IOM, 2001). The publication was dedicated to the improvement of the health of the population through health promotion programs.

The first recommendation in this report stated

"Funding agencies should direct resources toward interdisciplinary efforts for research and intervention studies that integrate biological, psychological, behavioral, and social values." (IOM, 2001, p. 16).

This recommendation is heavily influenced by an understanding of the many factors that may influence behaviors in a community. The report supports a well-developed **needs assessment** prior to the development of a new health promotion effort. The needs assessment allows the expansion of the public health model to better understand the various determinants that surround a community and ultimately determine the health of that community. This assessment will define the major **community health problems** and the health behaviors that are responsible for those problems.

Needs Assessment

A needs assessment is a method of discovering, evaluating, and prioritizing the health needs of a population.

The needs assessment is probably the most important component of the health planning and health promotion process. The assessment of what is required by those who utilize our service allows us to develop appropriate programs to meet their needs. Luck, Chang, Brown, and Lumpkin (2006) argue that local health information is a prerequisite to the improvement of community health, because it is capable of exposing both the problems and the potential solution to these problems in the community. The needs assessment is capable of giving us the local health information which is necessary to program planning.

Obtaining factual information about the frequency and causes of community health problems is an essential first step in solving the problem. Community health problems, small and large, require a dedicated planning process in order to achieve success in the abatement of these problems. We must always keep in mind the necessity of separating the real health problem from the symptoms that surround them.

Over the last several years, the role of a needs assessment has increased in importance in the planning process for health promotion efforts. In fact, the majority of individuals attempting to improve the health of a school, workplace, or community insist on a comprehensive needs assessment as the first step in the development of any new health promotion initiative.

Anspaugh, Dignan, and Anspaugh (2000) define needs assessment as a process of collecting and analyzing information to better understand the health problem before developing a program to prevent the problem. McKenzie, Neiger, and Smelzer (2005) argue that need assessment of the priority population is critical because it provides objective data in order to better determine the real health problem and to be able to measure progress toward solving the health problem.

These definitions sound very similar to the process followed by an epidemiologist when investigating an outbreak of disease—in other words, determining those at risk and why they are at risk for a health problem. Better health data usually means better decision making when designing programs that attempt to prevent high-risk health behaviors.

Needs assessment has also been called **problem assessment** by some researchers. Laverack (2004) points out that community problem assessment must involve community members who are empowered to be part of the decision-making process in determining the wider health issues in their community. Needs assessment can provide direction to a community, workplace, or school as community members prepare to intervene in an identified health problem. It also allows for the prioritization of the use of scarce resources.

The entire planning process for health services in any area is going to fail without a comprehensive needs assessment very early in the development phase. If you are aware of the needs of the consumers of health services and the providers of these services very early in the development of health promotion programs, you have increased the chances of success in your venture. The needs assessment is a continuous process that changes as more information is gathered from credible sources. The advantage of completing this process early allows a clear understanding by everyone involved in the health promotion effort and makes it possible to attract a greater level of resource commitment as the process goes forward.

According to the CDC (2009), the formal needs assessment process requires the collection, analysis, and interpretation of the health-related needs of a school, community, or workplace at a given point in time. Because these needs are constantly changing, it is imperative that an assessment of current needs be obtained before developing a new health promotion effort.

The needs assessment can be conducted on an informal or a formal basis. The informal needs assessment consists of data gathered from conversations with people familiar with the community, but this discussion has no predetermined questions. It consists of discussions with clients and staff where services are being delivered. This informal assessment of met and unmet needs of current service offerings can be the starting point or preparation phase for the formal needs assessment process. The formal needs assessment is a very structured process that uses predetermined questions and one of the many models of community assessment that have been used with success in the previous gathering of health data.

Data Required for Needs Assessment

The completion of a needs assessment allows those assigned the responsibility to develop health promotion programs the ability to ask relevant questions of the members of a community. Examples of these questions include the following:

- What are the major health problems and issues that are found in the target group?
- Who in the target group are at risk for the health problems?
- What health behaviors place individuals at most risk for these health problems?

Target Population

The target population is the priority population for which the intervention is designed.

Major Data to be Acquired from a Needs Assessment

The data that needs to be obtained from a needs assessment include health outcome data, risk factor data, and community resource data. All of this data is necessary in the planning process for the development of a health promotion program.

Health Outcome Data

This data is available from local and state health departments and can be utilized to determine priority areas for the health promotion program. This data will be utilized to evaluate the success or failure of the health promotion program.

Health Outcome Data   This data allows the evaluation of the health status of the population for which the promotional effort is being developed. This data can be found in vital statistics data such as birth and death certificates, county health profiles, and various other public databases.

Risk Factor Data   Risk factors are the cause of various health problems. These factors include disease agents, personal characteristics, and environmental factors that predispose one to illness and disease. A great deal is known about how risk factors cause disease but very little is known about the reasons why individuals practice behaviors that place them at risk for illness and death. The needs assessment can be the mechanism to discover the risk factors of greatest importance in a given community and the demographics of those practicing the risky health behaviors.

Resource Data   This data includes the resources available in communities to treat disease or to stop the practice of risky behaviors. Resources can include health facilities, health professionals, clinics, exercise facilities, and any other resources that are available in a community to promote health. Resource availability data can help in the elimination of duplication of services in a given community. There is also the possibility of acquiring new resources from the community for the health promotion effort.

Demographic Data   The demographic data from every community is very helpful in addressing the need for health promotion efforts in various communities. Morbidity and mortality can differ by age, gender, marriage, and other demographic data and can be very important in the development of community-based health promotion programs.

Assessing Community Needs

McKenzie, Pinger, and Kotecki (2004) offer a step-by-step approach that is very useful in the assessment of the health needs of a workplace, school, or community. Figure 3-1 offers a model that demonstrates the sequence of steps that are required to complete a needs assessment.

Before starting the needs assessment, there needs to be a definition of the purpose and scope of the program. This part of the assessment is concerned with what will be accomplished by the process and the resources available to conduct the assessment.

McKenzie et al. (2004) argue that an assessment of needs should include the following components: determining the purpose and scope of the assessment, gathering data, analyzing the data, identifying factors linked to the health problem, identifying the program focus, and validating the prioritized need. These steps, if completed properly, should allow the development and implementation of promotion programs capable of reducing or eliminating many of the health problems under consideration. It is important to understand that even before the needs assessment begins there must be a determination of the questions that need to be answered as well as who needs to be interviewed.

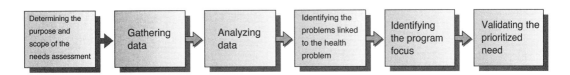

Figure 3-1 A Needs Assessment

Source: McKenzie, J. F., Pinger, R. R., & Kotecki, J. E. (2004). *An introduction to community health* (5th ed). Sudbury, MA: Jones and Bartlett Publishers.

Determining the Purpose and Scope

The first step in the assessment of needs is the determination of the purpose and scope of the assessment. Needs assessments can be used for a variety of reasons, and the scope of the assessment depends on the type of project being considered.

Gathering Data

There are a variety of ways to gather needs data when completing an assessment of the health of a community. The researcher will usually begin with an evaluation of secondary data that has been gathered by federal, state, and local health agencies. Then, primary data will be gathered from the population through a well-designed questionnaire.

Analyzing the Data

Data analysis is the third step in the assessment process. This step includes the application of statistical procedures in an attempt to describe the health of the population and, in some cases, validate the hypotheses generated as the needs assessment progressed. It must be assumed that the researchers have some understanding of statistics and access to some suitable statistical software packages. There is an excellent statistical program produced by the CDC and available at no cost in the public domain. It is titled *Epi Info* and can be found at the CDC website.

Identifying Factors Linked to the Health Problem

Once the health problems of the community have been determined, there is a need to obtain more data on the potential causes of these health problems. This is a very important step in the development of health promotion programs to abate the high-risk behaviors found in that community.

Leading Contributors to Death
- Tobacco
- Physical activity
- Diet
- Alcohol

There is a large amount of data available concerning the behavioral causes of high-risk health behaviors that predispose individuals to chronic diseases. This data can be made available at low cost and limited time involvement by utilizing various databases produced by various government agencies. There is a wealth of data available from the CDC, the "Wonder" program, and the *MMWR*.

Identifying the Program Focus

Fielding and Briss (2006) believe that participatory research is the key to better focus the relevance of research findings on the needs of a community—in other words, to include the opinions of those being affected by a new community program in the final research report. This requires going beyond data from questionnaires and inclusion of qualitative data gathered from community leaders and residents in the research effort. Because every community may be different, there needs to be a way to gather data concerning community priorities, beliefs, and cultures in order to improve the chances of success of the health promotion program.

Validating the Prioritized Need This rich data, gathered through a mixed approach of needs assessment that includes numerical data supported by qualitative data, can be extremely helpful in determining which strategies have a better chance of success in the improvement of health of a particular community. The needs assessment must be able to validate the community needs and to begin the process of assigning value to the various promotion efforts that need to be developed and implemented in the community.

Techniques for Collecting Information for Needs Assessment

The corner stone of public health practice is the ability to gather accurate and useful surveillance data. There is an enormous amount of health data available; in fact, there is so much available data that those charged with gathering the data have difficulty in determining what data is most valuable for the problem under consideration.

The primary consideration needs to be finding the real cause of the illness or disease. This step requires the definition of the real problem, not concentrating on the symptoms of the problem. McGinnis and Foege (1993) argue that discovering the real cause of chronic diseases is difficult because most of these diseases are multifactorial in nature. With many factors causing one disease, it becomes problematic to sort out the relative contribution of each factor in the disease process. McGinnis and Foege (1993) believe that the most prominent contributors to the development of chronic diseases are tobacco, diet and alcohol, microbial agents, toxic agents, and firearms, to name a few. These same contributors are very important in the development of the complications and loss of quality of life that come forth from having these diseases for a long period of time.

Luck et al. (2006) argue that local health information can be an invaluable component in the discovering of health problems and a potential solution to these health problems. This local data can be a very strong tool to open up opportunities for collaboration among businesses, government, and communities in the improvement of health. Therefore, the right data can help us better define the real problem and develop collaborative prevention efforts. This represents the starting point in the development of health promotion programs.

Community-Based Research

Because public health prevention programs are concerned about the health of the population, the interest is focused on communities, cities, counties, and states. McGinnis, Russo, and Knickman (2006) point out that there are at least five domains that shape health in the population: genetic and gestational endowments, environmental factors, behavioral choices, and the system of medical care available in the community. The result of the intersection of these domains is the finished health product. In the case of the community, this means the health of the population in that community.

Shi (1997) argues that health services research focuses on the health of populations rather than on the health of the individual. Blumenthal and DiClementi (2004) point out that community-based research can guide public health workers who are engaged in improving the health of the population. This type of research is a scientific inquiry involving human subjects and takes place in the community. It is capable of identifying health problems and issues and assessing them on a community-wide basis. It also allows public health prevention messages to be tested and evaluated by the community.

Shi (1997) points out that health services research is usually drawn from population surveys, community records, and direct observations of the population. In order to obtain valid and reliable data, the researcher may encounter tremendous cost and time in the acquisition of this data. Fortunately, there is a large amount of secondary data produced by the government every year. This data is found in the public domain, is readily available, and is a necessary adjunct to a community needs assessment. Another very good source of data is found in epidemiological research available from a number of government agencies, especially the CDC. A part of the CDC website, the *MMWR* provides a very large database on previous epidemiological reports and summaries that can aid the researcher in determining the causes of poor health indicators in a community.

Good data gathered from the community is very helpful in assessing the health of the population and aids in the search for the causes of disease, injury, and disability. This data is also very useful in measuring a community's progress in prevention and control efforts. By knowing the status of the health of a community at the beginning of a health promotion campaign, it is much easier to evaluate the success or failure when the effort is complete.

The Research Process

The process involved in gathering information about a particular health topic can seem like a daunting task to the health promotion specialist. It is very important to demystify the process of gathering research to better identify the problem and to improve the chances of a better problem definition before beginning health promotion planning. Gathering research data about a health problem resembles the epidemiological process of gathering data to form a hypothesis about disease causation. It is a long process, but if done properly, it is well worth the time and effort because of the value of the finished product.

Primary Data

McKenzie, Pringer, and Kotecki (2004) state that primary and secondary data are two important types of data that are utilized in the completion of a needs assessment. Primary data is new data gathered for a specific project by the researcher, while secondary data has already been gathered for another purpose.

Primary data is more relevant in health services research projects because it is up to date and gathered by the researchers for the current project. This is new data that has the capability of discovering the high-risk behaviors that should be addressed by the health promotion program. Primary data useful for the needs assessment is usually gathered by the health promotion specialist. It is useful in the development of a new or unique approach to the best way to promote a health prevention effort. It is also the appropriate method of gathering data when the researcher is unable to locate the relevant data from secondary research data. Unfortunately, the gathering of primary data is very time consuming and expensive to gather.

Quantitative Data

A survey can be an excellent way to help the researcher gain valuable data for the needs assessment. The survey can be designed to provide answers needed by health promotion specialists in the development of a health promotion program. Because the survey is used on only a sample of the population, great attention must be paid to bias in the sample selected.

Creswell (1994) argues that when using quantitative data the researcher remains distant from those being researched. The researcher is interested in the numbers only and not the reasons for the data. The interest includes counting people, behaviors, and conditions and classifying them into groups for analysis. Quantitative data gathered through a questionnaire makes it easy to reach a large number of respondents in a short period of time. This type of data gathering requires limited staff, can be gathered at low cost without bias, and can involve large numbers of respondents.

Qualitative Data

Qualitative data gathering relies on in-depth interviews and is a very practical way to design, conduct, and evaluate research in the area of public health and population-based services. Shi (1997) defines qualitative research as the gathering of data through observations and analysis that is less numerical and more an attempt to view the world from the eyes of the participants in the study. Green and Thorogood (2004) argue that the major difference between qualitative data and quantitative data is that qualitative data relies on language (written and oral) while quantitative data relies more on numbers and larger sample size. According to Creswell (1994), there is real interaction between the researcher and those being researched. The data gathered is used to offer an explanation to the why and how of health-related events.

Curry, Shield, and Wetle (2006) argue that research used for the development of public health programs can only be made better by the inclusion of qualitative methods in the study design. These researchers believe that a mixture of strong quantitative data supported by the use of qualitative data determining why the data on the problem occurred the way it did can offer a better explanation of the behaviors. There is a need to explain the reason why people behave the way they do with regards to healthy choices when developing and evaluating health promotion programs. The answer to this question cannot be obtained from quantitative data alone.

Qualitative researchers use interviews, **focus groups,** and observation in order to gather primary data. An interview is a one-on-one discussion with a survey participant. A focus group consists of personal interviews with a group of 8 to 10 participants that attempts to gain important data about the topic under consideration. **Observation** simply involves watching subjects and evaluating characteristics or patterns of behavior. This technique can also be accomplished with a mechanical device such as a camera. In needs assessment, there is use of open-ended questions looking for reasons why individuals believe that the high-risk behaviors occurred. There is also the use of unstructured interviews with key informants and focus groups representing the community. There is also the use of **probes**, which follow the lead of the informant while looking for additional details.

The use of a focus group format works very well when gathering qualitative data about the health of a community. The focus group is a technique that utilizes small groups of individuals that represent a target audience to collect information and opinions about specific subjects in a selected area. These groups are very helpful in developing hypotheses as to why high-risk health behaviors occur.

Secondary Data   Secondary data has been gathered by other researchers for other purposes but may be useful for the current health promotion effort. Secondary data has the advantage of being less expensive in terms of time to gather the data and the costs associated for the research and management of the data gathering project. The CDC has gathered health information for many years. This information is readily available and usually very easy to locate when developing answers to your research questions.

Secondary data is available from many government agencies, is found in the public domain so it is easy and inexpensive to use, and is usually of high quality following vigorous research studies. A complete listing of several sources of electronic secondary sources is available in Appendix A at the end of this text.

The Behavioral Risk Factor Surveillance System

The CDC (2009) conducts an ongoing, state-based surveillance system that provides information on health risk behaviors relating to the leading causes of death in the United States. The system that is used is called the Behavioral Risk Factor Surveillance System (BRFSS) and has been a source of data on high-risk behavior for the United States since 1984. It is a cross-sectional telephone survey that is conducted by all state health departments.

The BRFSS consists of three major components (CDC, 2009). They include the core questions, optional modules, and state-added questions. The core includes standardized questions that are asked of all individuals surveyed. The optional part includes questions that gather data relevant to health behaviors and health-related conditions. The state-added questions consist of questions of concern to the individual state completing the questionnaire.

The core questions look at demographics, health status, quality of life issues, health behaviors, disease status, screening tests, and firearms. The states add other health issues such as diabetes, asthma, secondhand smoke policy, binge drinking, and arthritis, to name a few.

The data is collected monthly by each state and then forwarded to the CDC for analysis. The survey, completed in 2004, utilized computer-assisted telephone interviewing (CATI) to collect the data from the states.

Completing a Needs Assessment

In order to complete a needs assessment, the starting point is the determination of the questions that need to be answered. These questions are instrumental in the determination of the health problems found in the community and the high-risk health behaviors that are prevalent in this community.

The Steps in Needs Assessment Revisited

Community needs assessment is a process that reveals the current situation in the community and determines how this situation can be made better in terms of a healthier community. Before the needs assessment begins there should be contact between those completing the assessment and the leaders within the community in order to alert them and to gain their support. The plan for a needs assessment should at a minimum include the following components:

- Sources of required data.
- Review of secondary data available from multiple sources.
- Contact of other agencies in the community to gain support for the project and secure additional data for the project.
- Interview of key informants in the community who have interest and experience with the problem under consideration.
- Consult with local government agencies that may have data concerning the area and the problem being investigated.

Application of Continuous Quality Improvement in Needs Assessment

Health promotion efforts have the overriding goal of improving the quality of life for the school, workplace, or community. All too often we rely on the experts to analyze the situation and to offer recommendations on how the current state of affairs can be improved. We look to experts in health care delivery to improve the quality of the system of care. We look to physicians to improve the medical quality of treatment, and we look to finance and economics people to improve the quality of health care at a price we can afford.

It seems like it might be time to consider getting greater input from the individuals affected by health services delivery to determine what quality care is for the patient. Perhaps it is not cure of disease that is the answer for the patient. It may be more emphasis on preventing disease in the first place that the consumer of care really wants. Taking this one step further, perhaps the patient or consumer can tell us what is needed for a health promotion program to work. It may be time for the application of continuous quality improvement to be applied to the way the most important part of health promotion programs, the needs assessment, is completed.

According to McLaughlin and Kaluzny (2006), experts in health care already have the knowledge about the subject matter but do not know how to improve the system of quality. How do we build a new theory that not only works but gains the respect of those who observe the process?

Figure 3-2 shows the FOCUS-PDCA cycle in quality improvement. This approach was fostered by W. Edwards Deming and is concerned with what he termed "profound knowledge" when dealing with systems. It has been utilized by many hospitals and is a very useful model for systems in health care.

This approach can also offer guidance to individuals working with a system involving health promotion activities. Because the health professionals involved in health promotion already have a good understanding of the subject matter, they can use the Deming model to improve the health promotion effort. Better data coming forth from a well-planned and implemented needs assessment is quite capable of allowing us to focus resources on the abatement of the real problem and improving the quality of life of the program customers.

The upper portion of Figure 3-2 consists of the acronym FOCUS, which stands for Find, Organize, Clarify, Understand, and Select. This model can be utilized to improve the process of health promotion programs. You start the process by finding a part of the health promotion program that requires improvement. You then move to a team that understands the process of the health promotion program, then evaluate what we know about the process, and learn what the cause of process variation is. You conclude FOCUS by selecting the process improvement.

The lower portion of the figure, PDCA, helps in the planning process for action in the health promotion process. The planning consists of data collection and improvement. Then, there is movement into data collection and analysis about the program process. The data is then utilized for process improvement using customer outcome as a result of the health promotion program. Finally, there is movement to hold the gain and to continue the improvement process.

This process forces health promotion specialists to attempt to discover what they are trying to accomplish and to question how they will know when they have accomplished their goal. The answers to these questions are usually found in the evaluation of the process of needs assessment. These are

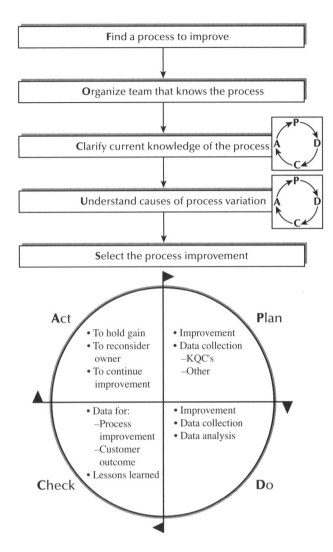

Figure 3-2
The FOCUS-PDCA
Cycle

Source: McLaughlin, C. P.,
& Kaluzny, A. D. (2006).
*Continuous quality
improvement in health care
theory, implementations,
and applications* (3rd ed.).
Sudbury, MA: Jones and
Bartlett Publishers.

the hard facts and this is why we think they are happening. Why do people practice high-risk behaviors even when they know the probable outcome of their actions? There is a mixed approach of data gathering and analysis required of the entire health promotion process.

An Example of the Needs Assessment Process

There are several good planning programs available to help with the development and implementation of a needs assessment. A good example of this type of program has been made available by the National Association of County and City Health Officials (NACCHO). They developed a program called

Mobilizing for Action through Planning and Partnerships (MAPP). The MAPP process offers a very good example of how the needs assessment fits into the overall planning process for the improvement of community health. This process, which will be discussed at length in the last chapter of this text, offers an excellent procedure for gathering data for a community needs assessment.

MAPP Process
Mobilizing for Action through Planning and Partnerships
A six-phase approach designed to improve the health of a community through mobilizing partnerships.

Community Health Status Assessment
The Community Health Status Assessment identifies priority issues related to the health of a community and quality of life.

The CHSA process allows comparison of peer communities in order to determine why one community is healthier than another community (see Figure 3-3). The entire MAPP process will be explained in great detail in the last chapter of this text.

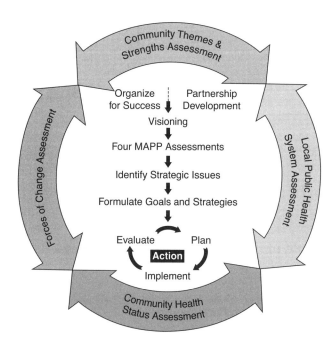

Figure 3-3
The MAPP Overview

Source: Courtesy of the National Association of County and City Health Officials (NACCHO).

CONCLUDING REMARKS

The starting point for a well-developed health promotion program involves the completion of an assessment of the needs of the target population for the promotion effort. The needs assessment allows those charged with the responsibility of health promotion activities the ability to offer the recipients the information they need to prevent or at least reduce high-risk health behaviors.

Those completing the needs assessment need to understand the primary research process and the use of a questionnaire to obtain accurate data from many sources regarding the research problem. They also need to appreciate the value of secondary data that has already been gathered through reputable sources for other reasons.

According to Curry et al. (2006), the planning and implementation of interventions in the health of a community is enhanced by the use of qualitative research methods that involve key stakeholders. These authors also call for the use of mixed research methods in community needs assessment that will provide a rich texture of response supported by quantitative data commonly found in program evaluation.

There is a need to constantly evaluate and improve the process of needs assessment. This can be accomplished through the use of continuous improvement programs discussed at great length in this literature.

There are also a variety of very good models available to make the job of gathering data a much easier process. The MAPP process has been tested and offers health promotion specialists a great planning tool to make the data gathering process a much easier task. It seems evident that health promotion programs can be improved by first improving the assessment of needs of the community. MAPP is a community-wide strategic planning and performance improvement tool. The step-by-step process is driven by four assessments to improve the way the local public health system conducts community health planning and programming.

DISCUSSION QUESTIONS

1. Name and explain the most important steps in the completion of a needs assessment for a community health promotion program.
2. What are the advantages and disadvantages associated with the collection of primary data?
3. Explain the use of a focus group to gather data to develop a comprehensive health promotion for a community.
4. What type of data can be gathered by a needs assessment of a community?

REFERENCES

Anspaugh, D. J., Dignan, M. B., & Anspaugh, S. L. (2000). *Developing health promotion programs.* Long Grove, IL: Waveland Press.

Blumenthal, D. S., & DiClementi, R. J. (2004). *Community-based health research.* New York, NY: Springer Publishing Company Inc.

Centers for Disease Control and Prevention. (1999). Framework for program evaluation in public health. *Morbidity and Mortality Weekly Report, 48*(11), 1–40.

Centers for Disease Control and Prevention. (2004). *Behavioral risk factor surveillance system.* Available at http://www.cdc.gov/brfss/index.htm. Accessed May 12, 2008.

Centers for Disease Control and Prevention. (2009). Available at http://www.cdc.gov/epiinfo. Accessed May 13, 2008.

Centers for Disease Control and Prevention. (2009). *Behavioral risk factor surveillance system: Turning information into health.* Available at http://www.cdc.gov/brfss. Accessed May 13, 2008.

Centers for Disease Control and Prevention. (2009). *Healthier worksite initiative.* Available at http://www.cdc.gov/nccdphp/dnpa/hwi/program_design/needs_assessment.htm. Accessed May 13, 2008.

Creswell, J. W. (1994). *Research design qualitative and quantitative approaches.* Thousand Oaks, CA: Sage Publications.

Curry, L., Shield, R., & Wetle, T. (2006). *Improving aging and public health research qualitative and mixed methods.* Washington, DC: American Public Health Association.

Fielding, J. E., & Briss, P. A. (2006). Promoting evidence-based public health policy: Can we have better evidence and more policy? *Journal of Health Affairs, 25*(4), 969–977.

Green, J., & Thorogood, N. (2004). *Qualitative methods for health services research.* Thousand Oaks, CA: Sage Publications.

Institute of Medicine (IOM). (2001). *Health and behavior: The interplay of biological, behavioral, and social influences.* Washington, DC: National Academy Press.

Laverack, G. (2004). *Health promotion practice power and empowerment.* Thousand Oaks, CA: Sage Publications.

Luck, J., Chang, C., Brown, E. R., & Lumpkin, J. (2006). Using local health information to promote public health. *Journal of Health Affairs, 25*(4), 979–991.

McGinnis. J. & Foege. W. (1993). Actual causes of death in the united states. *Journal of the American Medical Association, 270*(18), 2207–2212.

McGinnis, M., Russo, P. W., & Knickman, J. (2006). The case for more active policy attention to health promotion. *Journal of Health Affairs, 21*(7), 78–93.

McKenzie, J. F., Pinger, R. R., & Kotecki, J. E. (2004). *An introduction to community health* (5th ed.). Sudbury, MA: Jones and Bartlett Publishers.

McKenzie, J. F., Neiger, B. L., & Smeltzer, J. L. (2005). *Planning, implementing and evaluating health promotion programs: A primer* (4th ed.). San Francisco, CA: Pearson Benjamin Cummings.

McKenzie J., Neiger B., & Thackeray R. (2009). *Planning, implementing and evaluating health promotion programs: A primer* (5th ed.). San Francisco, CA: Pearson Benjamin Cummings.

McLaughlin, C. P., & Kaluzny, A. D. (2006). *Continuous quality improvement in health care theory, implementations, and applications* (3rd ed.). Sudbury, MA: Jones and Bartlett Publishers.

National Association of County and City Health Officials. (2004). *Achieving healthier communities through MAPP. A User's Handbook.* Washington DC: National Association of County and City Health Officials.

Shi, L. (1997). *Health services research methods.* Albany, NY: Delmar Publications.

Program Development

Bernard J. Healey, PhD
Robert S. Zimmerman Jr., MPH

OBJECTIVES

After reading this chapter, you should

- Understand the use of theoretical models in the development of health promotion programs
- Become aware of the components of the best intervention strategies for developing a health promotion program
- Understand the contributing factors to high-risk health behavior
- Become aware of the advantages and disadvantages of the PATCH program
- Be capable of explaining the various types of intervention strategies to produce a healthy community

KEY TERMS

Behavioral theory
Enablers
Evidence-based intervention strategies

PATCH
Process objectives
Theoretical constructs

Introduction

The major reason for the advances in the life span for most Americans over the last several years has been the discovery of the real causes of illness by public health and the use of health education and health promotion programs designed to stop the problems from occurring. These public health intervention strategies worked very well with communicable diseases, and the results have been proven by a longer life expectancy. Unfortunately, the new public health epidemic involves chronic diseases, not communicable diseases, caused for the most part by high-risk health behaviors that are difficult to change. These diseases can be prevented by well-developed health promotion programs.

Once the needs assessment has been completed and the mission statement, including goals and objectives for the health promotion effort, has been developed, it is time to choose the intervention strategies to attempt to reduce the problem. This is by far the most challenging part of the development of health promotion programs. It is a time-consuming process that requires the full attention of the health promotion program manager, stakeholders, and program staff. Fortunately, there is a large amount of research available to help in the development of an intervention strategy that can help achieve program goals and objectives. The starting point for building a database on intervention

---

Intervention Strategies

An intervention strategy is a plan of action for affecting a health-related problem. It is quite common to utilize multiple behavioral strategies in order to produce successful change.

---

strategies is an evaluation of the more popular theories about behavior change.

This part of the development of a health promotion program involves decision making about how to best achieve program goals. It involves choosing one type of intervention from a set of alternatives for dealing with the health problem. Because the health promotion manager is dealing with uncertainty, it makes sense to gather as much secondary data as possible about other programs that have dealt with similar health problems. Discussion with other health promotion managers can lead to a wealth of data that is already in use.

The program manager needs to consider interventions that have been tested while at the same time consider other creative options. Information needs to be obtained from colleagues, the public, and peer-reviewed literature. The best source of information can usually be obtained from **evidence-based intervention strategies** that have been successful elsewhere and made available by government agencies and foundations.

McKenzie, Neiger, and Smeltzer (2005) point out that interventions are activities or treatments received by the program participants that will help to achieve program goals. An intervention is a completed activity that should be instrumental in achieving the outcome that was proposed in the program goals and objectives. It is really an experience that will be provided for the participants of the health promotion program.

The Use of Theoretical Models

The major goal of health promotion programs is to help individuals convert poor health behaviors to healthy behaviors. Successful health promotion programs are developed through the use of solid planning techniques that utilize a theoretical base to develop their intervention effort. A theory consists of a set of concepts that are related that allows a better understanding of the situation under consideration. The theory of a behavior is the underlying cause of the behavior.

The understanding of **behavioral theory** is helpful when one is attempting to change the behavior. Those involved in the development of health promotion programs need to have a good understanding of why such behaviors exist.

A theory is very useful in offering the program manager a step-by-step approach to understand why people behave the way they do when it comes to their health and to look at possible ways to change that behavior.

Anspaugh, Dignan, and Anspaugh (2000) argue that a better understanding of the theories behind behavioral change can help to make health intervention programs more effective. McKenzie, Neiger et al. (2005) point out that utilizing theory allows a basis for understanding the various theories that are available concerning why things happen the way they do. These theories become useful when they are used to explain the relationship between the many variables that affect behavioral change. In the case of health promotion and behavioral change, it is very important to understand the theory behind human behavior. It is essential that the reasons for practicing high-risk health behaviors be studied and then **theoretical constructs** be used to formulate how best to attempt to change these behaviors through health promotion programs.

Intervention Models

There are numerous intervention strategies to consider in our quest to reduce or eliminate the high-risk health behaviors responsible for disease and death. Health promotion managers are looking for an effective program, but they also are working with limited resources to accomplish the goals and objectives put forth for the intervention effort. The IOM (2000) argues that the behavioral and social sciences are using new research to create strong theoretical models for interventions into health behaviors that predispose individuals to poor health.

Transtheoretical Model

Individuals usually move through a series of stages toward change before they complete the change. These stages include the following:

- Precontemplation
- Contemplation
- Preparation
- Action

The effectiveness of the model depends on sound theory and empirical evidence that supports the conclusions of the theoretical model. It is very important to attempt to develop the best intervention strategy that accomplishes goals while conserving the use of scarce resources. Interventions designed to promote healthy behaviors and to eliminate unhealthy behaviors have produced several theoretical models over the years. It is important to realize that the interventions are dealing with behaviors that are difficult to change.

McKenzie, Neiger et al. (2005) point out that very few individuals alter their behavior based on a single intervention. Rather, there is strong evidence that many different types of interventions are necessary to be successful in changing individuals behaviors. McKenzie, Pinger, and Kotecki (2005) also argue that interventions to change health behaviors usually are more successful if they are employed frequently and consist of more than one activity.

Table 4-1 shows a number of objectives, potential outcomes, evaluation methods, and health promotion program objectives. McKenzie, Pinger et al. (2005) point out that health promotion programs may be designed to achieve several objectives. These objectives may include **process objectives**, learning objectives, environmental objectives, and program objectives, as shown in Table 4-1. The numbers of objectives that need to be achieved to make progress against one high-risk behavior demonstrate the importance of good planning in dealing with health behaviors.

The Best Interventions   The U.S. Department of Health and Human Services (DHHS, 2003) defines a comprehensive intervention plan as one which

- includes the use of multiple strategies, such as educational, policy, and environmental strategies, within various settings, such as the community, health care facilities, schools, and work sites;
- targets the community at large as well as subgroups within the community; the community support is necessary to support the behavior change;
- addresses the factors that contribute to the health problem; and
- includes various activities to meet your audiences' levels of readiness.

> **Increase Chances of Success**
> The program should be
> - appropriate,
> - culturally sensitive, and
> - meet the needs of the target audience.

The interventions or health promotion programs that have the best chance of success must be appropriate, culturally sensitive, and meet the needs of the target audience. In order to ensure that these factors are present in the

Type of Objective	Program Outcomes	Possible Evaluation Measures	Type of Evaluation	Example Objective
Process–administrative objectives	Activities presented and tasks completed	Number of sessions held, exposure, attendance, participation, staff performance, appropriate materials, adequacy of resources, tasks on schedule	Process (form of formative)	On June 12, 2006, a breast cancer brochure will be distributed to all female customers over the age of 18 at the Ross grocery store.
Learning objectives	Change in awareness, knowledge, attitudes, and skills	Increase in awareness, knowledge, attitudes, and skill development–acquisition	Impact (form of summative)	When asked in class, 50% of the students will be able to list the four principles of cardiovascular conditioning.
Action/behavioral objectives	Change in behavior	Current behavior modified or discontinued, or new behavior adopted	Impact (form of summative)	During a telephone interview, 35% of the residents will report having had their blood cholesterol checked in the last 6 months.
Environmental objectives	Change in the environment	Protection added to, or hazards or barriers removed from, the environment	Impact (form of summative)	By the end of the year, all senior citizens who requested transportation to the congregate meals will have received it.
Program objectives	Change in quality of life (QOL), health status, risk, and social benefits	QOL measures, morbidity data, mortality data, measures of risk (e.g., HRA)	Outcome (form of summative)	By the year 2006, infant mortality rates will be reduced to no more than 7 per 1,000 in Franklin County.

Table 4-1
Hierarchy of Objectives and Examples of Each

Source: Adapted from Deeds, S. G. (1992). The Health Education Specialist: Self-study for Professional Competence. Los Alamitos, CA: Loose Canon; Cleary, M. J., and B. L. Neiger (1998). The Certified Health Education Specialist: A Self-Study Guide for Professional Competence, 3rd ed. Allentown, PA: National Commission for Health Education Credentialing; and McKenzie, J. F., B. L. Neiger, and J. L. Smeltzer (2005). Planning, Implementing, and Evaluating Health Promotion Programs: A Primer (4th ed.) San Francisco, CA: Benjamin Cummings.

intervention(s), it is imperative that program planners involve members of the target audience in the planning process. These individuals can give us many reasons for real world failure in changing these high-risk health behaviors. These same individuals can help us find creative ways to educate the high-risk groups about the behavior that the program is attempting to change.

The needs assessment has already provided program planners with the leading causes of morbidity and mortality for the target population to be addressed by the new health promotion program. The development of the program now needs to gather more information on not only the risk factors that are responsible for these health problems but the reasons why individuals practice these behaviors. This knowledge can help us put forth program objectives that if achieved will help to change the health behaviors that cause the health problems.

This information needs to include the reasons why some individuals begin practicing these behaviors and others do not. It is also important to find out why some people continue to practice these behaviors even when they become aware of the danger of these behaviors to their health. Secondary data from the literature is helpful, but discussion with members of the target group is probably of greatest value. Health planners call this information gaining knowledge of the contributing factors to the health problem. The more we know about the contributing factors, the more likely we are to develop successful interventions to change these behaviors.

In fact, information about the contributing factors to the health problem is the most important component in the development of a successful health promotion program. The CDC (2007) recommends that the contributing factors be grouped into three categories in order to not miss any significant factor. The categories include the following:

Motivators: factors motivating a person to take action. This group includes attitudes, beliefs, values, and knowledge. Motivating factors exist within the individual but can be set in motion through various parts of the health promotion program.

Enablers: factors enabling a person to take action. This group includes availability and accessibility of resources to make the change. Enablers include individual and environmental factors. The enablers can be set in motion through various parts of the intervention.

Rewards: factors rewarding a person's behavior. This group includes the attitudes and climate of support from providers of services, families, and community organizations that reinforce the behavior of a person. Included are social as well as physical benefits and tangible, imagined, or vicarious rewards. Approval or punishment for a behavior also fits into this category. The rewards can be included in a well-designed intervention strategy.

Those charged with developing health promotion programs need to appreciate and enhance the large theoretical base available for their use in trying to change human behaviors. They must also realize that behaviors are influenced by multiple factors, making it very important to have a good understanding of many of the theoretical approaches to behavioral change.

The CDC (2007) argues that a useful theory makes assumptions about a behavior that are:

- logical;
- consistent with everyday observations;
- similar to those used in previous successful programs; and
- supported by past research in the same area or related ideas.

Intervention Strategies

There is a great deal to be learned about health behaviors before moving to this stage of the health promotion program. A good understanding of behavioral theory allows the health promotion specialist the opportunity to better comprehend what is necessary to change human behavior. Without this knowledge, an intervention program may be targeting the wrong motives for the target audience practicing the high-risk behaviors that need to be changed. The intervention(s) need to be well planned and reviewed before they are actually implemented. All too often health promotion programs are implemented without adequate planning, and the results are short of expectations. The greater the time and effort that is spent in the program development stage, the better the chance of success in changing high-risk health behaviors for individuals and communities.

There are a variety of strategies that may be used in order to accomplish the program objectives. The type of intervention is dependent on the goals of the program and the availability of resources. Review of the literature and knowledge of best health promotions can also be helpful in the decision to utilize a specific intervention. They include health communication interventions, health education interventions, health policy interventions, health engineering interventions, health-related community interventions, and community organization interventions. A definition of each type of intervention would include the following:

Educational Interventions

This strategy involves the use of communication and training methods.

Communication Methods

There are a variety of communication methods that can be utilized to assist in the health promotion effort. The most used method is usually a classroom or seminar lecture and discussion methodology. Other effective communication methods include printed materials, audiovisual aids, educational television, and programmed learning. There have also been tremendous improvements in recent years in the use of information technology as a health communication tool using e-mail and dedicated websites.

Training Methods

There are several very effective training methods depending on the characteristics of the group that you are attempting to educate. These methods include, but are not limited to, skill development classes, game playing, inquiry learning methods, small group discussions, modeling, and behavior modification. These methods require an understanding of how individuals learn and the resources available to the health promotion program.

Health Policy Interventions

Recent research has been helpful in assisting health promotion managers to understand the value of health policy in changing health behaviors. Policies, regulations, and laws can be very effective in restricting or limiting unhealthy behaviors. Examples of these policies and regulations include no smoking ordinances, prohibition against the sale of tobacco and alcohol to minors, and laws against drunk driving. There can also be policies that can encourage healthy behaviors. Examples would include work time set aside for physical activity and requirements for employees to have an annual physical.

Environmental Strategies

The CDC (2007) argues that environmental strategies that include attention to the physical and social environment can be quite helpful for the health promotion manager. These strategies would include efforts that are supportive to health but discouraging to actions that are not supportive of health and support of normative changes in attitudes and behaviors that support healthy lifestyles.

Community Organization Interventions

There are several well-developed community-based health promotion interventions.

The Planned Approach to Community Health (PATCH)

The Planned Approach to Community Health (**PATCH**) emerged as a community approach to priority health problems in 1983. This widely used approach can still be used effectively today. This program recommends a comprehensive intervention plan to change high-risk health behaviors that include the following:

- Using multiple strategies within multiple settings, such as the community, health care facilities, schools, and work sites.
- Targeting the community at large as well as subgroups within the community.
- Addressing the factors that contribute to the health problem.
- Conducting various activities to meet your audience's levels of readiness.

The recent research concerning changing health behaviors strongly supports the fact that the health educator must understand the readiness of the target audience to change health behaviors.

Mobilizing for Action through Planning and Partnerships (MAPP)

MAPP is a strategic approach to the improvement of the health of the community. MAPP is a community-wide planning tool that leads communities to prioritize important public health issues and to be able to identify community resources necessary to eliminate the problems.

The MAPP program is concerned with strengthening the entire community health system rather than concentrating on separate parts of the system. The program has had tremendous success at being the catalyst to collaboration among multiple agencies to better community health. The MAPP program will be discussed at greater length in Chapter 17. Several case studies involving the use of the MAPP program will be provided in Appendix D of this book.

Application of Theory to the Intervention Process

In order to increase the chance of success in changing high-risk health behaviors, attention must be given to the behavioral models that have worked in previous health promotion programs.

Behavioral Models
- Health Belief Model
- Transtheoretical Model
- Theory of Planned Behavior

Three of the more popular behavioral models will now be explained and evaluated in terms of their application to health promotion programs. These models include the Health Belief Model (HBM), the Transtheoretical Model (TTM), and the Theory of Planned Behavior (TPB). These theories were chosen because they are logical and have been used frequently in numerous health promotion programs. They also offer a starting point to develop even better health promotion interventions.

Novick et al. (2008) believe that behavior can affect the health of individuals in direct and indirect ways. These effects have to be considered when designing the health promotion program. The health promotion manager must consider both types of effects when developing the intervention in order to provide for the potential indirect effects and also to include these variables in the program evaluation. This is demonstrated in Figure 4-1.

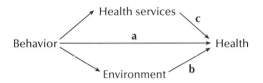

Figure 4-1
Behavior of Lifestyle Can Have a Direct Effect (A) or an Indirect Effect on Health
Through Exposure to the Environment (B) on the Use of Health Services (C)
Source: Green, L. W., & Kreuter, M. W. (1999). *Health promotion planning: An educational and ecological approach* (3rd ed.). Mountain View, CA: Mayfield Publishing Co.

Health Belief Model   One of the very first theories of health behavior ever introduced was the HBM. According to McKenzie, Neiger and Thakeray (2009), it was developed in the early 1950s by a group of individuals from the U.S. Public Health Service and is still one of the most widely respected theories in use today. These psychologists were interested in why so few individuals were concerned about disease detection and prevention programs.

McKenzie, Neiger et al. (2005) point out that HBM is a value expectancy theory that can be used to offer an explanation for many health behaviors. In this model, theorists were concerned with whether or not individuals perceived themselves to be susceptible to disease and whether or not they saw benefit in trying to prevent this disease. This is very important information to have when attempting to develop health promotion programs. According to Anspaugh et al. (2000), this model shed light on the complexity of behavior, especially when individuals are making decisions about their health. The HBM is concerned with one's perception of a situation as the basis for all behavior. For this reason, a better understanding of health behavior can be very useful in the development of successful health promotion programs. This model allows us to better understand the major influences on people's decisions with regards to becoming proactive about preventing or controlling illness.

The CDC (2007) believes that there are six main constructs that determine an individual's decision to take or not to take corrective action concerning their medical care. They argued that people are ready to act in a positive way if they

- believe they are susceptible to the condition (perceived susceptibility);
- believe the condition has serious consequences (perceived severity);
- believe taking action would reduce their susceptibility to the condition or its severity (perceived benefits);
- believe costs of action (perceived barriers) are outweighed by the benefits;
- are exposed to factors that prompt action (e.g., a television ad or reminder from one's physician to get a mammogram; cue to action); and/or
- are confident in their ability to successfully perform an action (self-efficacy).

This is a model for a health promotion program that focuses almost entirely on motivation.

The Transtheoretical Model   Another model that works very well with the development of health promotion interventions designed to promote behavioral change is the TM. According to Anspaugh, Dignan and Anspaugh (2000) this model, developed by Prochaska and DiClemente, focuses on change as a process rather than as an event. By considering change as a process, one can better identify the various stages of the change process.

Anspaugh et al. (2000) argue that people usually move through a series of steps as they attempt to change behaviors. In other words, the process of behavior does not just happen in a one-step process. Individuals move from state to state in a series of incremental steps before the behavior change is complete. McKenzie, Neiger et al. (2005) agree that there are several common steps followed as individuals proceed through the adoption and maintenance of behavior change, especially when dealing with a change in their health behaviors. The CDC (2007) describes this change process as having five important stages: precontemplation, contemplation, preparation, action, and maintenance. It is interesting to note that individuals may enter the process at any step in the process. They may also complete the entire process, change the behavior, and then relapse back to an earlier step in the process.

The change of one's behavior does not occur in rapid fashion. If change happens at all, it is a result of individual motivation, which cannot be rushed. In fact, in the first stage, pre-contemplation, individuals do not plan to change. It is an important stage because at least they are thinking about the various problems associated with their behavior. Once they become aware of the health risks posed by their behavior, they try to avoid thinking or even hearing about the issue from others.

The second stage of behavior change according to this theory is the actual contemplation stage. In this stage, the individual has become motivated to change behaviors and intends to take action within the next 6 months. They want to change, but they are not yet committed to making the required change at this point in time. These individuals have entered a stage where they have become motivated to make the health behavior change in the very near future.

The third stage involves actual preparation to make the behavioral change. Individuals in this stage of change are preparing to make the change in the next 30 days and are making preparation to do so. McKenzie, Neiger et al. (2005) believe that people at this stage of readiness have already taken steps to implement the change and need to be actively recruited to take part in the health promotion intervention. They are ready to change and need assistance from health educators in order to develop goals and time frames to make the behavioral change. This is the stage where they need continual motivation and reinforcement that this change in health behavior must be made as soon as possible.

The next stage of change is labeled the action stage and involves those who have changed their health behavior for less than 6 months. Anspaugh et al. (2000) argue that people at this stage of the change process encounter difficulty and often relapse into their former bad behavior patterns. They require social support, constant feedback, and reinforcement in order to maintain their previous success with behavior change.

The last stage in the change process involves maintenance and is defined by individuals who have changed their health behavior for longer than 6 months. A tremendous effort is required during this stage to integrate these new behaviors into every aspect of the individual's life. The health promotion manager must understand that these individuals require assistance with coping with the new behavior and discovering alternatives to the previous bad health behaviors. Relapse to the bad behaviors is always a very real possibility. These last 2 stages of the change process require constant reinforcement by the health promotion program staff.

Theory of Planned Behavior   The TPB explores the relationship between behaviors and beliefs, attitudes, and intentions. It is concerned with individuals' beliefs that they are able to control a particular behavior, including their health behavior. This model is very concerned with the attitudes toward the behavior and the outcome associated with the particular behavior. McKenzie, Neiger et al. (2005) point out that this theory is also concerned with perceived behavioral concerns and deals with the concept of self-efficacy.

Self-Efficacy

Self-efficacy is the competence to be able to accomplish desired tasks or behaviors. This requires an understanding of individuals' perceptions about their ability to be successful in accomplishing a task.

The concept of self-efficacy is of vital concern for those responsible for health promotion programs. Self-efficacy is defined as an individual's belief that they have the ability to control a certain function, which includes behaviors. In other words, they are in control of their behaviors and have the ability to change that behavior as they wish and without help from others. Because changing health behaviors is usually very difficult for most people, the health promotion manager needs to understand the concept of self-efficacy in the development of any health promotion program. Individuals with low self-efficacy, or those who believe that they have low self-efficacy, will need a great deal of help and support in changing the health behavior. The best way to help these individuals with the behavioral change process would be to show them how to make small behavioral changes rather than attempt to make large behavioral changes at one time.

Kreuter, Lezin, Kreuter, and Green (2003) point out that the most important components of this model include personal experience, observational experience, verbal persuasion, and physiological state. Kreuter et al. (2003)

offer a specific intervention strategy for dealing with safe sex, utilizing condoms. This step-by-step approach offers an excellent approach in dealing with low self-efficacy in the confrontation of a potential high-risk health behavior. This theory focuses on the individual's intention to perform the behavior under consideration. This intention to perform the behavior is influenced by the person's attitude concerning the behavior and a concern about the opinion of others concerning the behavioral change. Therefore, perceived behavioral control over the resources required to execute the behavior becomes critical.

Although the skill set by Kreuter et al. (2003) was specifically designed for learning how to discuss condom use with a sex partner, it is a very useful intervention for many other health behavior changes involving the concept of low self-efficacy. This is also a well-developed theory that is helpful when working with communities in the development of health promotion programs.

Community Coalition Action Theory

According to Kreuter et al. (2003), the Community Coalition Action Theory evaluates the processes and results from coalitions and discovers a step-by-step approach to the life of health-related coalitions. There are a number of agencies already offering health promotion programs in the community. These local community agencies include civic organizations, social agencies, and faith-based organizations, to name a few. Kreuter et al. (2003) point out that these coalitions are very common in the improvement of the health of the community and quite often arise out of a group's interest in a specific health topic. A very good example of this interest by a community group in a health topic is found in the interest by the Rotary in the eradication of polio (Rotary International, 2009).

Kreuter et al. (2003) argue that there are a number of dimensions that are common to the capacity of a community coalition to improve the health of the community. Just as individuals go through stages of change in behavior, communities go through various stages as they form coalitions. Kreuter et al. (2003) argue that these stages include formation, maintenance, and institutionalization. It is critical for health promotion managers to understand the value of community coalitions in obtaining the improvement of the health of the community. It is equally important for those in charge of health promotion efforts to understand the various stages of the development of community coalitions.

Work Site Wellness Programs

The work site has always been thought to be an excellent location for the development of health promotion programs. The work setting and co-workers are known to have a tremendous effect on one's health. Work site wellness programs also offer the employer the chance to reduce health care costs for their company and at the same time increase worker productivity.

A number of large employers have begun to offer employees the opportunity to improve their health while at work. According to the September 2007 issue of the *The Nation's Health*, employers that develop wellness initiatives for their workplace are finding the secondary effects of these initiatives to include higher employee productivity, less absenteeism, and heightened camaraderie among their workers.

According to Ron Davis, MD, president of the American Medical Association "the greater impact of healthy lifestyles lies in affecting 'presenteeism'—the level at which an employee functions when she or he is at work—not absenteeism." (APHA, 2007, p. 12). Although most employee wellness programs have had positive results, it is very clear that the effects of these programs require greater research. More will be said about workplace wellness programs in Chapter 8.

CONCLUDING REMARKS

The process of developing health promotion programs that have a chance of achieving their goals and objectives is a time-consuming process that requires a large knowledge base of behavioral theory and information about best practices in the health promotion area. Successful ventures do not just happen; they are well planned and include input from all stakeholders.

Health behavioral change requires an excellent understanding of how individuals learn. This is why the use of secondary data, especially related to theoretical models, is so helpful in the design of health programs. The more knowledge available to program planners, the better the chance that the new health promotion program will be properly designed to achieve desired outcomes.

The concept of self-efficacy is also a very important piece of information to be considered by program planners. Kreuter et al. (2003) argue that even though self-efficacy is not a theory, the process of change becomes easier to negotiate with a target audience that believes they are capable of taking the recommended action towards a desired health state, and they are usually more successful in making the change.

Successful health promotion programs are usually the result of using a strong theoretical base to better understand human behavior while also applying motivational techniques and incentives to the program design. Discussion in focus group format with potential program participants can only increase our understanding of the motivational aspects and required incentives for that particular group of participants. It is also necessary to understand the value of using multiple approaches to change the targeted behavior.

DISCUSSION QUESTIONS

1. Please offer a complete explanation of the necessary steps in the development of an intervention program to prevent high-risk health behaviors.
2. Why is the understanding of behavioral theory so very important in the development of a health promotion program?
3. Name and explain the various intervention strategies that can be used to prevent high-risk health behaviors.
4. Explain the value of the PATCH process.

REFERENCES

Centers for Disease Control and Prevention. (2007). Planned approach to community health. Available at http://wonder.cdc.gov/wonder/prevguid/p0000064/p0000064.asp. Accessed August 18, 2007.

Anspaugh, D. J., Dignan, M. B., & Anspaugh, S. L. (2000). *Developing health promotion programs.* Long Grove, IL: Waveland Press Inc.

Kreuter, M. W., Lezin, N. A., Kreuter, M. W., & Green, L. W. (2003). *Community health promotion ideas that work* (2nd ed.). Sudbury, MA: Jones and Bartlett Publishers.

McKenzie, J. F., Neiger, B. L., & Smeltzer, J. L. (2005). *Planning, implementing and evaluating health promotion programs: A primer.* San Francisco, CA: Pearson Benjamin Cummings.

McKenzie, J. F., Pinger, R. R., & Kotecki, J. E. (2005). *An introduction to community health* (5th ed.). Sudbury, MA: Jones and Bartlett Publishers.

American Public Health Association (APHA). (2007). Employers making room for health promotion in the workplace: Incentives, support yield health results. *The Nation's Health.*

Novick, L. F., Morrow, C. B., & Mays, G. P. (2008). *Public health administration principles for population-based management.* Sudbury, MA: Jones and Bartlett Publishers.

Rotary International. (2009). Available at http://www.rotary.org/en/Pages/ridefault.aspx. Accessed January 2009.

5

CHAPTER

Health Promotion Program Marketing Techniques

Bernard J. Healey, PhD
Robert S. Zimmerman Jr., MPH

OBJECTIVES

After reading this chapter, you should

- Understand the difference between a need and a want
- Become aware of the value of using a marketing strategy in a health promotion program
- Understand the various steps required in the development of a marketing plan for the health promotion program
- Become aware of the need to market to the stakeholders of the health promotion effort

KEY TERMS

Marketing mix	Social marketing
Marketing research	SWOT
Need	Want

Introduction

The major threat facing our health care system in the twenty-first century is the epidemic of chronic diseases resulting from the practice of high-risk health behaviors by a growing number of individuals. Those working in public health are being asked to reduce the incidence of these high-risk health behaviors by using public health tools from the past. This strategy is doomed to fail because the tools are antiquated and the resources to support public health programs are dwindling.

Because of limited resources, public health programs must become more creative. Social change is necessary to protect the public's health in this new century. The new tools being developed in promoting healthy behaviors can only be enhanced by the use of marketing principles applied to the very new and dangerous unhealthy behaviors. The understanding of marketing principles is extremely important for those involved in health promotion programs. This marketing knowledge offers the health promotion specialist additional skills to assist in health promotion program development and attracts those practicing high-risk health behaviors to take advantage of the health promotion programs.

Marketing is normally thought of as a series of steps that are directed at need and want satisfaction of the consumer through an exchange process. According to Berkowitz (2006), a **need** is nothing more than a condition where there is a deficiency of something while a **want** requires a wish or desire for something useful. This exchange process can involve a tangible good or an intangible service. As long as a need is being satisfied in exchange for something of value, the marketing process has occurred. This means that marketing principles may work with health promotion efforts.

Although the vast majority of marketing activity is found in for-profit business activities, it is also an acceptable process in the nonprofit sector. In the last few decades, government agencies have started using marketing techniques to improve their budget allotments and to obtain better relationships with their clients and their suppliers of resources, usually the government.

The health sector has increasingly begun to understand the value of developing a marketing orientation as they go about delivering health services to their patients. In recent years, public health has also begun to understand the use of marketing techniques to more effectively and efficiently exchange health-related information to audiences.

Health services, especially public health services, include the components of needs and wants that require an exchange process in order to be satisfied. In this type of exchange, there may also be a nonmonetary price, such as effort or time. There are several uses of the marketing concept in the development of health promotion programs, including the development and implementation of new promotion efforts and a realization that they are attempting to market an intangible service.

Marketing has been an unknown concept when it comes to public health departments and the programs developed by these departments. The marketing process has not been appreciated by public health professionals because the subject was not covered in schools of public health. It has always been thought that public health programs are too important to use marketing techniques to advance the goals of public health agencies. Siegel and Lotenberg (2006) point out that when public health workers encourage the adoption of individual behavior and lifestyle changes, they are actually in the business of marketing. The development of a marketing approach to doing business has produced successful results for businesses and government agencies for many years; it can certainly aid public health agencies in the accomplishment of their goals.

> **Value of Marketing Health Promotion Efforts**
>
> In order to continue and expand funds devoted to health promotion efforts, the success of health promotion efforts needs to be marketed to those who fund these efforts.

Bernhardt (2006) argues that it is time to apply health marketing strategies to health promotion and health protection programs. Marketing principles can be the answer to the problems encountered in the development and success of many health promotion efforts. The use of marketing techniques may very well mean the difference between success and failure in the health promotion effort. The use of marketing skills can aid the health promotion specialist in the development, implementation, and even the evaluation of the promotion effort.

Social Marketing

Social marketing is the use of marketing techniques to achieve behavioral goals. This concept began in the 1970s and requires heavy use of the social sciences in the development of a marketing campaign. Kottler and Zaltman (1971) first used the term *social marketing* as the use of marketing techniques to solve social and health problems. Anspaugh, Dignan, and Anspaugh (2000) argue that social marketing has been used to market attitudes and a healthier lifestyle. The concept is very useful in developing a promotional effort that is designed to get individuals to change high-risk health behaviors.

> **Social Marketing**
>
> Social marketing is the application of marketing tools to produce social change. This concept is applicable in our effort to get people to change to healthy behaviors.

The term social marketing has been defined by Siegel and Lotenberg (2006) as the utilization of marketing principles to influence the voluntary behavior of individuals in a positive way. It is possible to market products, services, people, ideas, and behaviors.

The CDC identifies social marketing as a practice allied with health education and health promotion. It is the type of marketing that benefits the target group of individuals, not the one doing the marketing, by attempting to improve the health of the target market. The ultimate objective of this type of marketing is to influence the action of the targeted market. According to the CDC (2009), the health product needs to be made attractive, reasonably priced, and readily available.

Bryant, Kent, and Lindenberger (1998) also maintain that social marketing can be an effective tool for public health leaders in securing continued government support of their popular health and social programs in the midst of increasing threats of public spending cuts.

Those working on health promotion programs have to understand that they are actually selling healthy behavior. In order to market healthy behavior, social marketers have to segment the market into groups with common high-risk health behaviors. They can then use the strategy of reaching their target market with the "four Ps" of marketing to facilitate the exchange. The four Ps of marketing are the product, price, place, and promotion. According to Berkowitz (2006), the four Ps of marketing are the controllable variables that can be utilized in the definition of a marketing strategy. Also known as the **marketing mix**, they can be very useful in marketing intangibles like healthy behaviors.

The major objective of marketing is to get the consumer to take action. This action occurs when the majority of the target audience believes that the benefits of the action outweigh the costs of the action for the individual. It is a social process involving the activities that facilitate exchanges of goods and services among individuals and organizations. In social marketing, the consumer remains the primary focus. There needs to be a real effort to research what the consumer desires and then to deliver an answer to satisfy those consumer needs.

Health Marketing Research

According to the CDC (2009), there is a need to discover the best method for individuals to assess their own health status. This would entail an evaluation of the various models available, including the medical model, public health model, wellness model, and community model impact on individuals in their search for health-seeking behavior and their response to public health messages. In other words, answer the question of how to best develop health promotion efforts with helping the consumer best understand the message and respond in a positive way.

> **Marketing Research**
> Marketing research consists of several steps of gathering information about the consumer. The process is extremely useful in the development and expansion of health promotion programs.

Siegel and Lotenberg (2007) believe that **marketing research** is a vital component of every stage of the marketing process. Mullins et al. (2005) point out that marketing research has great value in defining marketing problems while also discovering opportunities. The research process is also useful in gathering data necessary to solve a particular marketing challenge like the development of an effective health promotion campaign.

According to Lefebre and Flora (1988), marketing research can be very useful in determining the needs and desires of the priority population in a health promotion program because the major goal of health promotion programs is behavior change. The more you know about the target market the better able you become in facilitating the process of behavior change. Research is also needed in the area of health promotion efforts in how best to provide information to health professionals. How do we best distribute new knowledge to health professionals and get them to use this information in their practice?

Green and Kreuter (2005) argue that those involved in health promotion activities have a strong base of evidence demonstrating the strength of a risk factor and a specific outcome(s) associated with the practice of that risk factor. These authors call for a behavioral risk diagnosis in order to focus resources on the elimination or, at the very least, the control of that dangerous risk factor.

Siegel and Lotenberg (2007) call for taking the concept of risk behavior a step further by developing a behavior mapping process in order to better understand the actions of the target market. Lifestyle choices such as smoking, obesity, poor nutrition, alcohol use, and a sedentary lifestyle are related to the development and aggravation of chronic disease. Behavior is a collection of activities influenced by various factors like values, attitudes, and culture. In public health, there is concern with high-risk health behaviors that can predispose us toward the development of life-threatening diseases. The overriding concern of public health is why individuals begin practicing the high-risk health behavior and how to intervene by changing behaviors.

In Figure 5-1, Siegel and Lotenberg (2007) point out the dimensions of behavior by illustrating both the frequency of behavior and the complexity of various behaviors. This matrix allows us to evaluate the various steps in a behavior and then map the behaviors and either use health promotion programs to reinforce the good behaviors or to make an attempt to change the bad or high-risk health behaviors. By thinking of behaviors in terms of frequency and complexity and mapping the behaviors, we have increased our chances of developing an innovative approach to replacing that behavior with a behavior that is more conducive to a healthy life.

This matrix also allows health promotion specialists the opportunity to evaluate the motivational aspects of continuous or frequent high-risk health behaviors. Why do some people practice these high-risk behaviors and even increase their intensity when they know the ultimate result of their actions will mean poor health and, quite possibly, death?

	One-Time or Episodic	Continuous or Frequent
Simple	Getting a flu shot Getting screening tests performed at routine exams	Using condoms Not smoking Not driving after drinking Fastening safety belts
Complex	Getting a colonoscopy Preparing a household for natural disasters and other community emergencies Obtaining and installing a child restraint system in a car	Changing eating habits Engaging in physical activity Lowering risk of contacting communicable diseases

Figure 5-1
Dimensions of Behavior

The health promotion program is then not only able to target the audience but target the motivation for the bad behavior when they develop their health promotion campaign. Obtaining an objective, detailed, evidence-based understanding of these factors is critical to effective marketing decision making.

It is very important to obtain feedback from the market as a basis for continuing improvement in the products or services offered by the business. Research is the most important variable in the success of health marketing initiatives. This research has the ability to ensure the best way to disseminate the information needed by consumers to make informed health decisions.

Marketing Strategies

The research leads to the development of marketing strategies to help the health promotion program achieve its goals. A *marketing strategy* is the approach taken to reach a predetermined goal. Siegel and Lotenberg (2007) argue that marketing strategies are rather abstract and may be both long term and short term in execution. Once the target market for the health promotion program has been determined and segmented according to need, the marketing mix can be developed to fulfill the strategic plan objectives in order to ensure a successful promotional effort.

The utilization of a marketing strategy in the development and delivery of a health promotion program relies on a decision-making approach. Mullins, Walker, Boyd, and Larreche (2005) argue that the success or failure of any strategy is very dependent on an accurate assessment of the external environment that surrounds the target audience for the new program.

Siegel and Lotenberg (2007) argue that the key stakeholders need to be involved in the long-term goal of sustaining behavior change in a community. How can the health promotion effort be continued on a long-term basis once success is achieved in the community health improvement project? It must be realized by those involved in the project that closure in the project goals will never be achieved. Health promotion is a continuous process that never ends.

Anspaugh et al. (2000) believe that because of changing technology and the ability to receive information rapidly, health promotion strategies need to change in order to adapt to the new external environment. This is the major reason for a strong research component being present in the health promotion effort from the development phase to the evaluation phase as the program concludes and becomes revitalized. Better data usually means better decision making and that should mean successful health promotion programs.

Marketing Management

The process of marketing is a never ending dynamic process of making decisions about marketing the product or service and managing all aspects of the effort. Mullins et al. (2005) believe that marketing management is the process that works to make an exchange happen. It involves all aspects of planning and control of a marketing campaign. A health promotion program needs to use the various elements of the marketing management approach to aid in the development of a better control process for the entire promotion process.

The planning process is the driver for the process of marketing management. Siegel and Lotenberg (2007) argue that the planning process is the most important piece in marketing a policy, a health behavior, or a social change. In order to develop a planning process that facilitates the development and implementation of a successful health promotion program, attention needs to be paid to research concerning the problem.

Figure 5-2 shows the many activities that need to occur in the marketing process in order to ensure the best chance of success in the new venture. These activities are all very important in the understanding of the marketing process surrounding the development of the health promotion program.

It is important to understand that the consumer is not really buying the health promotion program but rather he or she is purchasing the benefits thought to flow from the health promotion product. In order to appropriately manage the marketing process, those responsible for the program must understand the benefits desired by the program and the cost to the consumer to achieve these benefits. Mullins et al. (2005) believe that marketing management involves the process that brings the exchange process to a successful conclusion. This process can be adapted to health promotion programs in order to achieve a greater success rate in achieving healthy communities.

Planning
- Step 1: Analyze the situation:
  - Identify problems and populations affected.
  - Analyze current and possible replacement behaviors.
  - Outline all components of a solution (education, law, marketing).
  - Assess the environment in which change will occur.
- Step 2: Select approaches and determine the role of marketing.
- Step 3: Set goals and objectives: Specify behaviors, conditions, or policies to be changed.
- Step 4: Segment and select target audiences:
  - Determine the target populations for each desired change, and within each population, the audience segment(s) on which you will focus.
  - Identify current and competitive behaviors and how they satisfy needs, desires, and values.
  - Identify barriers to the public health behavior.
- Step 5: Design public health offering(s):
  - Product: Identify and develop a bundle of benefits that you can deliver that differentiates the desired behavior from competitors. Develop any necessary supporting goods and services.
  - Price: Determine how to make costs manageable for target audience members.
  - Place: Determine how you will access channels that deliver the product so that it is easily available to target audience members at prices (financial, time, psyche, social, etc.) they are willing and able to pay.
  - Promotion: Develop a communication strategy to position the public health offering as something consistent with the audience's core values that delivers a key benefit
- Step 6: Plan evaluation.

Development
- Develop budgets and distribution and promotion plans.
- Develop prototype products, services and/or communication materials.
- Pretest with target audience members.
- Refine as necessary.
- Build in process evaluation measures.

Implementation
- Produce offerings and materials.
- Coordinate with partners.
- Implement intervention.
- Use process evaluation to monitor implementation.
- Refine offerings, promotions, and distribution channels as needed.

Assessment
- Conduct outcome evaluation.
- Refine intervention as needed.

Figure 5-2
Stages of the
Marketing Process

SWOT Analysis

Another marketing tool that can provide help to those developing health promotion programs is the use of **SWOT** analysis in the planning phase of the new program. The SWOT analysis (also known as TOWS analysis) begins after a clear program objective has been identified. This acronym stands for strengths, weaknesses, opportunities, and threats analysis and is actually a very good strategic planning tool.

This exercise for planners of programs is nothing more than performing an analysis of your program's strengths, weaknesses, opportunities, and threats. It allows the program manager to be prepared for any future problems or opportunities by better utilizing the strengths of the current program and by attempting to improve on the weak areas of the current promotion initiative.

This analysis attempts to uncover the key internal and external factors that will help achieve the ultimate program objective. The internal factors usually include the strengths and weaknesses found inside the department attempting to achieve the objective. The threats and opportunities are usually found external to the department. The results are usually presented in a matrix format to the program planners for decision-making purposes. This type of strategic analysis has been used in nonprofit agencies and should work very well in the planning and development of a health promotion program. It allows health promotion specialists the opportunity to critically evaluate their own efforts in an attempt to continuously improve on their program inputs and outcomes.

Use of Marketing Mix

Application of the marketing mix is a necessary component of the launch of any new product or service. The components of the marketing mix are not only useful but become a necessary adjunct to the development of a successful health promotion program. They are the core of the marketing strategy and include product, price, place, and promotion. They are independent variables that marketers and health promotion specialists can use to influence the behavior of the targeted audience.

You are asking recipients of the health promotion program to exchange one health behavior for another. Siegel and Lotenberg (2007) believe that in order for a successful exchange to occur, the recipient must realize an incentive to exchange behaviors. The product being offered through the health promotion program must be designed in such a way that the new behavior is clearly differentiated from the competitive behavior as adding greater life value to the recipient. This promotion package must also offer easy and cost-efficient delivery of the product to the recipient.

> **Marketing Mix in Public Health**
> The four Ps of marketing—product, price, place, and promotion—are very useful tools in marketing the health promotion programs to clients and funders.

According to the CDC (2003), these same components can be used in social marketing. It is important to realize that when attempting to sell healthy behaviors the product becomes what the individual is being asked to purchase—a healthy lifestyle obtained by practicing healthy behaviors.

The price is the cost associated with the purchase of the product. In the case of a healthy lifestyle, it is the cost associated with changing unhealthy behaviors to healthy ones. Siegel and Lotenberg (2007) argue that the price of the behavior change may include monetary costs or nonmonetary costs. The time, effort, and energy involved in the behavior change are examples of nonmonetary costs and may be quite high when individuals first attempt to make changes in their high-risk health behaviors. The economist would consider the cost of behavior change an opportunity cost in terms of having to give up one type of behavior, probably practiced for a long time, for a different type of behavior that may not be as attractive to the individual.

There can also be a monetary cost associated with healthy behaviors. Examples of these costs would include the cost of better nutrition, joining a health spa, or paying for a smoking cessation program not covered by your insurance plan. There are a variety of methods that can be used by the health promotion program to reduce these monetary and nonmonetary costs to program participants. These methods can include incentives provided by the health promotion program or the health insurance programs.

The place is where the product is available to be purchased by the consumer. The role of placement or distribution of the product plays a critical role in the success or failure of a health promotion program. The placement decision makes it convenient for the consumer to purchase the product.

Mailbach, Duyn, and Bloodgood (2006) argue that the most important opportunity for delivering evidence-based prevention information to the consumer is through sustainable distribution channels. Siegel and Lotenberg (2007) believe that the reason health promotion campaigns fail is because those marketing bad behaviors are more creative in their development of new channels of distribution for their bad behavior products.

An example of the importance of the effect placement can have on the costs associated with healthy behaviors is found in the offering of wellness programs in the school or the workplace. Both the monetary and nonmonetary costs to the consumer are reduced when the positive behavior change is made available where they go to school or work. The environment of these places can become conducive to wellness.

The promotion is the way in which information about the product is disseminated to the consumer. Promotion involves informing the customer about the availability of the product. Marketing managers often refer to the promotional mix as advertisements, personal sales, sales promotion, and public relations. There are advantages and disadvantages found in the use of each of these components in meeting the company or department objectives. Siegel and Lotenberg (2007) point out that once the health promotion product is developed, it is important to develop a communication strategy that has a complete description of the target market. There also needs to be a plan to promote the value of the behavior change and a way to motivate the target market to begin practicing the new behaviors.

Marketing Health Promotion Programs

It is virtually impossible to have a successful and sustainable health promotion program without the use of marketing tools that have worked so well in the private sector over the last 100 years. Most health promotion programs have good intentions but, unless they convince their audience to buy and use their product, their resources will dry up and their promotion efforts will fail.

A strong marketing effort can help health promotion programs increase their resources and also aid in achieving success in the outcomes attributed to their promotional effort. Marketing strategies can increase the number of program participants and increase successful and sustainable outcomes as a result of the health promotion program. The potential consumers of health promotion programs need to attend or witness the health promotion effort, and they also need to become convinced that the promoted behavior change is necessary for them.

Anspaugh et al. (2000) argue that promotion efforts are quite often cognitive change programs. The effort in this change process attempts to persuade consumers to use information about health that they have gained in a positive way. Therefore, the marketing effort uses the tools of marketing to develop an informative health package that is easily understood by participants.

Bernhardt (2006) argues that the time has come for public health to recognize the value of using a marketing approach for increasing the adoption of health promotion and protection information to better the lives of populations. He goes on to call principles of commercial marketing an underused resource by those given the responsibility to promote healthy lifestyles among Americans.

The ultimate goal of using these marketing principles in the development and delivery of health promotion is to provide greater opportunities for successful campaigns. The marketing process can be a very useful tool in the entire health promotion process. The tools of marketing, especially market research, can be applied to every aspect of the development, implementation, and evaluation of a new health promotion program.

Because a health promotion program involves the process of exchange, it can be heavily influenced by the marketing process. The health promotion process is an excellent example of what marketers call the process of exchange. Health promotion programs attempt to deliver value to customers by offering them ways to improve their health, and customers pay for the benefits of health promotion information with their time and effort in understanding the message that is being delivered by the health promotion program.

Siegel and Lotenberg (2006) argue that there needs to be a repackaging and repositioning of the public health product. They also believe that public health practitioners need to use the concept of a brand when developing their marketing approach to public health products. By using the branding concept, they are able to give the public health product a personality that can be acceptable to the consumer and then build a relationship with the target market.

McKenzie, Neiger, and Smeltzer (2005) argue that a marketing approach is something that does not require a long learning curve, but the process does require acceptance of the value of the process in the development of the new promotion program. Anspaugh et al. (2000) believe that marketing may be one of the most overlooked variables in the development of a health promotion program.

The use of marketing techniques in the creation of a healthy community is a population-based behavior management strategy. Public health agencies and especially health promotion programs define their target population as the entire school, workplace, or community rather than individuals segmented by age, gender, or race.

Although many of the marketing principles can be used in health promotion efforts, the components of the strategic marketing process for a public health product is different than the process used for a commercial product. Figure 5-3 displays four important components of the definition, position, package, and frame of the public health product. These components are product, promise, image, and support.

Siegel and Lotenberg (2007) define the product as the benefit that is desired by the target audience. The marketing process provides value by developing products or services that meet the needs of the target market of consumers interested in becoming and remaining healthy. The problem is that the customer needs to develop an appreciation for the value offered by the health promotion program; in this case, good health and better quality of life.

It is difficult to appreciate good health when you have never experienced poor health. Because the majority of chronic diseases and the bad health associated with these diseases manifest themselves later in life, it is difficult for the individual to appreciate the value of practicing healthy behaviors when they are young. The chronic diseases have a very long incubation period (20 to 40 years). How do we get young people motivated to prevent something from happening that far in the future?

The promise offers ways that the product will satisfy the needs of the target market. Most consumers are unaware of the fact that regaining good health after practicing high-risk health behaviors for years will take months if

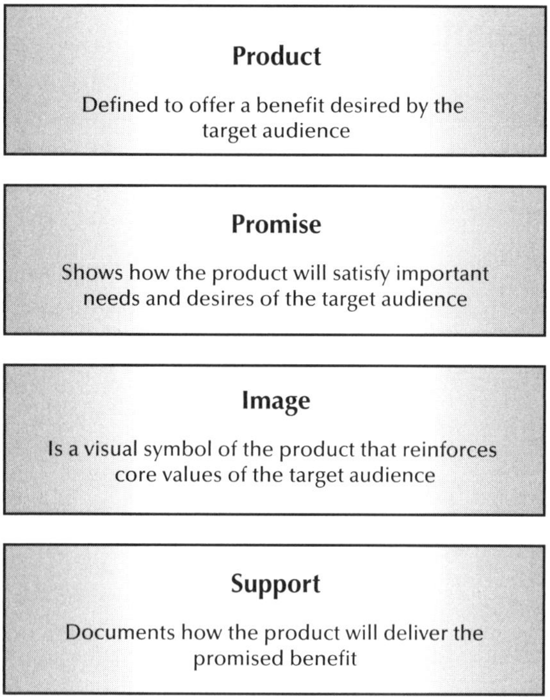

Product
Defined to offer a benefit desired by the target audience

Promise
Shows how the product will satisfy important needs and desires of the target audience

Image
Is a visual symbol of the product that reinforces core values of the target audience

Support
Documents how the product will deliver the promised benefit

Figure 5-3
Components of the Strategic Marketing Process for a Public Health Product

Siegel, M., & Lotenberg, L. D. (2007). *Marketing public health strategies to promote social change* (2nd ed.). Sudbury, MA: Jones and Bartlett Publishers.

not years of changed behavior with little noticeable betterment of health in the short run.

The image is the visual symbol of the product that aids in the need satisfaction of the target audience. Individuals are eager to be a part of the image of the given health product. This part of the branding process can also be utilized as part of the promotional process of the health product. Finally, support tells the target audience how the product will satisfy the consumer by delivering the benefit as promised by the product.

Siegel and Lotenberg (2007) argue that the brand of the product being delivered by public health has to develop a personality or identity that large groups of the public can identify with as their own product. The process of becoming healthier has to become the major motivating force in an individual's life. The vision of a healthier person has to become the overwhelming goal of the individual. Only then will healthy behaviors become the norm and replace the old unhealthy behaviors that may have been practiced for years by the individual.

The use of marketing principles can become the catalyst in the development of successful health promotion programs. It will take time and understanding of those engaged in health promotion, but marketing may very well be the missing ingredient that is needed to sustain the long road to a healthier nation.

CONCLUDING REMARKS

Those engaged in health promotion activities need to have a firm grasp of the principles of marketing in order to better develop their attempt at changing individual health behaviors and sharing the value of healthy behaviors with the target population. Knowledge of marketing techniques is also very helpful in making funders of such projects aware of what the projects are attempting to accomplish and the need for continued financial support of their mission. The correct use of marketing concepts can be the difference between successful and well-funded health promotion campaigns or the failure in meeting program objectives and program cancellation due to budget reductions.

The success of marketing principles has been demonstrated in the for-profit sector, but these same principles have only been tried on a limited basis in public health programs. In public health and health promotion campaigns, we are dealing with social marketing. With social marketing, you are working with an intangible product like an attitude or a lifestyle. The unhealthy lifestyles that health promotion programs are attempting to change are the result of the practice of high-risk health behaviors. These behaviors are complicated and difficult to understand and difficult to change once they have been practiced by individuals for a long period of time.

It is only in recent years that policy makers have begun to understand the economic value of keeping people healthy and free from the complications and costs that are a result of the epidemic of chronic diseases. Resources are becoming available for health promotion activities, but these programs must be able to demonstrate results.

The use of marketing principles in the development of a health promotion program allows the developer to abstract from the normal paradigm of health promotion. This abstraction allows for the possibility of developing a creative solution to the problems associated with behavior change.

The use of the marketing mix, four Ps, allows those developing a health promotion program to think in terms of the design, price, and placement, as well as how best to promote the product to program recipients. This again allows creativity and innovation to enter the planning process for the new health program. It is time to use every possible discipline, including marketing principles, to develop innovative approaches to the promotion of good health and the achievement of the goals put forth by the Healthy People 2010 initiative.

DISCUSSION QUESTIONS

1. Explain the value of using a marketing strategy for the target market to gain awareness of the health promotion program.
2. How do you use the marketing mix variables to attract attention and support for the health promotion effort?
3. Explain the various stages of the marketing process as they relate to health promotion programs.
4. How would you conduct a SWOT analysis of a health promotion program?

REFERENCES

Anspaugh, D. J., Dignan, M. B., & Anspaugh, S. L. (2000). *Developing health promotion programs.* Long Grove, IL: Waveland Press Inc.

Berkowitz, E. (2006). *Essentials of health care marketing* (2nd ed.). Sudbury, MA: Jones and Bartlett Publishers.

Bernhardt, J. M. (2006). Improving health through health marketing. *Preventing Chronic Disease, 3*(3), 1–3.

Bryant, C., Kent, E. B., & Lindenberger, J. (1998). Increasing consumer satisfaction. One social service and public health initiative shows social marketing can increase consumer satisfaction. *Marketing Health Services, 18*(4), 4–17.

Centers for Disease Control and Prevention. (2003). Designing and implementing an effective tobacco counter-marketing campaign. Atlanta, GA: CDC, National Center for Disease Prevention and Health Promotion, Office on Smoking and Health.

Centers for Disease Control and Prevention. (2009). Social Marketing. Available at http://www.cdc.gov/nccdphp/dnpa/socialmarketing/training/basics. Accessed February 26, 2009.

Green, L. W., & Kreuter, M. W. (2005). *Health program planning an educational and ecological approach* (4th ed.). Boston, MA: McGraw-Hill.

Kottler, P., & Zaltman, G. (1971). Social marketing: An approach to planned social change. *Journal of Marketing, 35,* 3–12.

LeFebre, R. C., & Flora, J. A. (1988). Social marketing and public intervention. *Health Education Quarterly, 15*(3), 299–315.

Mailbach, E. W., Duyn, M. A. S. V., & Bloodgood, B. (2006). A marketing perspective on disseminating evidence-based approaches to disease prevention and health promotion. Prev Chronic Dis {serial online} 2006 Jul {February 27, 2009}. Available at http://www.cdc.gov/pcd/issues/2006/jul/05_0154.htm.

McKenzie, J. F., Neiger, B. L., & Smeltzer, J. L. (2005). *Planning, implementing, and evaluating health promotion programs: A primer* (4th ed.). San Francisco, CA: Pearson Benjamin Cummings.

Mullins, J. W., Walker, O. C., Boyd, H. W., & Larreche, J. C. (2005). *Marketing management a strategic decision making approach* (5th ed.). Boston, MA: McGraw-Hill.

Siegel, M., & Lotenberg, L. D. (2007). *Marketing public health strategies to promote social change* (2nd ed.). Sudbury, MA: Jones and Bartlett Publishers.

Program Evaluation

Bernard J. Healey, PhD
Robert S. Zimmerman Jr., MPH

OBJECTIVES

After reading this chapter, you should

- Understand the value of evaluation of health promotion programs
- Define and explain the components of a well-developed evaluation procedure
- Become aware of the value of the development of an evaluation process early on in the development of a health promotion program
- Understand the various steps required in the logic model

KEY TERMS

Evaluation design	Program goals
Evaluation process	Stakeholders
Program evaluation	Systems model

Introduction

Very few people look forward to the process of evaluation. On a personal note, I am not comfortable being critical of individuals or of the programs that they represent. I also do not enjoy the process of being evaluated by others or by organizations. Over the years, I have learned that evaluation must be done in order for improvement to occur. I have also learned that the **evaluation process** can be a source of great opportunity to help the program get better and to attract additional resources that are necessary for program expansion.

Evaluation is one of the most important components of a health promotion program, but it is also the most difficult component to complete. There has to be an established methodology to prove that the goals and objectives of the program established before the program began were achieved. If the program has failed in meeting the specified goals and objectives, there needs to be a way to uncover the reason(s) why the program failed and to correct the deficiencies.

One of the major problems with health promotion programs is the inability to prove that a particular promotion effort made a difference. Edberg (2007) argues that continued funding for health promotion is dependent on evidence and accountability. In other words, health promotion programs are dependent on being able to prove that the program in question had an impact on what it was trying to achieve. This ability to prove success or failure in a health promotion effort may be the difference between program continuation or cancellation. Bartholomew, Parcel, Kok, & Gottlieb (2006) argue that it is important to evaluate health promotion efforts in order to improve these programs and also to conserve scarce resources allocated to health promotion programs. There needs to be more attention paid to not only program outcomes but also to the process of program implementation of the health promotion program. In other words, all of the components of the program need to be evaluated in order to determine any deviation from the program plan.

Evaluation consists of a series of steps to determine the value of an effort. One of the most important components of the health promotion process is the evaluation of the program accomplishments. This can also be one of the more challenging parts of the health promotion program because we encounter several difficult questions that require answers even before we begin designing the evaluation approach. These questions include the following:

- What is the cost of the evaluation in terms of dollars, time, and resources?
- How do we evaluate each separate part of the program process, methods, consumer reaction, or outcomes?

Anspaugh, Dignan, and Anspaugh (2000) argue that evaluation needs to be concerned with achievements of the program compared with the goals and objectives developed at the start of the planning process for the program. The question becomes What was produced by our effort? More importantly, are the results of the effort worth the costs compared to alternative ways of accomplishing the same objectives?

Changing Disease Patterns

According to Jack et al. (2006), the diseases contributing to the greatest morbidity, mortality, and disability in this country have become the chronic diseases. Cardiovascular disease, cancer, and diabetes are the most prevalent, costly, and preventable. Approximately 7 out of 10 Americans who die each year die as a result of a chronic disease.

The only way to prevent chronic diseases and their complications is through health education programs. These educational programs are not hard to develop but offer tremendous challenges in program evaluation. There is a need for a different type of **evaluation process** for health promotion programs whose goal is the reduction of the burden from chronic diseases in the country.

Chronic diseases generally have a long incubation period and are caused by multiple factors. These causative factors complicate the program development process, making evaluation of program success or failure extremely difficult.

The payoff for reducing the incidence of chronic diseases in this country is enormous. Jack et al. (2006) points out that the medical costs for individuals with chronic diseases account for 75% of the total health care costs in the country. More important than the monetary costs of these diseases are the years of potential life lost for people under the age of 65 years.

It is important to have a well-developed evaluation program in place before the implementation of chronic disease health promotion programs. Public health needs to have a good understanding of which health promotion program yields the greatest return before expending large amounts of resources on poorly designed programs that do not work.

Evaluation Process

Evaluation is the planned investigation of the worth of something and should involve as many **stakeholders** as necessary to uncover the merits of a particular program. The CDC has developed a document titled *The Framework for Program Evaluation in Public Health*, published in 1999, that is very useful in developing an evaluation process for public health efforts. This document recommends the following step-by-step process to be used in **program evaluation:**

1. Engage **stakeholders**
2. Describe the program
3. Focus the **evaluation design**
4. Gather credible evidence
5. Justify conclusions
6. Ensure use and share lessons learned

These six steps of the evaluation process are shown in a circular model in Figure 6-1. This is an excellent model to begin a discussion concerning the evaluation of a health promotion program.

Partners in Evaluation
- Those involved in program operations
- Those served by the new program
- Those who will be using the results of the evaluation

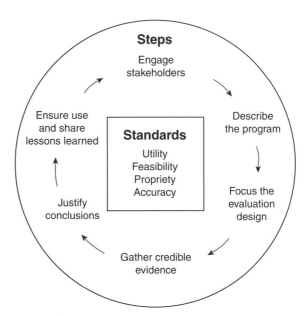

Figure 6-1
The Interrelationship of
Evaluation Approaches

Source: Centers for Disease
Control and Prevention.
(1999). Framework for program evaluation in public
health. *Morbidity and Mortality Weekly Report,* 48(11).

Figure 6-1, produced by CDC in 1999, offers a systematic way to justify the continuation or expansion of a health promotion effort and also to add the feature of continuous improvement of the program being evaluated. This guide was produced by the CDC to be utilized by public health officials when they are attempting to evaluate a public health program or intervention.

This well-developed evaluation tool is meant to guide evaluators through a series of steps designed to perform consistent evaluations as they attempt to help communities improve public health initiatives. This process also consists of a set of 30 standards organized into 4 distinct groups for the evaluation purposes.

The first step in this evaluation process requires the engagement of the stakeholders in the development and implementation of the proposed public health program. In order to make any health promotion program successful, there must be a concerted effort to develop partnerships.

The second step in the evaluation process would include a description of the program, including its mission, **program goals,** and objectives. By describing the program, everyone is able to get a better understanding of the goals of the program, enabling them to compare the program with other programs and to connect program components to their effects.

The third step in the evaluation process involves the focusing of the evaluation design. This step allows the evaluation to address the issues of greatest concern to stakeholders. This part of the evaluation process requires the use of an evaluation strategy that has the best chance of being useful and accurate for the evaluators.

The fourth step in the evaluation process developed by the CDC involves the gathering of credible evidence concerning the health promotion program being evaluated. This credibility needs to be intended for the primary users of the program. The CDC believes that having credible evidence of the success of a health promotion program strengthens the recommendations that flow from the program. This is why it is so important to use multiple approaches for gathering, analyzing, and interpreting the data produced by the evaluation.

The fifth step consists of linking the conclusions of the evaluation with the evidence gathered through the entire evaluation process. It is extremely important at this stage for the stakeholders to agree that the conclusions generated from the evaluation process are justified. The process of justifying the conclusions of the evaluation process includes standards, analysis and synthesis, interpretation, judgment, and recommendations.

The last step involved in the evaluation process involves sharing the results of what was learned in the evaluation process. The CDC calls for five steps that are critical to ensuring appropriate and continued use of the results of the evaluation of a public health program. These steps involve design, preparation, feedback, follow-up, and dissemination.

The multistep evaluation process developed by the CDC is an excellent process to assist a health promotion program to add value to the lives of community residents. The process also allows those who are part of the evaluation team to clarify their own understanding of the program goals. This allows all of the team members to become creative and innovative in their recommendations of how to better achieve the goals of the program while considering resource utilization.

Program Goals

Goals and objectives are very different, even though many people think they are the same. The goal is usually defined as a future event or outcome that we are attempting to achieve through actions taken in the past or the present. In a health promotion effort or activity, the goal is something that provides direction to the program. The program goal is longer term, requires simplicity, and will include those who will be affected by the health promotion effort.

> **Example of a Goal of a Health Promotion Program**
>
> By September 30, 2009, the use of tobacco at the XYZ company will be reduced from the current level of 26% of the workforce to 20% as reported by the annual company health survey.

Program Objectives

Objectives are usually stated as smaller steps to be taken toward achievement of the larger goal(s). They are measurable movements toward the accomplishment of the ultimate goal(s) of the health promotion program. Objectives should include who is involved, what is the desired outcome, how progress will be measured, and the time frame for achievement.

Once the objective is properly defined, it becomes the foundation of your evaluation procedure. The goal is what we wish to accomplish with the health promotion effort. The objectives are the various steps to get us to goal accomplishment.

Examples of Objectives for a Health Promotion Program

- Workers will be able to comprehend the dangers of tobacco use.
- Workers will understand the steps necessary to reduce their addiction to tobacco products.
- Workers will agree to attend smoking cessation programs sponsored by the XYZ company.

Evaluation Models

The process of performing an adequate evaluation of the proposed health promotion program must begin very early in the design of the new program. Ideally, this process should involve all stakeholders and should be considered while developing the goals and objectives that flow from the mission statement of the new program.

The **systems model**, which includes input, process, and output, is the simplest way of considering the process of performing program evaluation. An example of using the systems model for a program designed to evaluate an obesity intervention program can be seen in Figure 6-2.

This figure shows the program plan to be the input to the obesity intervention health promotion program. This part of the plan needs to include a

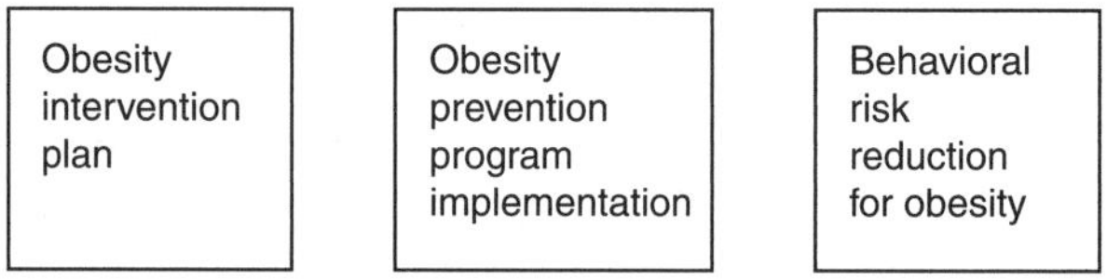

Figure 6-2
Obesity Intervention
Program

| Obesity intervention plan | Obesity prevention program implementation | Behavioral risk reduction for obesity |

mission statement along with the various goals and objectives to be achieved by this particular intervention effort. The process followed by the program is looked at in terms of the various components of the implementation phase of the program. The output of this health promotion effort should be the output that results from the effort and should include reduction in the habits that predispose one to obesity. This very simplistic approach at a health promotion program evaluation demonstrates that the evaluation process needs to be built into the program at a very early stage in the program development. It also demonstrates that thought must be given at an early stage in program development about what it is we want to evaluate in order to determine program success or failure.

Evaluation Models

There are numerous components in health promotion programs to evaluate and many different types of evaluation processes that can be utilized in the evaluation of health promotion initiatives.

Logic Model   One of the better models utilized to evaluate public health programs by the CDC is a logic model. The CDC (1999) describes this model as a way to look at the various events of a program in terms of a flowchart that leads to program results. The various logic models may look different, but they all include inputs, activities, and outputs. In terms of a health promotion program, the inputs could be a trained health education staff; the activities could include an educational program to prevent a high-risk health behavior; and the output could be a reduction in the practice of the high-risk health behaviors. The CDC (1999) argues that the use of a logic model will allow those responsible for the program to clarify the program's strategies and to better focus the program in terms of effectiveness (achieving program goals) and efficiency (keeping costs to a minimum).

Figure 6-3 shows the operational aspects of the basic logic model used frequently in evaluating public health programs. This evaluation model includes inputs, outputs, short-term impact of the program, and long-term outcomes of the program and relates all of the steps back to the goals of the program. This model allows program evaluators to look at each of the steps of the health promotion program separately to discover if deviation from program goals occurred and, if so, to fix the problem so that the program becomes successful.

Figure 6-4 shows the various components of a basic logic development template. These components are all considered necessary for a health promotion program to be successful. This model can be utilized to evaluate

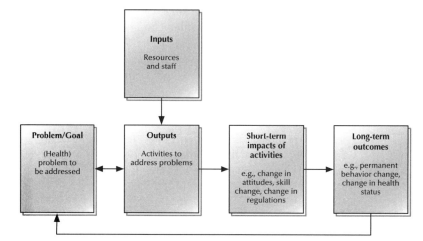

Figure 6-3

Example of a Basic
Logic Model

Source: Edberg, M. (2007).
*Essentials of health behav-
ior and social and behav-
ioral theory in public
health.* Sudbury, MA: Jones
and Bartlett Publishers.

any effort that is dedicated to preventing adverse health outcomes among populations.

The great value of this template is that it offers excellent definitions of each step in the evaluation process. The model also allows the evaluator to begin with program goals and go forward to outcomes or to reverse the process and go backwards from outcome to goals in order to discover the reasons for success or failure of the effort. If the initiative failed, it becomes easier to discover the reasons for failure, and if the program was successful, the initiative needs to be shared with others and written as a best practice for future use by other health promotion programs.

Figure 6-5 demonstrates the use of a logic model for a tuberculosis control program. It allows the evaluation of the entire process from the occurrence of a new case of tuberculosis to the outcome of improved status of the health of the population. This particular example includes the service components and the infrastructure components underlying the improved health status of the population. The model allows program managers to move forward or backward in the program evaluation process of a tuberculosis control program. This offers managers the opportunity to evaluate all components of the program in order to improve effectiveness and efficiency of the program.

Figure 6-6 shows the interrelationships of the various types of evaluations. Christoffel and Gallagher (2006) point out that there are several different types of evaluation processes to consider for each type of health promotion intervention program. Each of these processes has the capability of complementing one another, depending on the situation. These processes are also capable of answering different questions about the success or failure of the various components of the health promotion program.

Components of a comprehensive effort to improve child passenger safety outcomes:

Input/ Resources	Activities	Outputs	Short-term Outcomes	Medium-term Outcomes	Long-term Out-comes	Impact

Input/Resources: In order to accomplish our activities for our planned work, we will need the following: child passenger safety seats, trained staff, volunteers, protocol for clinic office visits, educational materials, funders, partners, research on best practice.

Activities: In order to achieve results, we will conduct the following activities: recruit clinic offices, develop an office protocol with clinic staff, provide on-site training for staff and volunteers, develop parent education materials, facilitate access to child passenger safety seats, obtain seats, identify locations for loaner programs, develop press releases for the media and for clinic newsletters.

Outputs: Once completed, these activities will produce the following evidence of service delivery: number of clinics participating, number of staff and volunteers trained, number of parents receiving counseling, number of prescriptions for car seats disseminated, number of loaner programs established, number of lists of loaner programs disseminated, number of times information on the clinic program appears in newsletters, number of times other publicity is generated for the program.

Short-term outcomes: We expect that if completed or ongoing, the activities will lead to the following changes in 1 to 3 years: parents will understand the risks in not using child passenger safety seats, parents will gain skills in correctly installing child passenger safety seats, parents will know where to obtain loaner seats, clinics will know where to refer low-income parents for child passenger safety seats, clinics will routinely provide prescriptions to parents for child passenger safety seats, a cadre of trained volunteers and clinic staff will be available, newsletter will provide reinforcement and reminders to participating clinics, the media will reinforce child passenger safety messages to parents.

Medium-term outcomes: We expect that if completed or ongoing, the short-term outcomes will lead to low-income parents getting seats from loaner program sites, parents putting children in the seats, parents putting children in the seats correctly, parents telling their friends and family about the program, observations showing an increase in children in car seats, checkpoints showing an increase in children correctly restrained, every rural clinic participating in the program, media reports publicizing the improved use of child safety seats.

Long-term outcomes: We expect that the medium-term outcomes will lead to a fundamental change in 5 to 7 years, including a reduction of motor vehicle-related injuries in young children.

Impact: We expect the final impact will be a fundamental change in community child passenger safety outcomes.

Figure 6-4
Basic Logic Model Development Template

Source: Christoffel, T., & Gallagher, S. (2006). *Injury prevention and public health practical knowledge skills and strategies* (2nd ed.). Sudbury, MA: Jones and Bartlett Publishers.

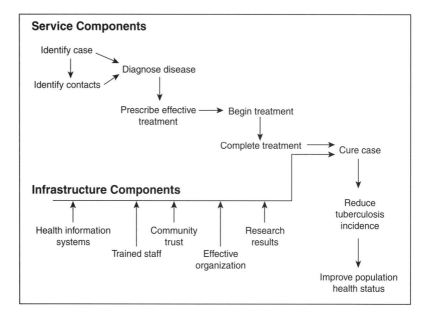

Figure 6-5

Logic Model for Tuber-
culosis Control Program

Source: Centers for Disease
Control and Prevention.
(2007).

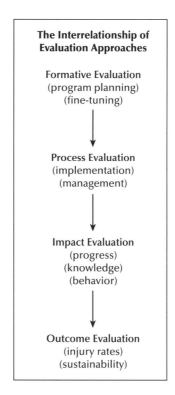

Figure 6-6

The Interrelationship of
Evaluation Approaches

Source: Christoffel, T., &
Gallagher, S. (2006). *Injury
prevention and public health
practical knowledge skills
and strategies* (2nd ed.).
Sudbury, MA: Jones and
Bartlett Publishers.

Types of Evaluation

Evaluation methods are the tools that need to be utilized to determine if a program is accomplishing its stated objectives. There are several different types of evaluation techniques that can be utilized depending on what part of a program needs to be evaluated.

Formative Evaluation   This type of evaluation occurs while the program is under development. The information that is gathered in this form of evaluation is given back to program developers in terms of feedback designed to help the developers with important information to aid in the final design of the program. This information is used to help program managers refine and, perhaps, refocus their program. This allows greater creativity in the design of the program and continuous improvement in the process.

Christoffel and Gallagher (2006) argue that formative evaluation is a way of testing program appropriateness early on in its implementation in order to improve the program quality. This type of evaluation may uncover problems with program implementation, which are usually a result of inadequate training for program staff, poorly developed materials, or any number of unforeseen barriers encountered when the program was originally conceived.

These types of issues are often encountered when a new health promotion initiative is first introduced to the target audience. This type of evaluation includes obtaining feedback from others through personal interviews or focus groups. This feedback is concerned with program activities and not with program outcomes. It is much better to receive constructive criticism very early in the life of the health promotion effort because at this time the program can be adjusted in order to get the program back on track and be in a position to better achieve program goals.

The focus group is usually an excellent way to get opinions from small groups of people about program objectives, materials being used by the program, and other reactions about the new health promotion initiative. These opinions allow the program managers the opportunity to make changes that may ensure program success and even help to reduce program costs.

Process Evaluation   Edberg (2007) argues that a process evaluation concentrates on how a particular program was implemented. It is a process that allows a comparison of what was actually accomplished by the effort with what was specified in the original program plan.

Outcome Evaluation   This part of the evaluation process is concerned with the achievement of objectives and goals of the program or intervention. In the case of a health promotion program, the evaluation will be concerned with the documentation of program effectiveness in achieving the goals and objectives put forth in the planning phase of the program.

There should always be great concern about the impact or outcome of any health promotion program. The major questions to be answered in this type of evaluation center on the short-term and long-term effects of the program being evaluated.

The CDC (2007) argues that outcome evaluation assesses change in knowledge, attitudes, and behaviors about a specific health care topic or issue as a result of individuals' exposure to the promotion campaign. Outcome evaluations can be accomplished through the use of a well designed pre- and post-test of the population that has participated in the health promotion program.

Christoffel and Gallagher (2006) point out that there are many ways to measure outcomes that may include questionnaires, observation, or even a complex epidemiological study. The best long-term indicator of program success will be a reduction in morbidity and mortality from the disease associated with the high-risk health behaviors that the program is trying to reduce. The results from this evaluation will take years to compile.

According to the CDC (1999), outcome evaluations, also called summative evaluations, are not suitable for every program. The CDC believes that outcome evaluations are appropriate only when

1. the intervention has been implemented as planned (determined by the intervention plan and process data); and
2. there are ways to collect reliable data about the population receiving the intervention.

It is also important for health promotion managers to realize that outcome evaluation usually requires the collection of baseline data. This means that some data needs to be collected from program participants before they are exposed to the promotion program. Therefore, it makes sense to include the potential outcome evaluation process into the very early piece of the program plan. It is the responsibility of health promotion managers to gather solid baseline data about program participants during the needs assessment portion of the program development process.

Impact Evaluation

Impact evaluation is a type of evaluation that is very close to outcome evaluation. The main difference between the two is that impact evaluation is concerned with the effect from several interventions while outcome evaluation is concerned with only one intervention. The other noticeable difference between the two types of interventions is found in the fact that outcome evaluation is also interested in intermediate goals while impact evaluation is most concerned with the ultimate goals of the public health program.

An excellent measure of an impact evaluation would be a change in high-risk health behaviors caused by a specific health promotion initiative. According to Christoffel and Gallagher (2006), this type of evaluation needs to be accomplished by direct observation rather than self-reported behavioral change. A good example of an impact evaluation would be observing the number of people using seat belts in an area after an intensive educational campaign concerning the value of seat belt usage was conducted.

With an impact evaluation, the logic model tells you what should have happened because of the intervention. In other words, what were the short-term or immediate effects of the program?

Enhancing the Credibility of the Evaluation Process

The most important component of the **evaluation process** is the ability to gather credible evidence that the program works. The CDC (1999) recommends that data credibility can be improved by utilizing multiple procedures for gathering data and by involving stakeholders in the design and interpretation of the data gathering process. Bartholomew et al. (2006) point out that the most important stakeholders may very well be the beneficiaries of the new promotion program. The beneficiaries would include persons, households, and even communities that are intended to receive the benefits of the health promotion program. Another very important stakeholder in the health promotion effort would be policy makers and decision makers involved in continued funding of the program. These stakeholders are critical in supplying input in how to best evaluate the program in order to prove its worth and continue or expand funding.

It is also helpful to gather data from multiple sources in order to obtain different perspectives on the program's success in achieving its objectives. The quality of the data gathered for the evaluation also increases the credibility of the results being reported about the program's achievements. The more the program receives critical evaluation, the greater the chance for program improvement and continued success.

Health promotion managers should also be very interested in providing a credible evaluation process for the program in order to generate new knowledge. It is a very exciting process to develop a new health promotion effort, to be able to prove its value, and then to share the results with others. The program can then be recognized as a best practice and shared with others to increase the number of successful program outcomes throughout the country.

The Evaluation Plan

The interest in the improvement in health promotion programs continues to grow in government and private and nonprofit sectors. In order to receive initial or continued funding for a health promotion program, the program manager must have built into their proposals or actual program an evaluation plan. The CDC (1999) points out that evaluation is the only way to separate programs that can be successful at preventing injury, disease, or disability from those that do not, and therefore, evaluation needs to become the driving force in the health promotion plan. The evaluation process has to be the critical factor that is considered when developing the program mission, goals, and objectives. The days of funding health promotion programs that do not work are over because resources available for such programs have become scarce.

According to Bartholomew et al. (2006) the evaluation approach should include questions, design, and outcome indicators that are required for a program to be successful. All of these components have already been discussed in the various models mentioned in this chapter.

The logic model has been used successfully with various public health promotion programs in the past and is an excellent starting point for a new health promotion effort. The use of a logic model helps program managers determine the data to be collected, who has the responsibility for data collection, and the costs associated with the evaluation process.

A great deal of thought has to be given to the intended outcome(s) of the health promotion program and how these outcomes will be reached by the inputs and processes used by the program. The logic model allows the program manager to see all of these components of the program. The model in effect becomes a causal map of the entire health promotion effort, allowing the ability for program managers to tweak the program components to reach intended outcomes. Time spent on the causal map or logic model is time well spent increasing the chances of program success and continued funding.

The evaluation plan needs to have an evaluation team that includes team members from within the organization and also members from partner organizations. By utilizing members from other organizations, there can be an increase in resources and enhanced credibility of the evaluation process.

It is also critical to allow sufficient time for the intervention to be able to achieve intended outcomes. The CDC (1999) argues that short-term outcomes should be attainable in 2 to 4 years, while longer-term outcomes may take 4 to 6 years and even longer-term outcomes may not be realized for as long as 10 years or more. It takes a long time to fully develop high-risk health behaviors and an even longer time to change these unhealthy behaviors because many of them may involve addiction to the behaviors by the individual.

New Outcome Measures for Health Promotion Programs

According to McKenzie, Neiger and Thackeray (2009) an outcome objective represents the change expected for a given health problem in a population during a specified time frame. Outcome objectives need to be realistic, measurable, and long term. They can be illustrated in terms of morbidity, mortality, or disability, or several behavioral measures may be utilized. An example of an outcome could be, "By July 1, 2010, the incidence of syphilis among residents of Luzerne County will be reduced from 11.9 cases per 100,000 in 2007 to no more than 7.5 cases per 100,000 populations." This is a realistic, measurable, long-term objective for a health education program for a county health initiative. This type of clarity in objectives is very important in dealing with health promotion programs developed to reduce the high-risk health behaviors associated with communicable and chronic diseases and their complications.

The major threat facing our health care system in the twenty-first century is the epidemic of chronic diseases resulting from the practice of high-risk health behaviors by a growing number of individuals. Those working in public health are being asked to reduce the incidence of these high-risk health behaviors by using public health tools from the past. This strategy is doomed to failure because the tools are antiquated and the resources to support public health are dwindling.

According to Morewitz (2006), over 25 million Americans have a chronic disease resulting in enormous costs that include reduction in quality of life, mortality, and huge expenditures on medical care. Well-designed health promotion programs are required to reduce the short- and long-term complications resulting from these chronic diseases. Therefore, it is very important that evaluation of program outcomes becomes a standard practice in the design of chronic disease educational initiatives.

The outcome measures that are specified in the plans for health promotion programs cannot be vague, or the program is destined to fail and eventually lose funding. This evaluation piece needs to be completed very early in the design of the health promotion program and needs to include the valuable input that can be provided by stakeholder expertise. It is much easier to establish your program outcomes to be measured at the time that you and the program stakeholders put forth the goals and objectives of the new health promotion initiative.

The outcome measures require clarity in order to be able to develop a technique to measure whether or not they were achieved as a result of the health promotion program. The longer-term outcome that is most important to the funders of many health promotion programs is the reduction in chronic diseases acquired by practicing high-risk health behaviors. The chronic health problems of Americans account for a very large percentage of the health care costs in this country. Morewitz (2006) argues that co-morbidities associated with chronic diseases can worsen disease outcomes and contribute greatly to the increasing cost of health care in the country. Therefore, chronic disease health promotion programs need to have a goal of preventing chronic diseases and reducing the complications from these diseases if they are developed.

CONCLUDING REMARKS

The most important component of the development of a health promotion program is program evaluation. Effective evaluation of health promotion programs is a systematic way to prove program success and offers continuous quality improvement of the program at the same time. It is a way to ensure program funding and, perhaps, increase the resources available to the health promotion programs.

There is no such thing as a perfect evaluation, but it is clear that we need to keep making the process better. Evaluation helps to chart a course for correction of flaws and better documentation of the successes of the program interventions. Edberg (2007) argues that evaluation remains a critical component in the determination of the effects of the program and the underlying theory that guides the program. In order to understand the evaluation process, several models of evaluation techniques have been developed. These models provide a structure for determining how an evaluation should be constructed. The model chosen for evaluation is dependent on what you are attempting to measure and how rigorous you want the evaluation to be.

The program outcomes of interest to evaluators could include quality of life, change in behaviors, or obtained predetermined program objectives. It is important to consider long-term program outcomes very early in the design of the health promotion program. The proposed outcomes need to be realistic given the resources available to the program and need to be stated in measurable terms.

The evaluation process needs to be looked at as an opportunity to make the health promotion program as close to a perfect model as possible. Critical evaluation of program design, process, and outcomes offers program managers the opportunity to continuously improve the health promotion effort.

DISCUSSION QUESTIONS

1. Name and explain the various steps in a sound evaluation process.
2. What role do objectives and goals play in the process of evaluation?
3. How do we measure the effects of health promotion programs on the development of chronic diseases?
4. Explain the process of a logic model of the success or failure of a health promotion program.

REFERENCES

Anspaugh, D., Dignan, M., & Anspaugh S. (2000). *Developing health promotion programs.* Long Grove, IL: Waveland Press Inc.

Bartholomew, L., Parcel, G., Kok, G., & Gottlieb, N. (2006). *Planning health promotion programs: An intervention mapping approach.* San Francisco, CA: Jossey Bass.

Centers for Disease Control and Prevention. (1999). Framework for program evaluation in public health. *Morbidity and Mortality Weekly Report,* 48 (No. RR-11).

Centers for Disease Control and Prevention. (2007a). Practical evaluation of public health programs. Public Health Training Network. Available at http://www.cdc.gov/phtn. Accessed June 23, 2007.

Centers for Disease Control and Prevention. (2007b). Chronic disease overview. Available at http://www.cdc.gov/nccdphp/overview.htm. Accessed June 23, 2007.

Christoffel, T., & Gallagher, S. (2006). *Injury prevention and public health practical knowledge skills and strategies* (2nd ed.). Sudbury, MA: Jones and Bartlett Publishers.

Edberg, M. (2007). *Essentials of health behavior and social and behavioral theory in public health.* Sudbury, MA: Jones and Bartlett Publishers.

Jack L Jr, Mukhtar Q, Martin M, Rivera M, Lavinghouze SR, Jernigan J, et al. (2006). Program evaluation and chronic diseases: methods, approaches, and implications for public health. *Prev Chronic Dis.* Available at http://www.cdc.gov/pcd/issues/2006/jan/05_0141.htm. Accessed June 23, 2008.

Morewitz. S. (2006). *Chronic Diseases and Health Care.* New York, NY: Springer Publications.

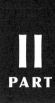

PART

Emerging Priorities in Health Promotion Programs

7

CHAPTER

Health Promotion in People with Disabilities

Jill D. Morrow-Gorton, MD

OBJECTIVES

After reading this chapter, you should

- Understand the concept of disability and the ways that disability is defined
- Recognize the importance of understanding the specific disabilities included in a population for planning health promotion programs
- Know how to identify the particular population of people with disabilities represented in a study in order to compare results of different studies
- Be aware of the similarities and differences in cardiovascular health and risk factors between the general population and groups of people with particular disabilities
- Understand how to apply public health strategies to health promotion issues for populations of people with disabilities using existing systems

KEY TERMS

Americans with Disabilities Act
Developmental disabilities

Disabilities
Healthy People 2010

Introduction

Health promotion is an important concept for all populations of individuals. A great deal is known about how to reach the general population through public awareness campaigns and other public health strategies. Less is known about how to reach certain subgroups of the general population, such as the group of people with **disabilities.** Often public health looks at people with disabilities as a single group, when in fact, there are many different groups of people with disabilities. Knowing more about specific disabilities and understanding how to modify approaches to public health activities, such as those to address health promotion, will help health departments and public health professionals more effectively reach these populations in order to impact their quality of health. This chapter outlines the differences in the categorization of different disabilities, what is known about disease and health conditions—in particular cardiovascular risks—in the populations of people with disabilities, and features some examples of how public health strategies addressing health promotion can be used to not only reach these populations but also to effectively influence health behavior.

Definition of Disability

Disability is a term frequently used but not always understood in its complexity. There are multiple definitions of the term, and it is used one way in public health—looking at the health issues affecting the population—and another in public welfare—determining the appropriate set of services for an individual person. The task at hand is to illustrate the diversity of the population of people with disabilities and to focus on how this population cannot be reached as a single unit.

Accardo et al. define a disability as "any restriction or lack of ability (resulting from an impairment) to perform an activity in a manner or within the range considered usual for a human being" (1996, p. 92). This definition is not specific to any particular impairment and involves sensory, physical, psychological, and cognitive disorders. It also includes an element of transience in that a disability may be temporary or permanent. This makes defining the population of people with disabilities for the purpose of studying its health and finding ways to establish health promotion programs difficult.

The World Health Organization (WHO) defines disability as part of a continuum involving impairment, disability, and handicap as illustrated in Figure 7-1 (Barbotte et al., 2001).

As the second level of this continuum, disability is usually referred to in the context of health and a health experience. It encompasses not only the person's individual characteristics but also the society or culture in which that person lives (Word Health Organization, 2007). This creates the possibility that what is considered a disability by one person or culture may not be in another, potentially making the comparison of health issues among people with disabilities difficult. Handicap, the third level of the continuum, is defined as a disability that affects the person's everyday life.

In addition, the concept of handicap complicates the matter as a person with a disability only has a handicap if society or lack of opportunity puts him

Figure 7-1
WHO Definition of
Impairment, Disability,
and Handicap

- An *impairment* is a physiological disorder or injury.
- A *disability* is the inability to do something related to an impairment.
- A *handicap* is the social result of a disability.

or her there. For example, a person who is near sighted and is able to see with glasses would have an impairment but not a handicap, unless he or she wanted to be an airplane pilot and needed to have perfect vision. Thus, one might choose to study the population of people with handicaps rather than those with disabilities.

Heterogeneity of Disability Subgroups

Studying health issues in the population of people with disabilities requires some categorization of different disabilities. While the issues of what is a disability versus a handicap complicate defining a population, variability in categorization and definitions of specific disability groups also make determining the size of the population of people with disabilities difficult. Different groups categorize disabilities in different ways, and public health professionals group disabilities differently from professionals involved in health care. Identifying what population group is being studied is important for both learning about the health conditions within that population and for applying health promotion strategies to what is learned in order to change health behaviors.

Medicine or health care divides disabilities into two broad categories: developmental disabilities and acquired ones. **Developmental disabilities** occur in the *developmental period*, which is defined by the Diagnostic and Statistical Manual of Mental Disorders published by the American Psychological Association in 1994 (DSM IV, 2000) as birth (or prebirth) to age 18 years, and by entities like the Commonwealth of Pennsylvania Office of Developmental Programs as birth to age 22 years (Office of Mental Retardation, 2002).

Developmental disabilities generally involve learning or cognition, movement, and/or behavior (Accardo et al., 1996; Batshaw & Perret, 1992). These include conditions like intellectual disabilities, cerebral palsy, learning disabilities, autism, and attention disorders. Developmental disabilities are mostly characterized by abnormalities in the brain, usually in the formation of the brain in utero caused by chromosomal abnormalities like Down syndrome (trisomy 21), exposure to toxins such as alcohol, or infections such as that caused by cytomegalovirus.

To further complicate things, different nomenclature is used for some developmental disabilities depending on the geographical area or time in history. For example, what is currently being called *intellectual disabilities* was called *mental retardation* a few years ago. Go back a few more decades in time and people with these disabilities were referred to as *imbecile* or *idiot*, obsolete terms that now have pejorative connotations (Accardo et al., 1996; Mondofacto, n.d.). Cross the Atlantic Ocean, and in England it is called a *learning disability*. The plurality of terms used for intellectual disabilities makes it difficult to compare populations in various geographic areas and from different time frames (O'Brien, 2001).

There are also disabilities that occur during the developmental period, such as the congenital lack of an extremity or phocomelia (Mondofacto, n.d.). This can result in a disability but does not involve a congenital brain abnormality. These might also be considered developmental disabilities, although they are not generally included with the disorders typically called developmental disabilities.

Acquired disabilities often result from an injury or a progressive neurologic condition. These include conditions like brain injury, spinal cord injuries, dementia, or Parkinsonism. Generally, these individuals were neurodevelopmentally normal prior to either an injury or the onset of a particular disease or infection (Accardo et al., 1996). Some injuries, like strokes, result in multiple disabilities, including speech and language problems and hemiplegias or paralysis of one side of the body, and most often affect older people.

In terms of definitions of disabilities, there is some overlap between developmental disabilities and acquired ones. For example, a child with typical development that contracts a viral encephalitis may incur a brain injury resulting in lowered cognitive functioning in the range of an intellectual disability or mental retardation. In this case, the child is considered to have an intellectual disability because the condition occurred during the developmental period even though it comes from an acquired condition.

Public services for people with disabilities organize types of disabilities in different categories from medicine. The Centers for Medicare and Medicaid Services (CMS) provides funding for groups of people with disabilities through 1915c waivers (Centers for Medicare and Medicaid Services [CMS], 2006), which require that the person have a condition that qualifies him or her to receive institutional services either in a nursing home or an intermediate care facility for people with mental retardation (ICF/MR) or other related conditions (ICF/ORC). Waivers offer people the opportunity to have supportive services in their home rather than an institution. These services include things like assistance with activities of daily living (ADLs), such as dressing, feeding, and grooming, as well as any specialized therapies, such as physical therapy to help with walking or mobility. Waivers are specific to individual states, and the specifics of a waiver are defined by the state. A state can define the population of people to receive funding from the waiver, i.e., which disability group to address as well as the particular services that are eligible to be paid for by the waiver (CMS, 2006). For example, Iowa's physical disability waiver provides funding for services for people with physical disabilities and who meet criteria for placement in a nursing home or an ICF (Iowa Department of Human Services, 2005). Physical disabilities can be developmental, like cerebral palsy or muscular dystrophy, or acquired, like a quadriplegia from a spinal cord injury of the cervical vertebra.

National programs like *Healthy People 2010* (Center for Disease Control and Prevention [CDC], 2000) put disability groups into different categories from the above. The Healthy People 2010 goals for people with disabilities describe two groups in particular. One is adults living in large, out-of-home facilities (congregate or institutional care), and the second is children with disabilities in regular classrooms. Neither of these two groups would easily be identified using any of the previously defined categories. Adults in congregate care might be elderly adults living in a nursing home or young adults with intellectual disabilities living in an ICF/MR. From the vantage point of health and health needs, these two groups do not have similar requirements.

The **Americans with Disabilities Act** (ADA, 1990) sets yet another definition for a disability—a legal one. The ADA defines a disability as "a physical or mental impairment that substantially limits one or more major life activities." This definition would include people that might not fit into some of the other categories or rubrics used. Other public health initiatives developed for the purpose of gathering health information about people with disabilities, such as the Survey of Income and Program Participation (SIPP; U.S. Census Bureau, 1994), define disabilities by functional level and not specific diagnosis or living arrangement. Functional activities in the SIPP include abilities to do things like walk 3 city blocks or carry 10 pounds. Difficulty with functional ability does not map to a particular clinical or programmatic diagnosis. A person with cerebral palsy clinically has a physical and developmental disability, but that person may be able to walk a mile and therefore would not meet the criteria for the functional limitations defined in the SIPP. Thus, information gathered about people fitting the legal definition of disability may differ from that derived from populations with clinical or programmatic definitions.

Evaluating literature studies involving populations of people with disabilities requires understanding the nature of the disability being studied. Health promotion will differ depending on the population that is being targeted, whether that is based on age or presence of cognitive disorders that interfere with the individual's ability to acquire and use health knowledge. Understanding the heterogeneity of disabilities allows for the study of different groups separately and identifies successful ways of reaching them to help maximize their health.

Demographics of Populations of People with Disabilities

Understanding the subpopulations of people with disabilities is instrumental to developing and implementing a public health promotion program. One set of important information includes the demographic characteristics of the group. Demographic characteristics consist of age, number of people estimated in the population, and health conditions important to the group. These characteristics help define who the populations are, which assists with determining the best way to reach each subpopulation.

Census Numbers

In 2000, the population of people with a disability over the age of 5 years from the U.S. Census Bureau was 49,746,248, which represented about 17.6% of the population (2000). These numbers exclude people living in institutions as well as people in the armed forces and children under the age of 5 years. In addition, the criteria for this data requires that 1 of the following 3 criteria be met: (1) They were 5 years old and over and reported a long-lasting sensory, physical, mental, or self-care disability; (2) they were 16 years old and over and reported difficulty going outside the home because of a physical, mental, or emotional condition lasting 6 months or more; or (3) they were 16 to 64 years old and reported difficulty working at a job or business because of a physical, mental, or emotional condition lasting 6 months or more.

The first census information about people with disabilities comes from the 1994 SIPP survey (U.S. Census Bureau, 1994). Comparing that data to the most recent census numbers from 2002, the proportion of the U.S. population with a disability as defined above is 18%. That proportion has remained stable over that 18-year period. In addition, the number of people with a severe disability as defined by the responding individual has changed slightly from 9% in 1994 to 11.5% in 2002. The SIPP acknowledges that it uses different definitions of disability when looking at populations of people with disabilities.

Age

The rates of disabilities increase with age and about 70% of people aged 80 years have a disability (U.S. Census Bureau, 2002). This is illustrated in Figure 7-2.

For children under age 15 years, the rates of disabilities are estimated to be 2% for children under age 3 years, 5% for children 3 to 5 years, and 6% for children 6 to 14 years of age. This likely reflects not only the development of disability related to acquired conditions like meningitis or traumatic brain injury but also the definitive diagnosis of disability in young children. Making a definitive diagnosis of a developmental disability is more difficult in younger children as the testing measures are less accurate and the less severe developmental disabilities are often not apparent at younger ages. For example, in the United States, the average age of diagnosis of a congenital hearing impairment of 50 dB or greater has been about 3 years of age, until recently (National Institutes of Health, 1993). The implementation of universal newborn hearing screening in many states has the potential to identify this hearing loss within the first year of life, possibly within the first few months (McCormick, 1995). This would increase the numbers of children

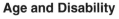

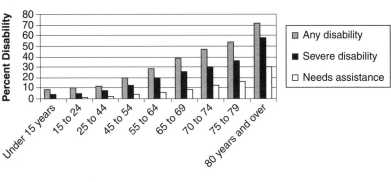

Figure 7-2
Prevalence of Disability
in Different Age Groups

identified as having a disability before age 3 years and change the rates of disabilities for particular age groups.

Many people with developmental disabilities are living longer as are people in the general population. Medical technology has also changed the survival rates for some individuals with disabilities, resulting in more older people with disabilities than ever before. The CDC studied causes and ages of death for people with trisomy 21 (Down syndrome), a common chromosomal problem associated with intellectual disabilities and congenital heart disease. The average age of death in this group rose from age 25 years in 1983 to age 49 years in 1997 (Roizen & Patterson, 2003). Contributing to this are the advances in treatment for congenital heart disease, as 40% to 50% of people with Down syndrome have some type of congenital heart disease. Other medical technology, such as feeding tubes for individuals with cerebral palsy who are unable to take in enough nutrition by mouth, has improved health as well as increased the life span for many people with disabilities (Sullivan et al., 2005).

Conventional wisdom often advised that many people with severe disabilities, especially those with severe cerebral palsy and/or intellectual disabilities, would not survive into adulthood. In addition to the data for people with Down syndrome, there is other data to show that many people do survive into adulthood (Hayden, 1998; Janicki et al., 1999; O'Brien, Tate, & Zaharia, 1991). Unpublished data from Pennsylvania (2001) reveals that the average age of death not adjusted for population for people receiving services in the mental retardation system was 56 years of age. The most common causes of death for people with intellectual disabilities were noncongenital or acquired heart disease (e.g., coronary heart disease), cancer, influenza, and pneumonia. The first two of these parallel exactly the causes of death for the general population (CDC, 2000). Chronic lung disease was lower on the list, but for those individuals dying of a respiratory cause, the average age was also lower at 45 years of age. Thus, people with disabilities have a greater life span than in the past, and many people are living to the age where they are at risk for acquiring additional disabilities related to chronic diseases, such as coronary heart disease, that are common in the general population as people age.

Specific Versus General Health Needs

Historically, health care for people with disabilities has targeted the specific needs of populations such as treatment of seizure disorders or orthopedic surgery for complications of cerebral palsy. Specialty medical care often included single condition, multispecialty clinics staffed by specific medical and surgical specialties. For example, health care for people with spina bifida, a disorder with spinal cord malformations and often hydrocephalous, includes neurosurgery, urology, orthopedics, various therapies such as physical therapy, and pediatrics to follow development. The goal is to address surgical shunt placement and management for the hydrocephalous as well as the initial repair of the spinal cord and back, urologic management of the neurogenic bladder, and orthopedic management of the spine and lower extremities. Therapies addressed the functional motor needs of individuals, and pediatrics typically looked at development and any acute health needs such as infections. If seizures were present, they might also be addressed through this venue.

Most states, including Pennsylvania, have specialty clinics for spina bifida located either in children's hospitals or at university settings. Various options for payment, including private insurance, public insurance, and services funded through grant money, make medical services for treatment of spina bifida and its complications accessible to most citizens (Spina Bifida Association, 2007a).

While these health care settings often address chronic medical problems, they may not provide health promotion or primary care. These centers tend to be regional in nature, often located in urban areas, and not convenient for primary care, such as immunizations or treatment of acute illnesses like ear and throat infections. This means that most primary care is more likely to be obtained closer to the home of the people rather at the urban clinic. Coordination of care between these two entities is often limited by time and distance constraints, sometimes leading to each assuming that the other is providing a particular service when in fact no one is doing it. This leads to holes in the medical care of people with disabilities because sometimes the less acute things, like screening hearing, get missed. As well, many people with chronic medical problems may have more physician visits for and more attention paid to the care of their chronic medical problems than they have for health promotion. Therefore, the health promotion may take a back seat to the other health issues even though people with disabilities and chronic medical problems can benefit from participation in health promotion activities. To combat this issue, the concept of a medical home for children and adults with special health care needs, including disabilities as well as some chronic conditions, has been developed to provide not only primary care but also care management to coordinate care between all of the health professionals involved in a person's medical care.

One example of where the medical home concept might be helpful is the monitoring of weight for individuals with spina bifida. In the model of health care before the medical home concept, monitoring the growth of children with spina bifida may be one of the things that takes a back seat to the ongoing urology treatment of bladder infections and other problems or neurosurgical management of their shunted hydrocephalous. Literature (Spina Bifida Association, 2007b) shows that children with spina bifida develop obesity at a higher rate than typical children. That proportion of obese individuals with spina bifida remains into adulthood. Obesity comes with substantial health risks for all individuals but has an additional impact on people with spina bifida. Extra weight tends to make walking more difficult in people with spina bifida, which in turn leads many to use a wheelchair for mobility. This serves to decrease the number of calories used and contributes to increased weight gain. An important goal in health promotion for the population of people with spina bifida should be the prevention and treatment of obesity to avoid its health complications. Until recently, however, there was little data to guide such health promotion recommendations.

Basic Health Information About People with Disabilities

The field obtains basic health information in two manners: surveys of health generally done through health departments and specific studies done by researchers to be published in the literature. Health information is an important driver of public health policy and programming as it allows targeting of funding and efforts toward those health issues with the most detrimental effects or toward those that have the highest prevalence. While much data is available for the general population, the body of knowledge for the population of people with disabilities and for specific disabilities is less robust. The next section looks at what is gathered and known about health for people with disabilities with a focus on health promotion related to prevention of obesity and promotion of physical activity.

General Population Surveys   A great deal is known about health and the prevalence of chronic disease in the general population. The CDC has studied not only the increase in life expectancy in the general population but also the impact of chronic disease, life style, and health behaviors on people as they age. The National Center for Health Statistics (CDC, 2007b) contains a plethora of data about all aspects of health including births, deaths, nutrition, hospital discharge, and ambulatory health data. The information for this data center comes from many different surveys that assess the health and nutrition of the general population as well as information from hospitals about utilization of health care services.

Behavioral Risk Factor Surveillance System (BRFSS)   One such survey, the Behavioral Risk Factor Surveillance System (CDC, 2007a), samples households in all 50 states as well as the District of Columbia, Puerto Rico, Guam, and the U.S. Virgin Islands. This survey has been used annually since 1984 and is administered by the health departments. The survey assesses information about health behaviors including alcohol and tobacco use, nutrition and physical activity, access to health care, use of screens like cancer screening, and certain disease conditions such as diabetes, asthma, and high blood pressure. This information is used to track and identify emerging trends in order to intervene and try to improve the health of the population. The data also provides information about the treatment of some conditions, which allows a look at the adequacy of the health care system as well as the presence of health risks. Some of the surveys described below accommodate and include people with disabilities, while others use methods that relative undersample that population. In addition, there are now surveys that concentrate on certain populations of people with disabilities.

The BRFSS is conducted by telephone and samples about 350,000 people per year, making it the largest health telephone survey in the world. The BRFSS (CDC, 2007a) was developed in 1984 by the CDC to provide a mechanism to gather information about personal health behaviors that research has shown contribute to premature mortality and morbidity. Demographic details gathered include age, gender, race and ethnicity, education level, marital status, employment, and number of children living in the household. The person answering the phone provides the information for the survey. States can add questions to the survey, and some include questions about disability and limitations of mobility in the survey. North Carolina includes a question about disability and uses that information to determine the prevalence of disability among adults living in that state. The prevalence of disabilities can assist in planning for services to support people with disabilities to live more independent lives.

In general, most surveys do not include information about people with disabilities and those that do generally use a single category labeled disability rather than looking at any of the subsets of people with disabilities. Phone surveys that capture information from the first person that answers the phone in private residences may not access people with disabilities, especially those with intellectual disabilities, deafness, or difficulties with speech. None of the survey strategies will access people living in other kinds of community living settings, like group homes or environments that provide support for people with intellectual or physical disabilities. These surveys also do not access health information about people living in institutions even though identifying the differences or lack of differences might help people live in more independent environments.

Behavior of School-Aged Children Survey

Kalnins et al. (1999) studied health behaviors in children with physical disabilities by using the Health Behavior of School-aged Children survey, which is a WHO survey. In completing the survey, they noted that they needed to modify the recommended protocol for administration of the instrument. The authors note that children with physical disabilities in Canada are rarely included in health behavior surveys; however, knowledge about risks for the development of secondary health conditions, especially those related to behavior, would contribute to the prevention of those secondary conditions. The prevention of obesity in children with spina bifida is one such area of health promotion that can prevent such secondary health conditions. The authors conclude that while there is a need for separate surveys of health behavior in children with physical disabilities, there is also a need to include questions about disabilities routinely in surveys used in the general population.

Survey of Income and Program Participation (SIPP)

The U.S. Census Bureau (1994) conducts SIPP, which includes a section that delineates disability using the ADA definition, on the general population. However, this survey does not include any information about health or health behaviors. Another survey conducted through the NCHS (CDC,

2007b)—the National Health Interview Survey (NHIS)—has periodically included special sections related to certain disabilities. In 1989, the survey collected data using a special questionnaire on mental health. A special questionnaire on disability was included in 1994 and 1995, which assessed limitations in activities and work and the need for personal assistance in activities of daily living. In the other years, the NHIS included information about chronic disease and limitations in activity.

In addition to population level surveys collecting information related to disabilities, there are some surveys that have been used with populations of people with specific disabilities. In the example given above, Kalnins et al. (1999) modified the Health Behavior of School-aged Children survey to apply to children with physical disabilities, like spina bifida or cerebral palsy. They conclude that not only can such surveys be applied to populations of children with disabilities, but the information derived from them can be used to reduce the risks of developing secondary conditions and to promote health and well-being as well. Steele et al. (1996) used the same survey and concluded that while children with physical disabilities were less likely than their peers to use alcohol, tobacco, or marijuana, they had less healthy diets and participated in less physical activity. The later behaviors put them at greater risk for obesity and the health risks for secondary conditions such as heart disease, diabetes, arthritis, and stroke, which come with obesity.

Disability Specific Surveys

National Core Indicators Project (NCI)

Other surveys were specifically designed for people with specific disabilities. The National Core Indicators project (NCI) was developed in 1997 by the Human Services Research Institute (HSRI), an organization developed in the 1970s to enhance the quality of services and supports for people with mental retardation and mental illness, in conjunction with the National Association of State Developmental Disability Directors (NASDDDS, 2007) to measure performance across the services offered to people with intellectual and other developmental disabilities. It targets states and the services provided by and/or funded by government entities with a goal not only to assess the quality of those services but also to gain knowledge about how to improve them and directions for future service development. Currently, 26 states and parts of another participate in the surveys collecting data about common performance indicators in the same manner. Participants work in a collaborative manner to identify important areas to survey and to modify the instrument to meet those information needs. Data collected includes information about consumer and family outcomes such as choice in a variety of aspects of life, cost, and health and safety outcomes and is analyzed to provide information that will help states and provider entities address the weaknesses in their programs.

NCI surveys are completed in a face-to-face interview on a sample of people within the service system (HSRI, 2006). Multiple surveys exist including consumer, family, and provider versions. Depending on the ability of the consumer to answer, some questions may not be used. Only a few health indicators exist, and they include the number of consumers that have had the following examinations in the last year: physical exam, women with an ob–gyn exam, and dental exam. Another health indicator looks at the number of people taking medication for anxiety or mood or behavior problems. Proposed indicators include a wellness measurement to assess the number of people with healthy behaviors in areas such as weight, physical activity, and unhealthy habits such as smoking. Another question in the current survey relates to participation in exercise or sports in the past month and does allow comparison to national public health data about the lack of participation in leisure-time physical activity, which is a Healthy People 2010 goal.

Pennsylvania Health Risk Profile (HRP)

Pennsylvania uses a unique electronic survey to assess health indicators in the population of people receiving mental retardation services in a licensed residential setting. This instrument, called Health Risk Profile (HRP; Office of Mental Retardation, 2001), collects health information annually on a random sample of people across the state. In the 2006–2007 fiscal year, 1,346 people were sampled—a number close to 10% of the residential population. Registered nurses visit the home and collect the information using the record from the residential provider agency. Questions cover three areas: (1) access to health care, (2) health promotion and disease prevention, and (3) disease management. Data from this instrument is used locally to address individual health issues and statewide to address broader health issues. Many of the questions asked directly relate to areas identified by the CDC's *Healthy People 2010* initiatives for the general population and include information about weight, nutrition, physical activity, and cancer screening as well as disease conditions and their treatment.

Healthy People 2010

In addition to its goals for health for the general population, *Healthy People 2010* (CDC, 2000) has specific goals for people with disabilities and secondary conditions, namely to eliminate disparities between people with and without disabilities, and to target these activities toward certain populations of people with disabilities. A sample of the groups described includes adults living in large, out-of-home facilities (congregate care) and children with disabilities in regular classrooms. *Healthy People 2010* uses existing sources of health data from established surveys such as NHIS and BRFSS. In the discussion of looking at data to determine disparities in groups of people with disabilities, the *Healthy People 2010* publication notes that few data systems identify people with disabilities. Some of the issues that have been identified to have disparities between the population of people with disabilities and those without are similar to those described by other authors, namely increased obesity and decreased physical activity. In addition, *Healthy People 2010* also found increased stress in people with disabilities and a lower proportion of women over 55 years of age who had an annual mammogram. In general, this initiative groups all individuals with disabilities into a single subpopulation of the general population, although there are specific goals related to certain subgroups of people with disabilities. These subgroups are often defined by where people live, such as adults living in congregate care (usually institutional living either in a nursing facility or an intermediate care facility), or children with disabilities that are in a regular classroom. These groupings will allow identification of some kinds of risks and some remedies based on the location of people but will not allow for looking at particular groups of disabilities.

Survey Methods   Surveys employ multiple methods to gather the needed health information. Phone surveys are common and generally use local phone listings to draw a random sample of the population in order to survey a statistically significant number of respondents. Some surveys are done with a combination of methods, such as phone and face-to-face interviews. Yet other surveys use a paper document that is sent through the mail, completed, and then returned by the recipient. Each of these methods has strengths and weaknesses. As well, some of them are more or less accessible to people with disabilities. The impact of these issues can determine whether or not a survey instrument will reach the population of people that is desired.

Phone Surveys

Phone surveys, like the BRFSS, have become a staple in the toolbox of health departments for monitoring health indicators in the population. Traditionally, these surveys have relied on landlines and accessing numbers that are published and public in nature. Emerging changes in technology may impact the ability to use this strategy to reach both the general population and the populations of people with disabilities. Estimates show that 25% of people aged 18 to 25 years and almost 33% of people aged 25 to 29 years live in a household without a landline (Landers, 2007). In addition, 32% of low-income young adults have only cell phones. These numbers do not appear in the local phone books making them more difficult to reach. This is also true for some populations of people with disabilities, especially those that live in small group homes in the community or people living in institutions that also do not typically have a phone number that is listed in the local phone directory. The lack of a listed phone number serves to bias the results of surveys that are done using randomly selected phone numbers, as these populations will not be surveyed. Given the prevalence of this in particular subpopulations, this could serve to underestimate behaviors that are more common in these age groups. These surveys also likely underestimate behaviors and conditions that are more prevalent in the populations of people with disabilities that make up almost 18% of the U.S. population, a substantial portion of the population (U.S. Census Bureau, 2000).

Face-to-Face Surveys

Most of the disability specific surveys, like the NCI project, use a face-to-face technique. This avoids the issues of people with intellectual disabilities not having the ability to read or write. It also avoids missing sampling people with physical disabilities that may not be able to answer the phone because of mobility limitations and therefore would not be the primary respondent to a phone survey. Even these methods cannot overcome the issues of the lack of ability to communicate—either to understand the question or to be able to answer—that impact some people with severe intellectual disabilities, despite special equipment or communication devices, to say the words for them. Instead, NCI uses surveys for caregivers and families to complete about the individual. This limits the ability to question about a number of things that are common questions used in health surveys in the general population, such as perceptions of health.

Mail Surveys

Postal questionnaires represent another strategy employed to monitor health indicators and risk factors. Mail surveys must be completed and returned by participants. The SF-36, or Short Form Health Survey, was developed for the Medical Outcomes Study and has been widely used to survey health status (Brazier et al., 1992). It has been used to estimate disease burden in specific diseases compared to the general population as well as to compare one disease to another. Application of the tool generally occurs by completing the written questionnaire in the physician or other health practitioner's office. For individuals that cannot self-administer the test because of a condition that prohibits them from being able to complete the forms, it may be administered verbally by a professional, such as a social worker (University of California at Los Angeles, 2007). Other researchers have applied the questionnaire by using it in a phone interview format. Interestingly, these interviews showed more positive impressions of the health quality of life questions than the written survey indicating a possible bias introduced by using a person to administer it. Garratt et al. (1993) assessed the possibility of using the SF-36 by mail instead of an in-person written format or a verbally administered questionnaire either by phone or in person. A Dutch study (Picavet, 2001) looked at the response rate between a survey done by interview and one done by mail. It discovered that the interview survey had a higher response rate, 58.5% to 46.9%, and women were more likely to respond to the mail survey. In addition, individuals with lower education levels did not respond as frequently to the mail survey.

The comparison of response rates as well as types of responses for surveys administered in different modalities adds an additional level of complexity and uncertainty in evaluating the results of different health surveys. In addition, some populations of people with disabilities will be unable to participate in some of the potential formats of surveys, which either leaves them out of the data pool altogether or uses a modification for them that might result in a different result than had they been able to use the same format. Individuals with disabilities have a lower education rate than their age peers without disabilities and are less likely to be employed. *Healthy People 2010* data (CDC, 2000) indicates that only 52% of people in the broad disability category are employed compared with 82% of the general population. Educational outcomes for youth with disabilities, as measured through the National Longitudinal Transition Study (Wagner et al., 2006), consistently show that individuals with disabilities achieve less educationally than youth in the general population. The subgroup of youth with intellectual disabilities and multiple disabilities typically score the lowest on all testing. This is consistent with their diagnosis of an intellectual disability but creates a barrier to using standard questionnaires about health related to lower abilities to either read or understand spoken language or to be able to communicate an answer. Therefore, measures that require giving a perception of health or using a multipoint, interval response scale, such as a Likert scale, may also be more difficult to administer to individuals that do not have the cognitive capacity to understand gradations of response related to a particular question. This makes comparison of some measures of health that are standard for the general population difficult with some subpopulations of people with disabilities.

Literature and Research

Research is another way that information is developed about health for people. Most research involves either the general population or groups of people with the same health conditions. Consequently, there is a relative paucity of research and information about health for many populations of people with disabilities. Many studies do not indicate whether or not the people in the study had any type of disability if the disability is not related to the health condition and not part of the study. The history of involving people with disabilities in medical research is a dark one, as illustrated by a CBS news article about Sonoma State Hospital. The report outlines a period in the late 1950s and early 1960s when children institutionalized there were reported to have been used in experiments involving radiation. This story is not unique and contributes to the barriers of researching health issues in this population (Mabrey, 2005). In addition, research assumes some risk, and informed consent related to those risks is difficult in some populations of people with disabilities who are unable to understand those risks.

Types of Research Studies

Information about health in people with disabilities comes from a variety of studies. Some are larger in size, involving thousands of individuals, and serve primarily to provide descriptive information about a particular population of people. Examples of this type of study are the mortality studies done in California by a variety of authors related to identifying risk factors for mortality in the population of people with intellectual disabilities living either in an institutional or a community setting (Chaney & Eyman, 2000; Eyman,

Call, & White, 1991; O'Brien et al., 1991). Others are relatively small in size and may study a single aspect of a particular disorder, such as a study of sleep disorders in individuals with neurofibromatosis type 1 done by Johnson, Wiggs, and Huson (2005). Most of the research is found in specialty journals, such as the journals published by the American Association on Intellectual and Developmental Disabilities (AAIDD formerly known as AAMR, the American Association on Mental Retardation) or *Developmental Medicine and Child Neurology*, the official journal of the American Academy for Cerebral Palsy and Developmental Medicine and the British Pediatric Neurology Association.

Cardiovascular Risks in Particular Populations of People with Disabilities

Although current knowledge about health conditions is limited, findings show some similarities to the general population. For instance, most studies of causes of mortality show that the causes of death for people with intellectual disabilities mirror those of the general population (Janicki et al., 1999; Patja, Molsa, & Iivanainen, 2001). The top cause of death is cardiovascular disease followed by cancer and respiratory diseases. Some studies have also shown a higher rate of cardiovascular disease in this population than in the general population (O'Brien, 1991; Pitetti, Campbell, 1991). Pitetti and Campbell (1991) relate this to the adoption of a sedentary lifestyle and eating patterns. As in the general population, lifestyle and health behaviors primarily related to nutrition and physical activity contribute greatly to the development of cardiovascular disease.

Other groups of people with disabilities have increased risks for cardiovascular disease. Individuals with spinal cord injuries have cardiac complications that occur early after their injury but also tend to have higher blood lipids, which are associated with cardiovascular disease leading to death (McKinley & Garstang, 2006). Approximately 20% of deaths of individuals with spinal cord injuries are due to cardiovascular disease. Increased incidences of not only high blood lipids but also obesity, physical inactivity, insulin resistance, and diabetes contribute to the higher risk for heart disease. Individuals with spina bifida have a similar pattern of increased risk factors for heart disease.

Certain disease conditions that put people at risk for disabilities may also bring risks of other disease conditions. Rheumatoid arthritis (RA) is one of these conditions in that it causes inflammation of joints that can lead to limitation in movement and difficulty with ambulation. A study done at the Mayo Clinic shows that people with RA have a higher risk for heart disease than the general population (Kaplan, 2006). Other researchers (Bacon et al., 2002; Kaplan, 2006) have corroborated this finding. Although some of this risk is likely specific to the inflammatory etiology of RA, traditional risk factors for cardiovascular disease do play some role (Del Rincon et al., 2001). Minimizing the general risks of heart disease as well as the disease-specific risks could help contribute to better health and to decreased mortality and morbidity due to heart disease in this group.

Two risk factors for heart disease include obesity and lack of physical activity (Hahn et al., 1986; McGinnis & Foege, 1993). Obesity contributes heavily to heart disease risk as well as predisposing an individual for diabetes, high blood pressure, and increased lipids, all of which are also risks for heart disease (Mensah & Brown, 2007; Pearson, 2007). In addition, obesity is a risk for the development of arthritis and orthopedic problems that may limit the ability to walk, providing an additional contribution to heart disease risk. On the other hand, physical activity reduces the risk of heart disease as well as reduces blood pressure, blood lipids, and obesity. (Kaplan et al., 1996; Kushi et al., 1997; Lee, Blair, & Jackson, 1999; Paffenbarger et al., 1993; Sherman, D'Agostino, & Cobb, 1994; Wei et al., 1999).

Obesity in People with Disabilities

Data about obesity and physical activity is more available for populations of people with disabilities than some of the other health measures used in the general population. Obesity is not only a risk for heart disease but also a contributor to disability in that it causes or complicates arthritis and diabetes (Iezzoni, 2003). This in turn complicates the use of physical activity to ameliorate obesity and to control weight. Obesity has been identified as a significant issue in a number of populations including people with Down syndrome or trisomy 21. Rubin et al. (1998) found that 45% of the men and 56% of the women followed in a large specialty clinic in the Chicago area were overweight. Other studies, including ones by Braunschweig et al. (2004) and Rimmer, Braddock, and Fujiura (1993), corroborate these results in the broader population of people with developmental disabilities.

Rhode Island has reported on their obesity results from the BRFSS surveys for the years 1998 to 2000 (Rhode Island Department of Health, 2000). Comparing the levels of overweight and obesity in the population of people with disabilities to those without reveals that the differences are minor (see Figure 7-2). As well, more than 50% of both populations are either overweight or obese. In a British study, Wannamethee et al. (2004) showed that the prevalence of overweight and obesity in a population of elderly men between ages 60 and 79 years was about 69%. The group of overweight and obese men had twice the risk of cardiovascular disease and twice the risk of mobility problems as the group that had weight in the normal range. A study of obesity in a cohort of people with spina bifida followed from birth to 35 years of age showed a 56% rate of obesity (Hunt & Oakeshott, 2003). In comparison to the prevalence of overweight and obesity within the general population, these results are not different and the problem of obesity is one that affects all members of industrialized society.

Participation in Physical Activity

One of the other components of risk for heart disease is lack of physical activity. Various authors have studied participation in physical activity in populations of people with disabilities. Physical activity is more difficult to study as it involves not only whether or not someone participates but also at what level of exertion and what frequency. The CDC has set guidelines for recommended amounts of physical activity (CDC, 2008); however, those are not necessarily the criteria used for participation in the research literature. Thus, rates of participation in the research literature may not reflect the recommended goals for physical activity. McGuire et al. (2007) note that physical activity is not very common in the population of adults with disabilities. *Healthy People 2010* data (CDC, 2000) indicates that slightly less than half of all people follow the CDC recommendations for physical activity. About 49% of people without a disability met the physical activity criteria compared to 37.7% of people with a disability. Multiple researchers have shown that rates of nonparticipation in physical activity for people with intellectual and developmental disabilities are similar to that of sedentary people without disabilities (Draheim, Williams, & McCubbin, 2002; Temple, Anderson, & Walkley, 2000). Messent, Cooke, and Long (1999) defined some barriers to participation for people with disabilities including limited access to activities and opportunities in the community.

Thus, there are two components of prevention for heart disease: normal weight and physical activity. Baseline data about the prevalence of both obesity and participation in physical activity for people with disabilities exists in the literature. Changes in personal behavior can impact both obesity and lack of physical activity, minimizing heart disease risk related to those factors. Changes in levels of obesity and physical activity in the population can measure the impact of public health interventions, making this a good example to illustrate how public health strategies can be used to improve health for populations of people with disabilities.

Using Public Health Strategies to Impact Obesity and Levels of Physical Activity for People with Disabilities

Public health has three core functions: assessment, policy development, and assurance (Figure 7-3).

Policy development provides a way to take scientific findings from the research studies to the real world to make meaningful improvements to the health of people. Policy development tools include public health law and voluntary practices and partnerships. These focus on development of systems and organizational change as well as changes in individual behavior. Although legislation often brings to mind Congress and the federal government, state and local legislation and regulation has a role in changing behavior and improving the health of the public. Partnerships for voluntary

Figure 7-3
Core Functions of
Public Health

1. Assessment
2. Policy development
3. Assurance

activities may also include state and local governmental entities in addition to academia and community groups. The case studies that follow focus on health promotion activities related to the issues around prevention of cardiovascular disease that were discussed in the last section. This section uses these cases to outline how public health tools can be used to impact people with disabilities.

National Initiatives

In general, all health promotion activities strive to move the science of the issue into practical application in the community or for the population to be able to change behavior. The CDC (2002) has identified prevention of cardiovascular disease as a national priority. Therefore, it is important to look at what is happening at the national level before discussing local initiatives in order to put the local activities in the context of the national ones. In 2002, the CDC developed a national public health action plan to prevent and decrease the rate of heart disease in this country. This plan takes a comprehensive approach to the issue in order to move the nation forward toward meeting the goals around prevention for heart disease and stroke set out in *Healthy People 2010* (CDC, 2000). The public health approach to this issue thus far has included assessment to identify the magnitude of the problem, policy development to address the knowledge gained from assessment, and assurance to continue to measure the impact and any changes in the magnitude of the problem. Citing the statistics that 39% of all deaths in Americans are due to heart disease and that there is growing disparities in people from racial or ethnic minorities and with lower income and education levels, the CDC (2002) has set out five areas to focus their activities. Figure 7-4 shows the five areas of focus outlined by the CDC.

Public Health Strategies

Public Awareness Campaigns

Numerous public health strategies have been used to address the epidemic of heart disease. These include public awareness campaigns, health information and education, materials that guide participation in activities, and

---

- **Taking action,** which turns current knowledge into effective actions from a public health vantage point to address the issues.
- **Strengthening capacity** by building and expanding partnerships and developing and sharing resources to implement and maintain the actions.
- **Evaluating impact** to monitor the prevalence of the disorders and to communicate the interventions that produce the best responses.
- **Advancing policy** to identify the most crucial issues, support the research to identify how to approach the issues, and develop the policies to support the findings of the research.
- **Engaging in regional and global partnerships** to share successes and failures and therefore to more effectively use resources.

Figure 7-4
CDC Five Areas
of Focus

development of partnerships including those between community organizations and government. Public awareness campaigns are a common tool used by public health not only to increase awareness of a particular health issue but also to generate interest in the issues. Radio and television spots about nutrition, articles in local newspapers and newsletters outlining local resources for obesity prevention, as well as the use of other paper media such as handouts, can generate interest in the need to both prevent and treat obesity. Some of the materials used in public awareness campaigns can also provide some health information to increase people's knowledge about the issue. For example, health information about the prevention of heart disease would include information about the relationship between obesity and sedentary lifestyle to the development of heart disease as well as its role in decreasing life expectancy. It also could include information about how to prevent obesity, such as ways to increase physical activity and improve eating habits. More detailed information would be included in a specific program that might be developed to address the needs of a particular population. For example, a program developed to prevent obesity in people with spina bifida would need to take into account the need to modify physical activities for people that either use a wheelchair for mobility or walk with crutches and braces. A partnership between a local department of health and a local chapter of the Spina Bifida Association could be used to create a program to prevent obesity in people with spina bifida. In this way, government and community can partner to address a common health issue.

Legislation and Regulation

In addition to the strategies above, the public health professionals also have legislation and regulation to add to their armamentarium related to health promotion. Although the concept of legislation often brings up the role of the federal Congress, there are multiple other layers of legislation and regulation that can have an impact on communities. State government has the ability to create legislation or regulation that assists in the monitoring of health problems such as obesity or to limit the access of the population to things that cause obesity. In addition, local ordinances can also be used to change behavior. One of the following case studies looks at a situation where a city health department with the ability to write legislation created a law to impact the intake of a particular type of fat in an attempt to decrease the problem of obesity and the risk of heart disease in that city.

Case Studies

Groups working with people with disabilities use the public health strategies to address the increasing problems of obesity and sedentary lifestyle with its increased risk of heart disease for people with disabilities. These strategies have been implemented in parallel with the national goals related to the prevention of heart disease through the prevention of obesity and increased physical activity. The strategies chosen represent different types of public health interventions to achieve the same result. Some of the strategies impact only people with disabilities, while other interventions address the general population and will impact people with and without disabilities. Each of the strategies provides a real life example of how public health interventions can be used to target certain populations of individuals to impact a public health problem such as the epidemic of heart disease

Case Study on Local Legislation   In October 2003, the Food and Drug Administration (FDA) published an edition of its consumer magazine noting that scientific evidence shows that not only saturated fat but also trans or partially hydrogenated fat contribute to heart disease. These compounds created by adding hydrogen to vegetable oil are found in margarines, cakes, cookies, french fries, and other foods made with vegetable oil. Trans fat increases the levels of low density lipoproteins, or LDLs, which increase the risk of developing heart disease. As of January 1, 2006, the FDA requires that the amount of trans fat in a food be included on the label on the nutrition facts panel. The scientific community recommends that people, especially those with heart disease or risk factors for heart disease, limit their intake of fat including trans fat in order to decrease their heart disease risk. Americans typically consume more fat than they need and on average consume 6 grams of trans fat although the American Heart Association (2007) recommends 2 grams per day. Because scientific evidence has shown a relationship between heart disease and trans fat, a diet that is low in fat is recommended to prevent the development of heart disease.

In New York City, the Board of Health can pass laws for the city related to public health issues. In response to the scientific information about trans fat and the epidemic of heart disease, they passed a law to ban trans fat from all restaurants (University of North Carolina, 2007). Trans fat must be removed from all foods by July 2008. The passing of the law comes after a trial period of voluntary removal of trans fat, which had no impact on the amount of the substance in foods. Although the legislation is controversial, it illustrates one strategy used in public health to effect change in behavior. This particular strategy impacts everyone that eats in a restaurant in New York City, helping to cut down on the amount of trans fat ingested by the general population. This in turn will help individuals with both weight and blood cholesterol control by decreasing the fat intake and decreasing their risk for heart disease based on LDL levels. It also affects all groups of people including those with disabilities that eat in restaurants in the city. It is an example of a way to reach people with disabilities through targeting a broader population.

The ultimate impact of this law on either the heart disease risk of the population or on the restaurant industry in New York City remains to be seen, especially as it relates to populations of people with disabilities. As this law impacts people only when they eat in a public restaurant, it may have more or less of an impact depending on the frequency of meals that are consumed out of the home. Although that is not known, specifically for people with disabilities, the more that people are out in the community and not in institutions, the more access they will have to the amenities that are used by the general population. This example shows how legislation or regulation offers public health a strategy to effect change in the population with the potential to reach subpopulations of people with disabilities.

Review Questions

1. How can legislation or regulation be used to support public health goals?
2. What populations of people does the New York regulation impact?
3. What other ways could legislation be used to address issues of obesity?
4. Would these have more or less of an impact on the populations of people with disabilities?

Case Study on State Level Program Development

Development of specific programs that target a population is another public health strategy to address a need. In this vein, the University of Illinois at Chicago (UIC) through the Rehabilitation Research and Training Center on Aging with Developmental Disabilities and the Center for Health Promotion used federal grant money to develop an exercise and nutrition program for adults with developmental disabilities (Heller, Marks, & Ailey, 2001). This program was tested using people from six different residential and vocational agencies and showed success in terms of increases in muscle strength and flexibility as well as improved knowledge and attitudes about exercise.

The UIC curriculum was developed by a number of specialists and includes an exercise program developed by an exercise physiologist, nutrition and cooking classes developed by a registered dietician, and health education classes (Heller et al., 2001). The design of the program involves 12 weeks' time and is recommended for 8 to 10 participants with disabilities. Each of the modules can be modified to meet people's specific interests as it is important that people choose what they do for physical activity in order to stick with it. For example, people are offered a choice of aerobic activities from walking or running to various types of cardio workouts available on videotape. They are then encouraged to choose their favorite activities in which to participate. It also includes concepts such as negotiation and compromise as well as social supports. This program provides materials to help people with developmental disabilities begin and maintain an exercise program with other people with developmental disabilities.

Review Questions

1. How might physical activities need to be modified for people with disabilities?
2. How does a state promote participation in a program like this?

Case Study on Local Implementation of Federal Program

The U.S. Department of Health and Human Services (DHHS) Office of Disabilities used another strategy for program development with its I Can Do It, You Can Do It program (Office of Disabilities, 2004). The Secretary of Health and Human Services, Tommy Thompson, set the goal of encouraging increased physical activity for the nearly 6 million children with disabilities in the country. The strategy pairs children with disabilities with physically fit mentors who may or may not have a disability. The goal of the pairs is to accumulate minutes of physical activity toward the goal of a series of awards starting with a Presidential Active Lifestyle Award (PALA) followed by a Presidential Champions Award with either a bronze, silver, or gold medal depending on the number of points accumulated. The outcomes included having children with disabilities adopt healthy life behaviors, including regular physical activity and health nutrition, and the adults in their lives not only recognizing the importance of this but also actively encouraging it. A long list of partners participates in this program and includes those representing children with a variety of disabilities from cognitive disabilities to physical ones. The program provides a series of materials for use in participation in the program, including daily activity logs.

In an extension of this program, the Adapted Physical Activity Program at Slippery Rock University of Pennsylvania (2007) applied the principle of using a mentor to adults with intellectual disabilities. This pilot, coordinated with the local and state mental retardation program offices, paired senior level undergraduate students studying adapted physical education with an individual with intellectual disabilities living in the area local to the University. The students acted as mentors, and the physical activity portion of the program occurred at local community resources such as the YMCA. Students used their knowledge from their didactic studies to adapt activities for their partners. Included in this was a brief component for education related to nutrition and food choice. Preliminary results of the pilot showed not only active participation throughout the program but also some positive gains in physical fitness for the people with intellectual disabilities.

Review Questions

1. Discuss other ways that the federal government could implement a program like I Can Do It, You Can Do It.
2. What other populations of people could act as mentors for this kind of program?
3. Consider the validity of a program studied in one population and applied to another such as this example where the program was originally designed to be implemented with children with disabilities and was extended to the adult population.

Case Study on Development of a State Level Program for Health Education

Health education such as that provided in the nutrition component of the I Can Do It, You Can Do It program constitutes an important public health tool. That, with the monitoring of a health issue, helps move a population forward to a particular health goal. The Commonwealth of Pennsylvania Office of Developmental Programs (ODP) developed such a program for people with intellectual disabilities receiving services through the state program. ODP and its stakeholders, including consumers of services, their families, advocates, service providers, and others, identified a lack of knowledge about health issues as a weakness in the program. In response to this realization, ODP developed the concept of Health Care Quality Units (HCQU) designed to provide training and technical assistance about health issues for the stakeholders of the system. The first HCQUs developed under this concept began operation in 2000 with the remainder beginning implementation within the next 2 years. There are 8 of these HCQUs across the state, and in fiscal year 2006–2007 (July 1 to June 30), they provided 4,000 health trainings to over 35,000 people. This modality of creating a special unit to provide training is not a unique concept, although most of such entities do not address health needs for people with disabilities. The strength of the HCQU approach is that they provide health information and education not only for consumers but also for their caregivers. From the standpoint of nutrition and eating habits, people that do not cook eat what is cooked for them. If their meals contain a high fat content and lots of calories, then they will more likely have difficulty with weight. The way to change that behavior is to increase the knowledge of the people cooking the meals so that they can provide more healthy foods. In addition to providing health information, HCQUs conduct a health survey to collect health indicators representative of the population of people living in licensed residential settings within the commonwealth. This serves as a way to follow health indicators related to topics of training in order to identify whether or not there has been a significant impact related to the increased exposure to health information. The instrument used is the health risk profile (HRP) (2001), and it gathers information related to weight, height, and physical activity among other health conditions.

Analysis of the HRP data from 2000 to 2001 showed that about 60% of the population of people in the random sample had a body mass index (BMI) in the overweight or obese range (CDC, 2004). This is not different from that found in the general population (CDC, 2007a). Over the time that the HCQUs have been providing training to the stakeholders of the ODP service system, nutrition was the most commonly presented topic. Subtopics within nutrition included healthy food choices, appropriate portions, and reading food labels. Included with this were trainings about physical activity and how to increase participation in physical activity. Individual service providers worked on developing physical activity opportunities or using existing programs, like that from UIC, in which people could participate. This provides specific guidance for implementing a program or information that was developed specifically for people with intellectual disabilities. In this manner, neither family members nor paid staff have to take information developed for the general public and modify it for this population. Because this approach is more individualized either to an individual or a small group of consumers, it may not reach as many people as the approaches used with the general public. However, with a population of people that are less able to access the tools provided to the general public, this may afford them the same impact. In fact, the data from fiscal year 2006 to 2007 shows that significantly more people had a BMI in the normal range than in the sample from 5 years prior in fiscal year 2001 to 2002 (ODP, 2007). In addition, there were significantly less people that participated in no leisure-time physical activity in the later sample. Without any other significant initiatives related to controlling weight and increasing participation in physical activity targeting this group in the state, the training provided by the HCQUs likely contributed to these positive changes in the population.

Review Questions

1. Who is the audience for health education for people with intellectual disabilities?
2. Would health education have more or less of an impact on this population as compared to the general population?
3. What modifications might need to be made to deliver this type of health education to a population of people with intellectual disabilities with limited or no reading abilities?

CONCLUDING REMARKS

Traditional public health methods of gathering health indicators in the general population may not access information about particular sub-populations, especially that of people with disabilities. As well, given the diversity between the groups of people with disabilities makes using a single category of people with disabilities a less useful activity. This is especially true because reaching different populations of people with disabilities depends on how they can both access and understand that information to increase their knowledge and to change their behavior. The population of elderly people with disabilities related to chronic diseases may not have the same needs or respond to the same strategies as the population of people with intellectual disabilities. Thus, not only do surveying techniques need to accommodate different groups of people with disabilities but so do the methods used to convey the information to each population.

As the population of the country grows older and people with and without disabilities are living longer, there will be an additional need to access the health status and issues for these populations. As well, reaching populations with disabilities through government and community partnerships, including the program offices where they receive services, may prove to be an effective strategy for public health officials to pursue. Using existing surveys and modifying them to address public health goals not only can gather information that can be compared to the general population but also can be used to improve the health of these populations.

Examples of public health interventions adopted by program services for people with disabilities include mechanisms to increase awareness for health issues; health education provision that is accessible to the population and their caregivers; adaptation of existing strategies to meet the particular needs such as those related to physical activity for people with disabilities; and judicious use of regulation or legislation. All can have an impact on the lives and health of people with disabilities. As particular groups of people within the general population occupy a larger and larger proportion of the population, public health focus on health promotion for these groups will become important to continue to make progress toward the health promotion goals for the country.

DISCUSSION QUESTIONS

1. What factors must be considered when developing a survey to assess health issues for people with disabilities?
2. How are groups of people with different disabilities the same? How are they different?
3. Where might you find information about health issues for people with disabilities?
4. How do you approach health promotion activities such as physical activity for people with disabilities?
5. Is legislation or regulation an effective way to promote health for people with disabilities? Why or why not?

REFERENCES

Accardo, P. J., Whitman, B. Y., Laszewski, C., Haake, C. A., & Morrow, J. D. (1996). *Dictionary of developmental disabilities terminology*. Baltimore, MD: Paul H. Brookes Publishing Company.

American Heart Association. (2007). Trans fats. Available at http://www.american heart.org/presenter.jhtml?identifier=3045792. Accessed December 3, 2007.

American Psychiatric Association. (1994). *Diagnostic and statistical manual of mental disorders* (4th ed.). Washington, DC: Author.

Americans with Disabilities Act. (1990). *Americans with Disabilities Act of 1990*. Washington, DC: Author. Title 42, Chapter 126, Section 12102, 2(A). Available at http://www.ada.gov/pubs/ada.htm. Accessed December 2, 2007.

Bacon, P. A., Stevens, R. J., Curruthers, D. M., Young, S. P., & Kitas, G. D. (2002). Accelerated atherogenesis in autoimmune rheumatic diseases. *Autoimmune Review, 1*(6), 338–347.

Barbotte, E., Guillemin, F., Chau, N., & Lordihandicap Group. (2001). Prevalence of impairments, disabilities, handicaps, and quality of life in the general population: A review of recent literature. *Bulletin of the World Health Organization. 79*, 1047–1055. Available at http://www.scielosp.org/scielo.php?pid=S0042-96862001001100008&script=sci_arttext.

Batshaw, L., & Perret, Y. M. (1992). *Children with disabilities: A medical primer* (3rd ed.). Baltimore, MD: Paul H. Brookes Publishing Company.

Braunschweig, C. L., Gomez, S., Sheehan, P., Tomey, K. M., Rimmer, J. H., & Heller, T. (2004). Nutritional status and risk factors for chronic disease in urban-dwelling adults with Down syndrome. *American Journal on Mental Retardation, 109,* 186–193.

Brazier, J. E., Harper, R., Jones, N. M., O'Cathain, A., Thomas, K. J., Usherwood, T., & Westlake, L. (1992). Validating the SF-36 health survey questionnaire: new outcome measure for primary care. *British Medical Journal, 305*, 160–164.

Center for Disease Control and Prevention. (2000). *Healthy people 2010.* Washington, DC: DHHS. Available at http://www.healthypeople.gov/. Accessed December 2, 2007.

Center for Disease Control and Prevention. (2002). *A public health action plan to prevent heart disease and stroke.* Washington, DC: DHHS. Available at http://www.cdc.gov/DHDSP/library/fs_state_healthcare.htm. Accessed November 30, 2007.

Center for Disease Control and Prevention. (2004). Behavioral risk factor surveillance system. Washington, DC: US Department of Health and Human Services. Available at http://www.cdc.gov/BRfss/technical_infodata/surveydata/2004.htm. Accessed December 2, 2007.

Center for Disease Control and Prevention. (2007a). Behavioral risk factor surveillance system. Washington, DC: US Department of Health and Human Services. Available at http://www.cdc.gov/brfss/. Accessed December 2, 2007.

Center for Disease Control and Prevention. (2007b). National Center for Health Statistics. Washington, DC: DHHS. Available at http://www.cdc.gov/nchs/surveys.htm. Accessed November 30, 2007.

Center for Disease Control and Prevention. (2008). *Physical activity for everyone: How much physical activity do you need?* Atlanta, Georgia: Division of Nutrition, Physical Activity and Obesity. Available at http://www.cdc.gov/physicalactivity/everyone/guidelines/adults.html. Accessed March 22, 2009.

Centers for Medicare and Medicaid Services. (2006). 1915c waiver application. Washington, DC: DHHS. Available at https://www.hcbswaivers.net/CMS/faces/portal.jsp. Accessed November 30, 2007.

Chaney, R. H., & Eyman, R. K. (2000). Patterns in mortality over 60 years among persons with mental retardation in a residential facility. *Mental Retardation, 38,*289–293.

Del Rincon, I. D., Williams, K., Stern, M. P., Freeman, G. L., & Escalante, A. (2001). High incidence of cardiovascular events in a rheumatoid arthritis cohort not explained by traditional cardiac risk factors. *Arthritis Rheumatology, 44,* 2737–2745.

Draheim, C. C., Williams, D. P., & McCubbin, J. A. (2002). Prevalence of physical inactivity and recommended physical activity in community-based adults with mental retardation. *Mental Retardation, 40,* 436–444.

Eyman, R. K., Call, T. L., & White, J. F. (1991). Life expectancy of persons with Down syndrome. *American Journal on Mental Retardation, 95,* 603–612.

Food and Drug Administration. (2003). Revealing trans fat. Washington, DC: Author. Available at http://www.fda.gov/fdac/features/2003/503_fats.html. Accessed December 3, 2007.

Food and Drug Administration. (2006). Trans fat now listed with saturated fat and cholesterol in the nutrition facts label. Washington, DC: Office of Nutritional Products, Labeling, and Dietary Supplements. Available at http://www.cfsan.fda.gov/~dms/transfat.html. Accessed January 1, 2006.

Garratt, A. M., Ruta, D. A., Abdalla, M. I., Buckingham, J. K., & Russell, I. T. (1993). The SF36 health survey questionnaire: an outcome measure suitable for routine use within the NHS? *British Medical Journal, 306,* 1440–1444.

Hahn, R. A., Teuesch, S. M., Rothenberg, R. B., & Marks, J. S. (1986). Excess deaths from nine chronic diseases in the United States. *Journal of the American Medical Association, 264*(20), 2554–2559.

Hayden, M. R. (1998). Mortality among people with mental retardation living in the United States: Research review and policy application. *Mental Retardation, 36*(5), 345–359.

Heller, T. Marks, B. A., & Ailey, S. H. (2001). *Exercise and nutrition health education curriculum for adults with developmental disabilities.* Chicago, IL: Rehabilitation Research and Training Center on Aging and Developmental Disabilities, University of Illinois at Chicago. Human Services Research Institute. (2006). National core indicators. Available at http://www.hsri.org/nci/. Accessed December 2, 2007.

Hunt, G. M., & Oakeshott, P. (2003). Outcome in people with open spina bifida at age 35: Prospective community based cohort study. *British Medical Journal, 326,* 1365–1366.

Iezzoni, L. (2003). *When walking fails: Mobility problems of adults with chronic conditions.* Berkeley, CA: University of California Press.

Iowa Department of Human Services. (2005). *Home and community based services physical disability waiver information packet.* Des Moines, IA: Author. Available at http://www.dhs.state.ia.us/MHDD/quality_assurance/hcbs_specialists.html. Accessed December 11, 2007.

Janicki, M. P., Dalton, A. J., Henderson, C. M., & Davidson, P. W. (1999). Mortality and morbidity among older adults with intellectual disability: Health services considerations. *Disability and Rehabilitation, 21,* 284–294.

Johnson, H., Wiggs, L., & Huson, S.M. (2005). Psychological disturbance and sleep disorders in children with neurofibromatosis type 1. *Developmental Medicine and Child Neurology,47*(4), 237–242.

Kalnins, I. V., Steele, C., Stevens, E., Rossen, B., Biggar, D., Jutai, J., & Bortolussi, J. (1999). Health survey research on children with physical disabilities in Canada. *Health Promotion International, 14*(3), 251–260. Available at http://www.heapro.oxfordjournals.org/cgi/content/full/14/3/251.

Kaplan, G. A. A., Strawbridge, W. J., Cohen, R. D., & Hungerford, L.R. (1996). Natural history of leisure-time physical activity and its correlates: Associations with mortality from all causes and cardiovascular diseases over 28 years. *American Journal of Epidemiology, 144*(8), 793–797.

Kaplan, M. J. (2006). Cardiovascular disease in rheumatoid arthritis. *Current Opinions in Rheumatology, 18*(3), 289–297. Available at http://www.medscape.com/viewarticle/530073_2. Accessed November 30, 2007.

Kushi, L. H., Fee, R. M., Folsom, A. R., Mink, P. J., Anderson, K. E, & Sellers, T. A. (1997). Physical activity and mortality in postmenopausal women. *Journal of the American Medical Association, 277*(16), 1287–1292.

Landers, S. J. (2007, October 15). Health survey dilemma: Can you hear me now? *AMNews*. Available at http://www.ama-assn.org/amednews/2007/10/15/hll21015.htm. Accessed December 2, 2007.

Lee, C. D., Blair, S. N., & Jackson, A. S. (1999). Cardiorespiratory fitness, body composition, and all-cause and cardiovascular disease mortality in men. *American Journal of Clinical Nutrition, 69* (3), 373–380.

Leung, R. (2005). *A Dark Chapter in Medical History*. Available at http://www.cbsnews.com/stories/2005/02/09/60II/main672701.shtml. Accessed February 9, 2005.

Mabrey, V. (Writer). (2005). A dark chapter in medical history. [Television series episode.] In J. Fager (Producer), *60 minutes.* New York: CBS News. Available at http://www.cbsnews.com/stories/2005/02/09/60II/main672701.shtml. Accessed December 11, 2007.

McCormick, B. (1995). *The medical practitioner's guide to paediatric audiology.* New York: Cambridge University Press.

McGinnis, J. M., & Foege, W.H. (1993). Actual causes of death in the United States. *Journal of the American Medical Association, 270*(18), 207–212.

McGuire LC, Strine TW, Okoro CA, Ahluwalia IB, Ford ES. (2007). Healthy lifestyle behaviors among older U.S. adults with and without disabilities: Behavioral risk factor surveillance system. *Prev Chron Dis., 4*(A09).

McKinley, W., & Garstang, S. V. (2006). Cardiovascular concerns in spinal cord injury. *WebMD.* Available at http://www.emedicine.com/pmr/topic20.htm. Accessed December 2, 2007.

Mensah, G., & Brown, D. (2007). An overview of cardiovascular disease burden in the United States. *Health Affairs, 26*(1), 38–48.

Messent, P. R., Cooke, C. B., & Long, J. (1999). Primary and secondary barriers to physically active healthy lifestyles for adults with learning disabilities. *Disability and Rehabilitation, 21,* 409–419.

Mondofacto. (n.d.) Online medical dictionary. Available at http://cancerweb.ncl.ac.uk/cgi-bin/omd?imbecile. Accessed December 7, 2007.

National Association of State Developmental Disability Directors. (2007). National core indicators (NCI). Available at http://www.nasddds.org/AboutNASDDDS/core_indicators.shtml. Accessed November 30, 2007.

National Institutes of Health. (1993). *Early identification of hearing impairment in infants and young children. NIH consent statement.* Washington, DC: DHHS. Available at http://consensus.nih.gov/1993/1993HearingInfantsChildren092 html.htm. Accessed November 30, 2007.

O'Brien, G. (2001). Defining learning disability: What role does intelligence testing have now? *Developmental Medicine and Child Neurology, 43,* 570–573.

O'Brien, K. F., Tate, K., & Zaharia, E. S. (1991). Mortality in a large southeastern facility for persons with mental retardation. *American Journal on Mental Retardation, 95,* 397–403.

Office of Developmental Programs. (2001). Mortality review data. Pennsylvania: Unpublished.

Office of Developmental Programs. (2007). Health risk profile. Pennsylvania: Unpublished

Office of Disabilities. (2004). *I Can Do It, You Can Do It.* Washington, DC: DHHS. Available at http://www.hhs.gov/od/physicalfitness.html. Accessed November 30, 2007.

Office of Mental Retardation. (1998). *Blueprint for Health Care Coordination Units*. Harrisburg: PA: Unpublished.

Office of Mental Retardation. (2001). *Health risk profile*. Harrisburg, PA: Commonwealth of Pennsylvania Department of Public Welfare.

Office of Mental Retardation. (2002). *Clarifying eligibility for mental retardation services and supports* (No. 4210-02-05). Harrisburg, PA: Commonwealth of Pennsylvania Department of Public Welfare.

Paffenbarger, R. S., Hyde, R. T., Wing, A. L., Lee, I. M., Jung, D. L., & Kampert, J. B. (1993). The association of changes in physical-activity level and other lifestyle characteristics with mortality among men. *New England Journal of Medicine, 328*(8), 538–545.

Patja, K., Molsa, P., & Iivanainen, M. (2001). Cause-specific mortality of people with intellectual disability in a population-based, 35 year follow-up study. *Journal of Intellectual Disability Research, 45,* 30–40.

Pearson, T. (2007). The prevention of cardiovascular disease: Have we really made progress? *Health Affairs, 26*(1), 49–60.

Picavet, H. S. L. (2001). National health surveys by mail or home interview: Effects on response. *Journal of Epidemiologic Community Health, 55*(6), 408–413. Available at http://jech.bmj.com/cgi/search?andorexactfulltext=and&resourcetype=1&disp_type=&sortspec=relevance&author1=&fulltext=dutch+survey&volume=55&firstpage=408. Accessed December 2, 2007.

Pitetti, K. H., Campbell, K. D. (1991). Mentally retarded individuals—A Population at risk? *Medicine and Science in Sports and Exercise, 23*(5), 586–593.

Rhode Island Department of Health. (2000). Behavioral risk factor surveillance system. Providence, RI: Author. Available at http://www.health.ri.gov/cjoc/statistics/data/overweight-disability.php. Accessed December 2, 2007.

Rimmer, J. H., Braddock, D., & Fujiura, G. (1993). Prevalence of obesity in adults with mental retardation: Implications for health promotion and disease prevention. *Mental Retardation, 31,* 105–110.

Roizen, N., & Patterson, D. (2003). Down syndrome. *The Lancet, 361*(9365), 1281–1289.

Rubin, S. S, Rimmer, J. H, Chicoine, B., Braddock, D., & McGuire, D. E. (1998). Overweight prevalence in persons with Down syndrome. *Mental Retardation, 36,* 175–181.

Sherman, S. E., D'Agostino, R. B., & Cobb, J. L., (1994). Physical activity and mortality in women in the Framingham Heart Study. *American Heart Journal, 128*(5), 879–884.

Slippery Rock University. (2007). *Adapted physical activity program*. Slippery Rock, PA: Author. Available at http://www.sru.edu/pages/7713.asp. Accessed December 7, 2007.

Spina Bifida Association. (2007a). Spina bifida clinics. Available at http://www.sbaa.org/site/c.liKWL7PLLrF/b.2642345/k.C49F/Clinics.htm#nh. Accessed November 30, 2007.

Spina Bifida Association. (2007b). Obesity. Available at http://www.sbaa.org/site/c.liKWL7PLLrF/b.2700287/k.C25F/Obesity.htm. Accessed November 30, 2007.

Steele, C. A., Kalnins, J. W., Jutai, J. W., Stevens, S. E., Bortolussi, J. A., & Biggar, W. D. (1996). Lifestyle health behaviours of 11- to 16-year-old youth with physical disabilities. *Health Education Research, 11*(2), 173–186. Available at http://her.oxfordjournals.org/cgi/content/abstract/11/2/173.

Sullivan, P. B., Juszczak, E., Bachlet, A. M., Lambert, B., Vernon-Roberts, A., Grant, H. W., Eltumi, M., McLean, L., Alder, N., & Thomas, A. G. (2005). Gastrostomy tune feeding in children with cerebral palsy: A prospective, longitudinal study. *Developmental Medicine and Child Neurology, 47*(2),77–85.

Temple, V. A., Anderson, C., & Walkley, J. W. (2000). Physical activity levels of individuals living in a group home. *Journal of Intellectual and Developmental Disabilities, 25,* 327–341.

U.S. Census Bureau. (1994). Survey of income and program participation. Available at http://www.census.gov/hhes/www/disability/publications.html. Accessed December 2, 2007.

U.S. Census Bureau. (2000). State and county quick facts. Washington, DC: Author. Available at http://quickfacts.census.gov/qfd/states/00000.html. Accessed December 2, 2007.

U.S. Census Bureau. (2002). *Survey* of income and program participation. Available at http://www.census.gov/hhes/www/disability/sipp/disab02/awd02.html. Accessed December 2, 2007.

University of California at Los Angeles. (2007). FAQ. Available at http://gim.med.ucla.edu/kdqol/page7.html. Accessed December 2, 2007.

University of North Carolina. (2007). *Cutting-edge legal preparedness for chronic disease prevention.* Chapel Hill, NC: Author. Available at http://www.public healthgrandrounds.unc.edu/legal/webcast.htm. Accessed November 27, 2007.

Wagner, M., Newman, L., Cameto, R., & Levine, P. (2006) *The academic achievement and functional performance of youth with disabilities: A report from the National Longitudinal Transition Study-2* (NCSER 2006-3000). Menlo Park, CA: SRI International. Available at http://www.nlts2.org/reports/2006_07/index.html. Accessed December 2, 2007.

Wannamethee, S. G., Shaper, A. G., Whinecup, P. H., & Walker, M. (2004). Overweight and obesity and the burden of disease and disability in elderly men. *International Journal of Obesity, 28,* 1374–1382. Available at http://www.nature.com/ijo/journal/v28/n11/abs/0802775a.html. Accessed December 2, 2007.

Wei, M., Kampert, J. B., Barlow, C. E., Nichamen, M. Z., Gibbons, L. W., & Paffenbarger, R. S. (1999). Relationship between low cardiorespiratory fitness and mortality in normal-weight, overweight, and obese men. *Journal of the American Medical Association, 282*(16), 1547–1553.

World Health Organization. (2007). Disabilities. Geneva, Switzerland: Author. Available at http://www.who.int/topics/disabilities/en/. Accessed November 30, 2007.

Health Promotion Programs in the Workplace

Bernard J. Healey, PhD

OBJECTIVES

After reading this chapter, you should

- Understand the value of workplace wellness programs
- Be able to define and explain the components of a well-developed workplace wellness program
- Become aware of the value of a workplace health needs assessment
- Understand the various steps required in the development of a comprehensive workplace wellness program
- Become aware of the need to evaluate workplace wellness programs

KEY TERMS

Health risk appraisal	Productivity
Incentives	Work site wellness
Needs assessment	

Introduction

The American health care system is very different than the health delivery system found in other industrialized countries in the world. It has developed over time with very little planning, and most major changes in the system seem to have occurred as accidents rather than with conscious thought. The system consumes over 2 trillion dollars each year, representing $7,000 dollars per person, and still allows people to become ill and die prematurely.

A large part of this enormous cost of health services is paid for by employers. According to Emanuel (2008), this employment-based insurance was a result of wage and price controls initiated after World War II. This is when the War Labor Board allowed employers to offer workers a 5% fringe bene-fits package to attract and retain needed workers. This massive allocation of resources to workers in the form of employer-paid health insurance did nothing to keep workers healthy but rather provided a way for employees to pay bills after they became ill.

The vast majority of the diseases that are responsible for the escalating costs of health care are the chronic diseases. These diseases have a very long incubation period (20 to 40 years); are very expensive, especially in terms of complications; and are quite often caused by personal health behaviors. According to Harris et al. (2008), employers can be a very important partner in the prevention of chronic diseases for at least 3 reasons: They have great power over the environment where workers usually spend one third of their day; the employers are being hurt by the escalation in health insurance costs and loss of **productivity** due to illness; and the employers have not done a good job at helping workers prevent illness.

The Escalating Costs of Health Insurance for Employers

The United States spends a large percentage of its gross domestic product (GDP) on a system of health care that is essentially not worth what it costs. That percentage of GDP given to the health care delivery is going to con-tinue to rise as the ranks of the elderly demanding health services increases dramatically over the next several years. The American health care system has definitely entered a state of crisis.

The best health care system in the world costs too much, does not allow the sickest members access, and does not sufficiently value prevention of ill-ness. It must be remembered that when a patient is in crisis, he or she may die or may return to better health than when they first became ill. Once a patient returns from illness, they are usually highly motivated to remain well. They usually start to practice better health behaviors that can keep them healthy. This same transformation needs to occur in the American health care system before people become ill. This will represent a major change in the way we as a nation think about how health care is delivered and received. There can be no more incremental improvement with a system that simply does not work.

According to the Health Affairs website (2006), health care spending will consume 18.7% of GDP by 2014. A study by the Robert Wood Johnson Foundation in 2003 found that there has been a 6% increase in the share of premiums paid by workers. Business owners contacted in the same survey indicated that there will be an increase in health care expenditures by employees every year. A study released by Price Waterhouse Coopers in July 2009 found that 75% of large companies may ask employees to pay more for health insurance and may also lower pay raises for current employees. The study also found that 20% of these employers plan to hire fewer workers this year because of rising health insurance costs.

As health care costs continue to rise above the inflation rate, everyone from state and federal legislators to the owners of businesses are struggling to reduce the costs associated with delivering health care services to their respective constituents.

Epidemic of Chronic Diseases in the Workplace

Chronic diseases—such as heart disease, cancer, and diabetes—are the leading causes of death and disability in the United States. According to Jack et al. (2006), as the ever increasing burden of chronic diseases in the United States continues, greater efforts will be made to identify and implement interventions that successfully reduce disease risk, especially in the workplace. These diseases account for 7 of every 10 deaths and affect the quality of life of 90 million Americans. Although chronic diseases are among the most common and costly health problems, they are also among the most preventable.

McGinnis and Foege (1993) point out that daily habits such as smoking, inactivity, diet and alcohol use, and their consequences contribute to the development of virtually all of morbidity and mortality in industrial nations. Adopting healthy behaviors such as eating nutritious foods, being physically active, and avoiding tobacco use can prevent or control the devastating effects of these diseases.

According to the CDC (2005b), years of potential life lost (YPLL) is the number of years lost when death occurs before the age of 65 years. When public health departments add up the cost of YPLL from poor health, they discover that the leading causes of mortality in this country are due to chronic diseases and injuries. They also immediately discover that these two areas are responsible for disability and days lost from work along with tremendous costs for incurable health problems. The employer also loses productivity from the ill employees taking sick time for their disability.

According to CDC (2005a) in 2005, 62% of adults 18 years of age or over reported excellent or very good health, 62% of adults never participated in any type of vigorous leisure-time physical activity, and 15% of adults did not have a usual place of health care. Twelve percent of adults had been told by a doctor or health professional that they had heart disease, and 22% had been told on 2 or more physician visits that they had hypertension.

Brownson, Remington, and Davis (1998) discovered that chronic diseases often affect the quality of life long before it affects the duration of life. Study after study, conducted by epidemiologists, implicate tobacco use, obesity, physical inactivity, and diet as the major causes of many of the most deadly and expensive chronic diseases. These diseases are developing during the working years and produce enormous economic costs for the worker and the employer later in life.

Recent surveillance data from the National Institute of Health (2006) indicates that 21% of all adults are current smokers and 21% are former smokers. Based on estimates of body mass index, 35% of adults are overweight and 24% are obese. These statistics do not make one optimistic about the success of helping people to understand the long-term ramifications of chronic diseases. It does indicate that our country needs to evaluate how we deliver health services and to try to understand why the current model of delivery has failed. There are many in public health that believe the entire health care system should be restructured to focus on prevention and not on cure.

The United States is experiencing one of the largest epidemics of disease in the workplace in the world, and it is growing in numbers of victims. It has the greatest costs in terms of disability, death, and cost of any other disease found in the workplace. The ironic part of this disease is that it is almost totally preventable, and it is being ignored by employers and employees. It is the rapid escalation of chronic diseases that are occurring as we grow older at work.

Because the young feel well, they tend to believe that their health will remain good even if they practice one or more high-risk health behaviors. Health is interpreted by them to mean that they are not now ill. They are unaware of the fact that the chronic diseases usually have long incubation periods (20 to 40 years), and once they develop, they are usually incurable. They also have no concerns about being injured because they believe that accidents and violence are someone else's problem. They enter the workforce and start or continue unhealthy behaviors, which increase because of peer pressure and eventually may result in the development of one or more chronic diseases or injuries. This scenario could have possibly been avoided for the young if they had received the required health information when they were younger, and it was reinforced as they went to work.

Tobacco Use, Secondhand Smoke, and the Workplace

The CDC (2005) argues that the use of tobacco is the leading cause of the development of many chronic diseases in this country. Smoking harms nearly every organ of the body, causing many diseases, and reduces life expectancy and quality of life for many Americans. The fact that the use of tobacco products is the most dangerous high-risk health behavior and it is practiced by over 20% of individuals in this country has been known for decades. Tobacco use is so very dangerous that one of the national health objectives for 2010 is to establish laws in all states to prohibit or restrict smoking in all public places and work sites.

Secondhand smoke has decreased in recent years due to fewer smokers, but research is uncovering more and more dangers from this so called "passive smoke." The U.S. Surgeon General of the United States, Richard H. Carmona, recently concluded that there is no risk-free level of exposure to secondhand smoke. He went on to argue that secondhand smoke at home or work increases the risk of developing heart disease by 25% to 30% and lung cancer by 20% to 30%. According to Surgeon General Carmona, "The scientific evidence is now indisputable: secondhand smoke is not a mere annoyance. It is a serious health hazard that can lead to disease and premature death in children and nonsmoking adults. Secondhand smoke contains more than 50 cancer-causing chemicals, and is itself a known human carcinogen" (U.S. Department of Health and Human Services, 2006, p. 23).

A report titled "Health Consequences of Involuntary Exposure to Tobacco Smoke: A Report of the Surgeon General" (2006) pointed out that nonsmokers who are exposed to secondhand smoke inhale many of the same toxins as smokers. According to the former Surgeon General, Richard H. Carmona, "as understanding increases regarding health consequences from even brief exposures to secondhand smoke, it becomes even clearer that the health of nonsmokers overall, and particularly the health of children, individuals with existing heart and lung problems, and other vulnerable populations, requires a higher priority and great protection" (USDHHS, 2006, p. 24). The country needs to pass laws or regulations that guarantee no exposure to secondhand smoke by everyone.

The workplace has been identified as a major source of secondhand smoke exposure for adults in this country. An epidemiological relationship has been established between secondhand smoke in the workplace and increased risk for heart disease and lung cancer among adult nonsmokers. Even with this overwhelming evidence, about 30% of workplaces are not covered by smoke-free policies. Those not covered by smoke-free policies are usually blue collar workers and restaurant employees.

Overweight, Obesity, and the Workplace

According to Lorentz (2005), the growing obesity problem in the United States can cut the average life expectancy of Americans by as much as 5 years unless an aggressive campaign is begun to reduce weight and to increase physical activity in this country. Studies show that the majority of Americans are overweight (61% overweight, 20.9% obese) and that overweight individuals use health care services at higher rates than those of normal weight (10% to 36% higher). Given this trend and the large investment in health insurance that employers make (second only to wages), it appears employer-sponsored weight management programs could yield significant cost savings for the workplace.

According to the CDC (2005c), over the last 20 years the percentage of overweight and obese individuals has increased dramatically. Overall, in the United States, 65% of adults are overweight and 30% meet the criteria for obesity. These two components are the triggers for hypertension, diabetes renal failure, and several forms of arthritis and cancers. The CDC reports that a very good estimate of the overweight problem in this country through random surveys is the best we have available.

Grossman (2004) argues that employees do not leave their increasing weight at home in the morning when they come to work. This extra weight is having serious ramifications relating to health care costs, productivity, morale, and potential employee discrimination.

Physical Inactivity

Tobacco use is a greater threat to our health than physical inactivity, but the prevalence of sedentary lifestyles makes physical inactivity a force to be dealt with by employers. The many benefits associated with daily physical activity cannot be overemphasized. This relationship between physical activity and disease prevention becomes extremely evident when evaluating the cause and prevention of chronic diseases such as heart disease, cancer, stroke, diabetes, hypertension, and even depression.

The CDC (2005) reports that two objectives of Healthy People 2010 are to increase the proportion of adults who engage in regular moderate or vigorous activity to at least 50% and to decrease the proportion of adults who engage in no leisure-time physical activity to no more than 20%. These goals can be achieved during leisure time at home or in the workplace. It does not matter where the physical activity occurs; it only matters that it should occur almost every day.

The CDC (2005) also reports that the nationwide prevalence of leisure-time physical inactivity for adults in this country has declined 0.6% per year over the last 11 years. In 2004, approximately 21% of men and 26% of women reported no leisure-time physical activity, which is the lowest reported prevalence in the past decade. Progress in this area needs to be made if the country is going to be successful in improving the health of Americans.

The barriers to physical activity have been found to be time, motivation, social support, and knowledge. All of these barriers can potentially be reduced or eliminated in the workplace. The employer needs to consider a physical activity program in the workplace for all employees because of the tremendous cost benefit results for this small investment. A recent cost benefit analysis concluded that over 4 billion dollars per year could be saved if all sedentary adults participated in a walking program at home or at the workplace.

The barriers to successful physical activity on a daily basis can be removed by the employer who encourages physical activity at work. Another major advantage of workplace physical activity programs can be found in the availability of a potential surveillance system to report progress and to further evaluate the cost benefit effects offered by this type of employee wellness program.

Nutrition in the Workplace

Dietary factors are associated with 4 of the 10 leading causes of death; coronary heart disease, some types of cancer, stroke, and type 2 diabetes. Health conditions related to dietary factors cost society an estimated $200 billion each year in medical expenses and lost productivity. According to the United Nations International Labor Office (2006), the annual economic costs of obesity (insurance, paid sick leave, and other payments) in the United States is 12.7 billion dollars, and the report also states that poor diet on the job is costing countries around the world up to 20% in lost productivity.

According to the Prevention Institute (2002), eating is a behavior that is greatly influenced by the workplace. Work is where many people spend the majority of their weekday waking hours. At least one meal is consumed at work, and snacks are often a means to relieve pressure and take breaks throughout the workday. Food available in employee cafeterias, vending machines, and at work-sponsored events frequently determines what people eat throughout the day. Many times, food provided by the workplace is not highly nutritious or is high in fat or sugar; for example, snacks or meeting foods often include cookies, pastries, and candy, all potential sources of extra fat and calories. The realities of the work environment can overpower the good intentions of workers to eat healthier. Employers should implement workplace policies that require nutritious food options in employee cafeterias and at work-sponsored events.

Rationale for the Expansion of Workplace Wellness Programs

American employers provide employment and income to workers and their families. Many employers also provide complete or partial health insurance coverage to their employees in an attempt to attract and retain the best workforce to earn high profits for their business. Unfortunately, the rising costs of health insurance premiums are forcing many employees to pay a share of the insurance premium or, in many cases, to eliminate insurance as an employer-paid benefit.

In response to the rising costs of health insurance, many employers are now beginning to offer their employees **work site wellness** programs. The work site offers an excellent opportunity for the development of a new health promotion program. There is no question that healthy employees are more productive employees earning even greater profits for the business owners. The major stakeholders, employers, and employees should have an interest in keeping employees healthy and productive while reducing the cost of health insurance for participants. According to Anspaugh, Dignan, and Anspaugh (2000), the workplace has been successful in reducing health care costs through injury prevention programs and work site wellness initiatives.

Value of Workplace Wellness Programs
- Lower health insurance premiums
- Increase worker productivity
- Increase worker morale and loyalty

Work Site Wellness Programs

The Institute of Medicine (IOM, 2003) argues that a strong relationship exists between modifiable risk factors of employees and the health care costs for the employer. These modifiable risk factors are also related to worker absenteeism and, therefore, to worker productivity. These effects can be measured before and after implementation of a work site health promotion program in order to prove the value of such a program. Examples of work site wellness programs that can be offered to employees include health screenings, including blood pressure and cholesterol measurements; health risk appraisals; cancer screenings; vision examinations; smoking cessation programs; injury prevention education efforts; and a variety of additional health education programs. It is the intent of this chapter to guide the reader through the necessary steps to develop, implement, and evaluate a comprehensive health promotion intervention effort for the workplace.

The Need for Planning for Workplace Wellness

The starting point for the establishment of a work site health promotion program is to appoint a planning committee consisting of management, workers, union representatives, and someone from the human resource management department. The establishment of a planning committee needs to be immediately followed by a meeting with all employees to explain the rationale for the development of a workplace wellness program at their place of employment. This is important because the support of the workers early on in the success of a workplace wellness program is critical to the success of this initiative.

This planning committee then needs to follow the sequential steps outlined in this text. The steps would include (1) development of a program rationale, (2) development of a complete health promotion program plan, (3) completion of a **needs assessment**, (4) development of a health promotion program to meet the identified needs, (5) implementation of the program, and (6) evaluation of the success or failure of the health promotion program. The majority of these functions are found in Figure 8-1, which offers a very logical way to develop a health promotion program for the workplace.

Benefits of Workplace Wellness Initiatives

It is not very difficult to make the case that healthy employees are less likely to use expensive health services and that they are also more productive employees. The employer not only wants but also needs healthy employees in order to remain competitive. According to Schulte et al. (2007) most of the research evidence supports the effectiveness of work site wellness programs in keeping employees healthy.

The majority of young workers have probably not seen a physician in a very long time, because they are generally in good health. Therefore, this group of individuals are prime candidates for preventive services and health education efforts. They are unaware of the fact that even though they feel well they may be incubating a chronic disease.

Educating the worker about his or her health is a mammoth task because the current system of health care has no incentives for the individual to be knowledgeable about their health. Fortunately, employers have many incentives to keep workers healthy, including increasing profits that result from lower health insurance premiums and greater employee productivity. Good

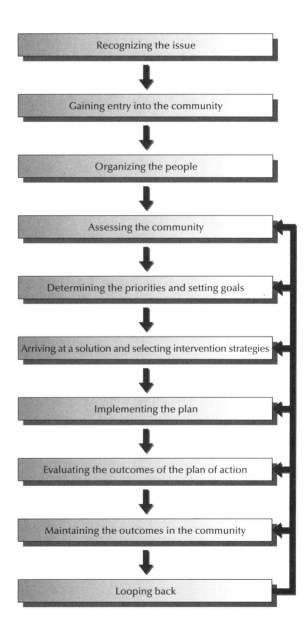

Figure 8-1
A Summary of Steps in Community Organizing and Building

Source: McKenzie, J. F., Pinger, R. R., & Kotecki, J. E. (2005). *An introduction to community health* (5th ed.). Sudbury, MA: Jones and Bartlett Publishers.

health is generally taken for granted in that we are usually healthy when we are born and remain that way as we grow older. Our thought process regarding illness develops around the occurrence of communicable diseases in which we see a doctor, take some medication, and rest until we get better. An example of this would be when we develop the common cold. We have also been conditioned to have health insurance to pay for the health problem. It is interesting to note that even if one has complete health insurance coverage, it does not guarantee good health. The health insurance alone does not guarantee that an individual has the knowledge to make the right choices about his or her personal health at the right time.

The workplace offers a place where everyone should have **incentives** to remain healthy. The employer desires a well-trained, healthy workforce that is capable of producing profits. The employee desires a fair wage and a benefit package that includes health insurance paid predominantly by the employer. Most employees desire to remain healthy as they grow older, allowing them to enjoy life to its fullest. These dual incentives offer a very unique opportunity for employer and employee to join forces in the focus on good health for everyone in the place of employment.

> "Over the next three to five years a majority of employees (88%) plan to make 'significant' investments in longer term solutions aimed at improving the health and productivity of their workers" (Hewitt Associates, 2008, p. 1).

There is also a need for strong leadership and dedicated followership in the workplace in order to achieve and maintain wellness. Top management needs to become convinced that workplace wellness programs are worth the investment of time and money necessary for the company to seize this opportunity to keep workers well. Workplace leaders of the future will be involved in building thick cultures that are capable of making a healthy workplace the norm.

There are many reasons for employers to offer wellness programs to their employees. These programs have been shown to improve morale, improve productivity, and decrease the use of health insurance. The number of organizations offering health promotion programs has grown exponentially since 1980 with over 80% of work sites offering some type of health promotion program. The problem has been the inability to prove the value of these programs. Evaluation of the success or failure of workplace wellness programs is extremely difficult for many reasons. Many work sites may offer wellness programs, but their sophistication is so low that it is difficult, if not impossible, to measure achievement. This is the reason why the evaluation process must be considered very early in the workplace wellness planning process. It needs to be determined early on what is going to be evaluated and how the evaluation is going to be accomplished.

If work sites want to offer quality programs, they usually do not have the resources to support theoretical research to document the program's outcomes. These facts make it very difficult to evaluate the success or failure of workplace wellness programs. Their mere existence is a testament to a belief that if given time and resources, employers could become a catalyst in helping to keep their employees healthy.

The Need for Primary Health Care in the Workplace

According to Cohen, Chavez, and Chehimi (2007), primary prevention requires action before a problem occurs in order to entirely avoid the problem. There is no reason for American businesspeople to look at prevention as an afterthought. It just makes sense that to reduce the incidence of health problems, especially costly chronic diseases, the company has to rely heavily on proactive steps with employees that involve some form of primary prevention.

American businesses are starting to see the workplace wellness as one health care reform that works. According to a survey conducted by Hewitt Associates (2008), businesses in America are seeing health and productivity as a business issue.

Despite the enormous volume of success stories that result from primary prevention efforts, there has always been reluctance by the majority to embrace primary prevention as the model of health care delivery for this country. It may be a result of greed by medical professionals, apathy by elected officials, or ignorance by consumers, but the nation usually deals with health problems "upstream," after they have happened and the damage is done. It is now time for all the players in health care delivery, including employers and employees, to embrace primary prevention as the health delivery model, especially in the workplace. The economic incentives are present to make this revolution happen now.

Prevention is probably our only hope for reducing unnecessary and wasteful demand on our health care system. It stands to reason that as a nation we will not be demanding expensive medical care interventions if we do not practice the behaviors that have been proven to cause the health problems that require these medical interventions. Former Surgeon General Richard Carmona believes that because of our current poor dietary habits and physical inactivity, this may be the first generation in decades to witness decreased life expectancy and poorer quality of life in later years of life. There is strong evidence that his prediction is already becoming a fact.

Development of a Comprehensive Workplace Wellness Initiative

The most important part of the development of a new health promotion program is the development of a comprehensive plan to obtain the goals and objectives of the new program. The starting point in this process involves obtaining the cooperation and input of the major stakeholders in the development of a mission statement for the health promotion initiative.

Needs Assessment   The IOM recommends the completion of a needs assessment of all of the participants that we plan to target in the new health promotion program.

> The needs assessment allows the health promotion program manager to better understand the health problems in the workplace and the behaviors that are practiced by the workers that place them at risk for the health problems.

It is very important to have a very good understanding of the determinants of good and bad health in the specific group for which a new intervention is being developed. The more information obtained about the target audience the easier it becomes to separate the real problems from the symptoms of the problem. For example, heart disease is reported as one of the leading killers of Americans. The real truth is that the leading killer of Americans is tobacco use, which causes 430,000 deaths every year. A well-developed needs assessment would allow the new program to concentrate on tobacco use, including passive smoke, and other high-risk health behaviors rather than on heart disease. Once the real problem is defined, the health promotion program can better measure progress toward solving the health problem. For example, how many employees stopped using tobacco because of the health promotion program?

Needs assessment is a process that never ends, because as new information is found, it should be included in the further development of the health promotion program. The CDC (2009) points out that a targeted needs assessment can help the program manager and the planning committee in the completion of the necessary activities during the development phase of a work site health promotion program.

These activities include the following:

1. The establishment of goals, objectives, and activities for the health promotion initiative
2. The definition of the purpose and scope of the program
3. The identification of social–behavioral attitudes, behaviors, and perceptions of the targeted audience
4. The provision of the basis for evaluation as part of formative and summative studies of interventions

---

Requirements of a Needs Assessment

- Identification of data sources
- Review of secondary data
- Survey of other agency data
- Interviews of key respondents

---

5. The establishment of workplace support for the proposed activities

These activities need to become a critical part of the mission statement, program development, and completion of the evaluation piece that needs to be put in place before the program is launched. A solid evaluation procedure developed in the program planning phase can go a long way in proving the worth of the intervention to management at a later date.

How to Conduct a Workplace Needs Assessment

The importance of the needs assessment is found in the fact that this assessment is a critical part of all of the other components of a health promotion program. This is especially true in the evaluation of the success or failure of the health promotion effort after the interventions have been accomplished. The CDC (2009) argues that if a program is to be evaluated, the ability of a particular promotion effort to address the important needs of the target audience must be the primary focus of the evaluation. For these reasons, significant time and effort must be part of the process of assessing the needs of the employees for which the new health promotion program is being developed.

Needs assessment requires an in-depth analysis of the real problem that we are trying to solve with the development and implementation of the new health promotion effort for the workplace. Once the needs assessment is started, it becomes easier for the business to obtain the necessary resources for the workplace intervention.

Questions to be Answered by the Needs Assessment

1. What are the major health problems that are found in this workplace?
2. Who in the workplace are at risk for the major health problems uncovered by the needs assessment?
3. What are the health behaviors that place our employees at most risk for these health problems?
4. What resources or changes in the workplace do employees believe are necessary to deal with the most important health problems found at our workplace?

By answering these questions, the company can then focus on the development of a work site wellness program to deal with the problems. Opinions of those being affected by a new work site wellness initiative should be included in the final report produced from the needs assessment. This requires going beyond data from questionnaires and inclusion of qualitative data gathered from workplace leaders in the research effort. Because every workplace is different, there needs to be a way to gather data concerning workplace priorities, beliefs, and culture in order to improve the chances of success of the health promotion effort.

This rich data gathered through a needs assessment utilizing a mixed approach of needs assessment that includes quantitative data supported by qualitative data can be extremely helpful in determining which strategies have a better chance of success in the improvement of the health of a particular workplace. The needs assessment must be able to validate the workplace needs and to begin the process of assigning value to the various promotion efforts that need to be developed and implemented in the workplace. Gathering research data about a health problem resembles the epidemiological process of gathering data to form a hypothesis about disease causation. It is a long process, but if done properly, it is well worth the time and effort because of the value of the finished product.

The use of a focus group format works very well when gathering qualitative data about the health of the workplace. The focus group is a technique that utilizes small groups of individuals that represent the target audience to collect information and opinions about specific subjects in a selected area. These groups can be very helpful in developing a hypothesis as to why high-risk health behaviors occur.

There are several good planning programs available to help with the development and implementation of a needs assessment. A good example of this type of program has been made available by the National Association of County and City Health Officials (NACCHO). They developed a program called Mobilizing for Action through Planning and Partnerships (MAPP). The MAPP process offers a very good example of how the needs assessment fits into the overall planning process for the improvement of community health. This process, which will be discussed at length later in this text, offers an excellent procedure for gathering data for workplace needs assessment.

Program Development or Intervention Phase

Once the needs assessment of the workplace is completed, the process of developing a comprehensive health promotion program for the workplace can begin. The majority of the health problems in the workplace should have now been identified along with many of the high-risk health behaviors responsible for the health problems and their complications. It is now time to move into the intervention phase of the workplace health promotion program. In this phase, there will be the expansion of a well-developed program to reduce the high-risk health behaviors that are responsible for the health problems in the workplace that were discovered in the needs assessment.

The workplace health promotion planning team needs to convene a meeting to review the results of the needs assessment and to design the intervention program. The starting point in this process will be the development of a mission statement including goals and objectives for the new program. The workplace health promotion program needs a mission statement to give it direction and focus as it moves from a plan to an actual intervention to reduce high-risk health behaviors in the workplace.

Mission Statement

The mission statement for the workplace health promotion program is a brief description of the program that is used to guide the development of program goals.

The mission, goals, and objectives represent the anchor for the planning process and give the team the ability to evaluate the intervention as it moves from a plan to a finished program. The goals and objectives of the program come forth from the mission statement and are future oriented. The mission statement should be a very clear representation of the workplace wellness planning team's reason for existence. The statement should include measurable components of what accomplishments the group is striving to achieve. The mission statement for the wellness program needs to closely align itself with the overall mission of the business that is developing the health promotion effort.

The goals of the health promotion program should be the desired long-term accomplishments expected from the program. The goals need to be realistic and acceptable to the major stakeholders of the program. The program goals must also be time bounded and measurable in order to be able to prove that they have been achieved by a particular work site intervention.

The objectives that come forth from the mission statement are expected short-term accomplishments that relate to one or more of the work site wellness program goals. Once the program objectives have been established, it is time to consider specific interventions to aid in achieving goals and objectives for the workplace health promotion program. It is at this point that specific responsibilities can be assigned to the health promotion manager and his or her staff.

Table 8-1 displays several possible intervention strategies that can be included in the development of a workplace health promotion program. McKenzie, Pinger, and Kotecki (2005) argue that a solution to intervening in the practice of high-risk health behaviors involves the selection of one or more of the strategies shown in Table 8-1. The choice of strategy is dependent on many variables including cost of the program, probable effects of the choice of program, and acceptance of the program by the stakeholders and the employees participating in the program.

There are several different types of interventions that may prove successful in a workplace wellness health promotion program. The focal point of each different type of intervention is the provision of understandable health-related

Table 8-1
Intervention Strategies
and Example Activities

1. Health communication strategies: Mass media, billboards, booklets, bulletin boards, flyers, direct mail, newsletters, pamphlets, posters, and video and audio materials
2. Health education strategies: Educational methods (such as lecture, discussion, and group work) as well as audiovisual materials, computerized instruction, laboratory exercises, and written materials (books and periodicals)
3. Health policy/enforcement strategies: Executive orders, laws, ordinances, policies, position statements, regulations, and formal and informal rules
4. Health engineering strategies: Those that are designed to change the structure of services or systems of care to improve health promotion services, such as safety belts and air bags in cars, speed bumps in parking lots, or environmental cues such as No Smoking signs
5. Health-related community services: The use of health risk appraisals (HRAs), community screening for health problems, and immunization clinics
6. Other strategies
    a. Behavior modification activities: Modifying behavior to stop smoking, start to exercise, manage stress, and regulate diet
    b. Community advocacy activities: Mass mobilization, social action, community planning, community service development, community education, and community advocacy (such as a letter-writing campaign)
    c. Organizational culture activities: Activities that work to change norms and traditions
    d. Incentives and disincentives: Items that can either encourage or discourage people to behave a certain way, which may include money and other material items or fines
    e. Social intervention activities: Support groups, social activities, and social networks
    f. Technology-delivered activities: Educating or informing people by using technology (e.g., computers and telephones)

Source: McKenzie, J. F., Pinger, R. R., & Kotecki, J. E. (2005). *An introduction to community health* (5th ed.). Sudbury, MA: Jones and Bartlett Publishers.

information to all employees. This information is aimed at helping each employee to understand how to avoid bad health behaviors and to offer reasons to begin practicing good health behaviors both in the workplace and in their community.

The most effective health intervention strategies include health communication strategies, health education strategies, health policy strategies, health engineering strategies, and health-related community services. Several examples of these strategies are shown in Table 8-1. It must be pointed out that there is no best strategy for a new workplace wellness program. Most businesses offer a combination of approaches until they discover what method works best for their employees. The cost to implement each strategy must also be considered as a determining factor in the choice of strategy. The program developers must be very concerned with effectiveness and efficiency of the new program.

Program Implementation

Program implementation involves putting the entire planning process into action with the launch of a developed work site health promotion program. It is probably best to begin the implementation process with activities that have a good chance of success and then move to less popular more difficult components of the program at a later point in time.

Implementation of a new health promotion program in the workplace includes training staff, marketing the new program to participants, and motivating employees to participate in the program. It is quite possible that all of these activities can happen at the same time in the implementation of a new workplace wellness program.

Marketing the health promotion program to all employees is probably the most important component of the implementation process. The marketing process can serve as an effort to make everyone aware of the fact that the program has begun and to help motivate employees to take advantage of the wellness initiative. The implementation phase of the program also offers opportunities to experiment with incentives to increase program enrollment, continued participation in the program, and completion of each cycle of the program. The CDC (2009) argues that well-conceived incentives can increase participation rates from 12% to 35%. One very important incentive to program participation is to remove barriers to program attendance. This can be accomplished by scheduling wellness activities at a convenient time during the employees work day.

Computer technology can be used very effectively and efficiently through Internet websites and tailored e-mails directed to all employees of the company. There are also community service strategies that include health risk appraisals, health screening programs, and provision of annual physicals for employees. Attention also needs to be paid to the workplace culture that has developed around the practice of poor health behaviors. There needs to be a change in culture development that expresses what is and is not considered important for this organization in terms of health behaviors while at work and at home.

The Need for Program Evaluation

You have to look at health indices of large populations over time. According to Cohen et al. (2007), even though it is extremely difficult to evaluate the results of primary prevention programs, it can be done. In order to make the evaluation process possible and more revealing, the program stakeholders need to be included in the evaluation process. According to the CDC (2009), the needs assessment is an extremely important component of the evaluation process.

The evaluation process needs to be considered during program development. This evaluation needs to consider both how well the program is working (process) and whether or not it is successful in achieving the predetermined results.

Evaluation is one of the most important components of a health promotion program, but it is also the most difficult component to complete. There has to be an established methodology to prove that the goals and objectives of the program established before the program began were achieved. If the program has failed in meeting the specified goals and objectives, there needs to be a way to uncover the reason(s) why the program failed and to immediately correct the deficiencies.

One of the major problems with health promotion programs has been the inability to prove that a particular promotion effort made a difference. Edberg (2007) argues that continued funding for health promotion is dependent on evidence and accountability. In other words, health promotion programs are dependent on being able to prove that the program in question had an impact on what it was trying to achieve. This ability to prove success or failure in a health promotion effort may be the difference between program continuation or cancellation. There needs to be more attention paid not only to program outcomes but also to the process of program implementation of the health promotion program. In other words, all of the components of the program need to be evaluated in order to determine any deviation from the program plan.

One of the better models utilized to evaluate public health programs by the CDC is the logic model. This evaluation model can be easily adapted to a workplace health promotion program. The CDC (1999) describes this model as a way to look at the various events of a program in terms of a flow-chart that lead to program results. In terms of a health promotion program, the inputs could be trained health education staff, the activities could include an educational program to prevent high-risk health behaviors in the workplace, and the output could be a reduction in the practice of the high-risk health behaviors by employees. The CDC (1999) argues that the use of a logic model will allow those responsible for the program to clarify the program's strategies and to better focus the program in terms of effectiveness (achieving program goals) and efficiency (keeping costs to a minimum).

Figure 8-2 shows the operational aspects of the basic logic model used frequently in evaluating health promotion programs. This evaluation model includes inputs, outputs, short-term impact of the program, and long-term outcomes of the program, and relates all of the steps back to the goals of the program. This model allows program evaluators to look at each of the steps of the health promotion program separately to be able to discover if deviation from program goals occurred and, if so, to fix the problem so that the program becomes successful.

The most important component of the evaluation process is the ability to gather credible evidence that the program works. The CDC (1999) recommends that data credibility can be improved by utilizing multiple procedures for gathering data and by involving stakeholders in the design and interpretation of the data gathering process. The beneficiaries are the employees that are intended to receive the benefits of the health promotion program.

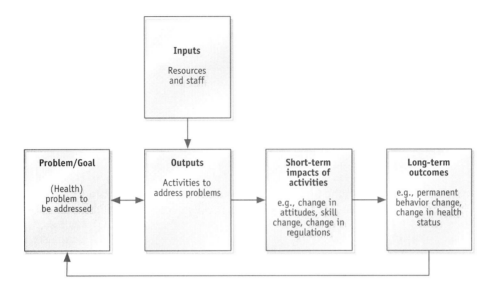

Figure 8-2
Example of a Basic Logic Model
Source: Edberg, M. (2007). *Essentials of health behavior: Social and behavioral theory in public health.* Sudbury, MA: Jones and Bartlett Publishers.

Health promotion managers should also be very interested in providing a credible evaluation process for the program in order to generate new knowledge. It is a very exciting process to develop a new health promotion effort, to be able to prove its value, and then to share the results with others. The program can then be recognized as a best practice and shared with other employers to increase the number of successful program outcomes throughout the country.

According to the CDC (2007), an outcome objective is "a statement of the amount of change expected for a given health problem–condition for a specified population within a given time frame." Outcome objectives need to be realistic, measurable, and long term. They can be illustrated in terms of morbidity, mortality, or disability, or several behavioral measures may be utilized.

> **An example of an outcome could be**
> "By July 1, 2010, the incidence of tobacco use among employees of Company X will be reduced from 42% to 35% of the workforce."

This is a realistic, measurable, long-term objective for a health education program for a workplace health initiative. This type of clarity in objectives is very important in dealing with health promotion programs developed to reduce the high-risk health behaviors practiced in the workplace.

The outcome measures that are specified in the plans for health promotion programs cannot be vague or the program is destined to fail and eventually lose funding. This evaluation piece needs to be completed very early in the design of the health promotion program and needs to include the valuable input that can be provided by stakeholder expertise. It is much easier to establish your program outcomes to be measured at the time that you and the program stakeholders are putting forth the goals and objectives of the new health promotion initiative.

The outcome measures require clarity in order to be able to develop a technique to measure whether or not they were achieved as a result of the health promotion program. The longer-term outcome that is most important to the funders of many health promotion programs is the reduction in chronic diseases acquired by practicing high-risk health behaviors.

Health Risk Appraisals

An excellent starting point in the development of a work site wellness program is found in the use of a **health risk appraisal** (HRA). According to the CDC (2009), a 1999 National Survey of Worksite Health Promotion activities indicated that among all companies, 35% offered HRAs. The use of an HRA has become more popular as a tool used in health promotion programs in recent years because of their ability to help participants understand their own high-risk health behaviors.

The completion of an HRA by employees can be a great tool to increase employee awareness of high-risk health behaviors that may predispose them to chronic diseases later in life. It can be administered to employees by personal interview, mail, or through the company website. The information must be kept confidential, and incentives should be in place to encourage employee's participation.

> The Task Force on Community Preventive Services (2005) describes HRA as a method to collect information from individuals in order to identify high-risk health behaviors for intervention.

The results of the HRAs should be presented to all employees in the aggregate by a medical consultant. Individual counseling with employees using health professionals needs to be available. A website should be built that includes information regarding the diseases and high-risk health behaviors uncovered by the HRA. This information should be made available to all employees and their family members.

Examples of Successful Work Site Programs

The current health care system in the United States is expensive because it spends too much money on treating illness rather than on preventive care. There is no better example of this problem than the way health insurance is handled by employers in this country.

The CDC (2007) reports some interesting statistics on workplace wellness programs that include the following:

- Coca-Cola reports savings of $500 every year per employee after implementing a fitness program, with only 60% of their employees participating.
- Pacific Bell reported that overall absenteeism decreased after implementing a wellness program.
- Coors Brewing Company reported that for each dollar spent on their Corporate Wellness Program, they saw a $5.50 return, and the employees who participated reduced their absentee rate by 18%
- Prudential Insurance Company reported that the benefits costs for employees participating in their program were $312, as opposed to $574 for nonparticipants.

Many employers are looking at their current health care benefit plans offered to employees as a way to integrate health insurance coverage and wellness programs in order to maximize their investment in their most important resource, their employees. This new attitude coupled with the fact that some health insurers are now starting to offer premium discounts to those who pay for insurance coverage when they participate in programs designed to reduce high-risk health behaviors will start a sustained attempt by purchasers and buyers of health insurance to reduce the costs of the health insurance product.

There needs to be a sustained attempt to link employee wellness to the design of the health insurance plan offered by employers. In a very competitive business environment, businesses lack the market power to raise prices to pay the costs for health insurance and to stay in business over the long run. This is why workplace wellness needs to become a business strategy that literally combines the goals of the employee health and the overall economic health of the business.

Many employers have moved past discussion of employer-sponsored wellness programs to the implementation and evaluation of these company-sponsored wellness initiatives. The majority of these companies are reporting excellent results from these programs that include better health for their employees, improved morale for all employees, increased productivity and reduced absenteeism, and workpeople's compensation claims for the business.

CONCLUDING REMARKS

The costs of supplying health insurance to workers in this country are increasing at such a rapid rate that many businesses are passing more and more of the costs of health insurance on to the employee. At the same time, the workers' productivity is decreasing because of poor health due to the effects of chronic diseases developed and manifested during the working years. These rising costs of providing health insurance to workers is increasing at such a rapid rate that many businesses are reconsidering whether they can pay these insurance costs and remain competitive with other businesses in the world.

Because the majority of chronic diseases develop during the working years and many employers suffer the consequences of these diseases in the form of lost productivity and higher insurance premiums, employers have a solid incentive to do everything in their power to keep their employees well. In a cost benefit analysis, increased investment in many work site wellness programs results in greater dollar returns to the business.

Goetzel (2004) reports that the rate of return on investment for these workplace wellness programs ranges from $1.40 to $13.00 in benefits per dollar spent on the program depending on what type of program is offered to employees. These programs are obviously a good investment and provide the opportunity to develop proactive planning for businesses in their quest to lower health insurance premiums and to provide their employees with better health, which should translate into increased productivity in the workplace. These programs are available as an appendix to this chapter (see Appendix B).

The number of businesses offering their employees a workplace wellness program are growing in number. Following the steps outlined in this chapter can benefit businesses in their attempt to develop, implement, and evaluate workplace health programs that benefit both the employer in terms of premiums for health insurance and the employee by having better health as they grow older.

DISCUSSION QUESTIONS

1. How do workplace wellness programs help to improve health and to reduce health insurance premiums?
2. Why has it taken so long for workplace wellness programs to be accepted by employers as a way to deal with the health insurance crisis in this country?
3. What is the value of conducting a needs assessment before beginning a workplace wellness program?

REFERENCES

Anspaugh, D. J., Dignan, M. B., & Anspaugh, S. L. (2000). *Developing health promotion programs.* Long Grove, IL: Waveland Press Inc.

Brownson, R., Remington, P., & Davis, J. (1998). *Chronic disease epidemiology and control.* Washington, DC: American Public Health Association.

Centers for Disease Control and Prevention. (1999). Framework for Program Evaluation in public health. *Morbidity and Mortality Weekly Report, 48*(11), 1–40.

Centers for Disease Control and Prevention. (2005a). Adult participation in recommended levels of physical activity—United States, 2001 and 2003. *Morbidity and Mortality Weekly Report, 54*, 1208–1211.

Centers for Disease Control and Prevention. (2005b). Annual smoking-attributable mortality, years of potential life lost, and productivity losses—United States, 1997–2001. *Morbidity and Mortality Weekly Report, 54*, 625–628.

Centers for Disease Control and Prevention. (2005c). Prevalence of obesity among U.S. adults by characteristics, 1991–2001. *Morbidity and Mortality Weekly Report, 54*, 765–768.

Centers for Disease Control and Prevention. (2005d). Trends in leisure-time physical inactivity by age, sex, and race/ethnicity—United States, 1994–2004. *Morbidity and Mortality Weekly Report, 54*, 991–993.

Centers for Disease Control and Prevention. (2009). *Components of a logic model.* Available at http://www.cdc.gov/nccdphp/dnpa/socialmarketing/training/pdf/logicmodelcomponents.pdf. Accessed February 22, 2009.

Centers for Disease Control and Prevention. (2009). *Healthier worksite initiative: Need assessment 101.* Department of Health and Human Services. Available at http://www.cdc.gov/nccdphp/dnpa/hwi/program_design/needs_assessment.htm. Accessed May 13, 2008.

Christoffel, T., & Gallagher, S. S. (2006). *Injury prevention and public health practical knowledge, skills, and strategies* (2nd ed.). Sudbury, MA: Jones & Bartlett Publishers.

Cohen, L., Chavez, V., & Chehimi, S. (2007). *Prevention is primary strategies for community well-being.* San Francisco, CA: Josey Bass.

Edberg, M. (2007). *Essentials of health behavior: Social and behavioral theory in public health.* Sudbury, MA: Jones & Bartlett Publishers.

Emanuel, E. (2008). *Health care guaranteed: A simple, secure solution for America.* Philadelphia, PA: Perseus Books Group.

Goetzel, R. Z. (2004). *Examining the value of integrating occupational health and safety and health promotion programs in the workplace.* Paper presented at the *Steps to a Healthier U.S. Workforce Symposium.*

Harris, J. R., Cross, J., Hannon, P. A., Mahoney, E., Ross-Viles, S. & Kuniyuki, A. (2008). Employer adoption of evidence-based chronic disease prevention practices: a pilot study. *Prev Chronic Dis, 5*(3). Available at http://www.cdc.gov/pcd/issues/2008/jul/07_0070.htm. Accessed May 2, 2008.

Hewitt Associates. (2008). *Two roads diverged: Hewitt's annual health care survey.* Available at www.hewiitt.com. Accessed February 21, 2008.

Institute of Medicine. (2003). *The future of the public's health in the 21st century.* Washington, DC: National Academies Press.

International Labor Office of United Nations. (2006). *UN Study Finds Better Nutrition Does the Workplaces Good.* Available at http://hr.blr.com/news.APIX?ID=17879. Accessed March 14, 2007.

Jack, L. Jr., Mukhtar, O., Martin, M., Rivera, M., Lavinghouse, S. R., Jernigan, J. (2006). Program evaluation and chronic diseases: methods, approaches, and implications for public health. *Prev Chronic Dis* (serial online). Available at http://www.cdc.gov/pcd/issues/2006/jan/05-014.htm. Accessed June 2006.

Lorentz, D. (2005). Childhood obesity: Epidemic spurs state attention: Will kids live shorter lives than their parents. *Council of State Government,* June–July, 2005, *4*, 12.

McGinnis, J., & Foege, W. (1993). Actual causes of death in the United States. *Journal of the American Medical Association, 270,* 2207–2212.

McKenzie, J. F., Pinger, R. R., & Kotecki, J. E. (2005). *An introduction to community health* (5th ed.). Sudbury, MA: Jones and Bartlett Publishers.

National Institutes of Health. (2006). State-of-the-Science conference statement. Tobacco Use: Prevention, cessation, and control. *Ann Intern Med, 145.*

Prevention Institute. (2002). *Workplace policies to offer nutritious foods.* Available at www.preventioninstitute.org. Accessed March 2006.

The Commonwealth Fund Commission on a High Performance Health System. (2009). *The Path to a high performance health system: A 2020 vision and the policies to pave the way.* Available at http://www.commonwealthfund.org/Content/Publications/Fund-Reports/2009/Feb/The-Path-to-a-High-Performance-US-Health-System.aspx. Accessed February 2009.

Robert Wood Johnson Foundation. (2009). *Employers provide health insurance benefits for practical, not ethical, reasons study fines.* Available at http://www.rwjf.org/pr/product.jsp?id=17119. Accessed January 12, 2008.

Rowitz, L. (2006). *Public health for the 21st century: The prepared leader.* Sudbury, MA: Jones and Bartlett Publishers.

Schulte, P. (2007). Work, Obesity and Occupational Safety and Health. *American Journal of Public Health. 97*(3).

Task Force on Community Preventive Services. (2005). *Preventive services: What works to promote health.* New York, NY: Oxford University Press.

U.S. Department of Health and Human Services. (2001). *Surgeon general's call to action to prevent and decrease overweight and obesity.* Washington, DC: Center for Disease Control and Prevention, National Center for Health Statistics, Health Behavior of Adults. Available at http://www.cdc.gov/nchs/. Accessed June 2006.

U.S. Department of Health and Human Services. (2006). *The health consequences of involuntary exposure to tobacco smoke: A report of the surgeon general—executive summary.* Washington, DC: Center for Disease Control and Prevention, National Center for Health Statistics, Health Behavior of Adults. Available at http://www.cdc.gov/nchs/. Accessed June 2006.

Wanjek, C. (2005). *Food at work: Workplace solutions for malnutrition, obesity and chronic diseases.* Geneva, Switzerland: International Labour Office.

Toward Health Equity: A Prevention Framework for Reducing Health and Safety Disparities

Rachel A. Davis, MSW

Larry Cohen, MSW

with assistance from Sharon Rodriguez, BA

OBJECTIVES

After reading this chapter, you should

- Be able to provide a framework for understanding how health disparities are produced and how they can be addressed and eliminated
- Have the ability to increase capacity to discuss an environmental approach to health disparities
- Have an understanding of the take two steps back model, from medical conditions to exposures and behavior to the environment

KEY TERMS

Community conditions	Equity
Community health	Norms
Disparity	Primary prevention
Environment	Resilience
Environmental approach	Root factors

Prelude

In 1965, H. Jack Geiger, physician and civil rights activist, opened one of the first two community health centers in the United States in Mound Bayou, Mississippi (Prevention Institute, 2007b). The invention of the double-row cotton-picking machine had recently replaced the need for an entire population of sharecroppers, causing massive unemployment and exacerbating poverty (Caplan & Rodberg, 1994).

To assess the needs of the community, the Mississippi health center began holding a series of meetings in homes, churches, and schools. As a result of these meetings, residents created 10 community health associations, each with its own perspective and priorities. In the beginning, the health center saw an enormous amount of malnutrition, stunted growth, and infection among infants and young children. Geiger and his colleagues linked hunger, a health issue, to acute poverty and linked poverty to the massive unemployment that had turned an entire population into squatters (Prevention Institute, 2007b).

Instead of just treating individual cases, Geiger and his colleagues addressed the problem of malnutrition, first by writing prescriptions for food. Health center workers recruited local Black-owned grocery stores to fill the prescriptions and reimbursed the stores out of the health center's pharmacy budget. "Once we had the health center going, we started stocking food in the center pharmacy and distributing food—like drugs—to the people. A variety of officials got very nervous and said, 'You can't do that.' We said, 'Why not?' They said, 'It's a health center pharmacy, and it's supposed to carry drugs for the treatment of disease.' And we said, 'The last time we looked in the [Physician's Desk Reference], the specific therapy for malnutrition was food (Geiger, 2005, p.7).'"

By addressing the roots of illness drawn from community concerns, these health centers pioneered an effective methodology for approaching health care in underserved communities. They explored environmental conditions such as housing, food, income, education, employment, and exposure to environmental dangers and linked them to health outcomes. Then, in an effort to prevent these poor health outcomes, they moved upstream to change the conditions that led to those illnesses in the first place.

Introduction

There are large, chronic, and increasing socioeconomic and racial and ethnic disparities in health in the United States (House & Williams, 2000). While the overall health of the U.S. population in general is improving, racial and ethnic minorities experience higher rates of morbidity and mortality than nonminorities (Institute of Medicine [IOM], 2003). Focusing attention and resources on **primary prevention** could significantly reduce this huge and unfair inequity. Specifically, attention to the broader environmental conditions that shape well-being could be life saving. **Environment** refers to the broad social, economic, and physical context in which everyday life takes place. Community action, changes in institutional practices, and policy change represent a tremendous opportunity to reduce health disparities through altering existing environmental conditions.

Health disparities are differences "in the overall rate of disease incidence, prevalence, morbidity, mortality, or survival rates in the population as compared to the health status of the general population." (Minority Health and Health Disparities Research and Education Act, 2000). They are generally not the result of people experiencing a different set of illnesses than those affecting the general population. Rather, the same diseases and injuries that affect the population as a whole affect people in low-income communities and communities of color more frequently and more severely.

Poor health is not only a burden to those directly affected but also to the entire population of a community whose health status is worsened by the poor health status of its least healthy members (IOM, 2003). A population that is not well is more susceptible to, and less able to ward off, infection, which can be transmitted to others. Poor health status also puts a disproportionate strain on the health care system. An excess of people with poor health overburdens the health care infrastructure, increases the spread of infectious diseases, and uses up public health and health care resources. Good health for all is precious; it enables productivity, learning, and building of opportunities. Poor health jeopardizes independence, responsibility, dignity, and self-determination.

The success of U.S. communities, society, and economy also depend on good health. Healthy workers and a healthy emerging workforce are critical for progress. As a nation, the United States spends 1 of every 7 dollars of its GDP on health care, and it is anticipated that proportion will soon rise to 1 of 6 dollars (California HealthCare Foundation, 2005a, 2005b). In fact, the United States spends double that of any other nation (Farley & Cohen, 2005). However, by spending primarily on the medical end—after people get injured or sick—the nation is expending and not investing. The strain is also taking a toll on government and consequently on taxpayers. When public money is used for medical care, there is less money available for other vital services, such as education and transportation.

There is a great risk that the prevalence of disparities may increase in the United States as the population becomes even more multicultural. As the country becomes increasingly diverse, the reality of a healthy and productive United States will increasingly rely on the ability to keep all Americans healthy and to reduce disparities.

Disparate health outcomes are not primarily due to one microbe or one genetic factor. A broad range of social, economic, and **community conditions** interplay with individual factors to exacerbate susceptibility and to provide less protection. These conditions, such as deteriorated housing, poor education, limited employment opportunities and role models, limited household resources, and ready availability of cheap high-fat foods, are particularly exacerbated in low-income neighborhoods where people of color are more likely to live. Research has now shown that after adjusting for individual risk factors, there are neighborhood differences in health outcomes (House & Williams, 2000). These neighborhood conditions are related to a history of bias directed against people of color. Therefore, it is not surprising that there are disparities in health; it is the relationship of place, race, ethnicity, and poverty that can lead to the greatest disparities.

This chapter provides a primary prevention framework for thinking about how disparities can be reduced. It begins with an overview of primary prevention, provides a framework for understanding the health disparities trajectory,[1] examines how social determinants enable an **environmental approach** to addressing health disparities, and describes what can be done to help close the persistent gap in health and safety outcomes in the United States.

Primary Prevention

Prevention is a *systematic* process that promotes safe and healthy environments and behaviors, reducing the likelihood or frequency of an incident, injury, or condition occurring. Ideally, prevention addresses problems *before* they occur, rather than waiting to intervene after symptoms appear or incidents occur. This is called primary prevention. Examples of primary prevention include ensuring availability of healthy, affordable food in communities to help reduce frequency of chronic disease and developing and mandating child safety restraints in vehicles to prevent injury and death of young children.

Prevention Continuum Example: Lead

Primary prevention: strives to ensure there is no lead in the environment through policies, laws, and organizational practices targeting new lead production and removal of existing lead

Secondary prevention: screens to establish the presence of lead and actions to minimize the consequences

Tertiary prevention: treats and rehabilitates those who have physiological damage and implements efforts to see that the damage does not advance

---

Effective primary prevention holds the promise of reducing needless suffering, premature death, and disparities. By utilizing primary prevention to address the underlying factors that contribute to health disparities, the quality of life for communities and individuals alike can also appreciate drastic improvement. Primary prevention employs systematic processes that enable a cost-effective use of resources while decreasing the pressure on the medical care system, in effect siphoning off cases that otherwise require treatment. In addition to decreasing the demands for medical services, primary prevention also reduces the need for other services such as mental health services, protection, criminal justice, and incarceration. It is this

---

[1] The health disparities trajectory is a model developed by Prevention Institute that diagrams the major components that contribute to poor health, safety, and mental health outcomes.

synergistic relationship of concurrently reducing the needs for costly services while improving the overall quality of life of a community that embodies primary prevention.

Prevention Continuum

Primary prevention is distinguished from secondary prevention because it explicitly focuses on action *before* there are symptoms. Secondary prevention relies on symptoms to determine action, focusing on the more *immediate* responses *after* symptoms have appeared. Tertiary prevention focuses on *longer-term* responses to ameliorate future negative health consequences. Efforts at all three levels are important, mutually supportive, and reinforcing.

Quality Matters: Ensuring Prevention is Effective

Despite its many benefits and successes, primary prevention practice is often misunderstood—resulting in it being viewed as tangential and underutilized. Many believe that prevention is delivered mainly through messages. Thus, health care providers add teachable moments to exams, educational brochures are made available for health fairs, or public service announcements are developed. Frequently employed as an add-on to treatment, prevention might be based more on what fits into the treatment or medical model than what is known to be effective prevention. This misunderstanding impinges on the potential for far-reaching, long-term impact and consequently reduces the enthusiasm and commitment for prevention efforts. Some organizations approach prevention more as a marketing strategy, in response to polls indicating that people want prevention as part of their health services, instead of utilizing prevention as a strategy to improve health and safety.

Defining prevention as simply education is not only inaccurate but does not effectively address the complexity and nature of problems such as health disparities. Behavior is complicated, and awareness about risk does not automatically result in protective action (Ghez, 2000). Further, in many cases when prevention is confused with education, practitioners and advocates jump from "What can we do *before* a problem," to "Here is some information *about* the problem." Although important, information about the magnitude of the problem or the availability and importance of treatment services does not foster healthy, equitable community environments and behaviors.

Educational efforts tend to focus on behavior change; changing the environment is often critical to support behavior change. For example, if it is important to walk regularly, an environment conducive to walking—an environment with safe, pleasant sidewalks, parks, business districts, stairwells, or trails—will maximize the likelihood of walking. Behavior change will not be as likely without comprehensive efforts that change environments in order to make the healthy choice the easy choice.

The Challenges of and Opportunities for Garnering Support for Prevention

Despite the advantages of primary prevention, it can be challenging to maintain as a focus. In the real world, priorities are based on criteria, such as urgency, time, funding, and achievability. To many, prevention can feel like a distraction given the urgency of ensuring that everyone has access to quality medical treatment.

Because the "big changes" may be hard to accomplish, it is critical to develop and identify interim markers that provide context for more modest efforts to assure that prevention strategies are on the right track. Prevention evaluation needs to be strengthened to garner this support. An evaluation myth is that prevention is invisible and therefore cannot be measured. This is not the case, as population-based evaluation strategies provide evidence of improvement. Nevertheless, the drama, and the human face of a problem, is better conveyed with an actual event than with data that show an event did not take place. Powerful advocacy movements tend to arise from victims and survivors. Therefore, for primary prevention, there is not the same constituency, because these efforts have resulted in people being able to go about their daily lives without experiencing the pain and trauma. All of this makes it harder to garner the legislative attention and to develop the political will. That is why primary prevention needs advocates who bear witness to the suffering and strongly assert that it is unacceptable for anybody to experience that suffering ever again.

Another challenge to garnering support is that in the past, economists have argued against the economic benefits of prevention, contending that accrued savings will be lost in end-of-life care costs. However, conventional economic models do not account for the many complexities at play in assessing the health of populations. As new models emerge that better account for the varied factors affecting health, they predict potential cost savings from prevention (Prevention Institute and the California Endowment, 2007).

Traditional models have been limited in three crucial respects. First, results are measured almost exclusively based on the effect of prevention measures on single conditions. This misses the impact that those measures have on other related conditions. Programs to lower the incidence of diabetes by increasing physical activity could also improve outcomes for stroke and cardiovascular disease.[2] Initiatives that reduce smoking affect cancer rates and also emphysema and childhood asthma. Policies aimed at improving mobility among senior citizens can reduce the incidence of falls as well as improve mental health and hypertension. Second, the models look chiefly at medical system costs, which, though a crucial measure of cost savings, are an incomplete measure because improved health results in savings beyond the health care sector. Therefore, one initiative could result in reduced costs in a number of different areas, including medical care, workers compensation payments, and disability claims. It could also result in improved worker productivity. Thirdly, the models generally focus on a short time frame — 2 to 6 years — while the benefits of prevention are likely to accrue over a much longer period. Illnesses and injuries typically

---

[2] David Chenoweth's Topline Report on the costs to California of physical inactivity and obesity clearly illuminates the ways in which addressing one factor influencing health, such as physical inactivity, increases costs across a wide spectrum of health issues including diabetes, hypertension, and cardiovascular disease (Chenoweth, 2005).

become more expensive the older the afflicted individual is and the longer the duration of the problem, so the greatest savings from prevention will accumulate not in the immediate future but further out as the individual remains disease free.

Emerging models are able to account for a broader range of possible savings from prevention measures. Researchers who have looked at the relationship between savings to the health care system and returns in other areas from improved health have concluded that the direct medical costs savings should be multiplied to account for the overall savings (see Figure 9-1). Estimates of the multiplying factor range from 2 to 12 times the medical cost savings (Colliver, 2007; Shiell & McIntosh, 2006).

The multiplier effects model shown here is based on a stock-and-flow conception of the health process. That is, it takes into account the number of people that are potentially at risk of a particular condition and the factors that influence whether the individual progresses to that condition over time. It then considers the influence of primary prevention on that process, the

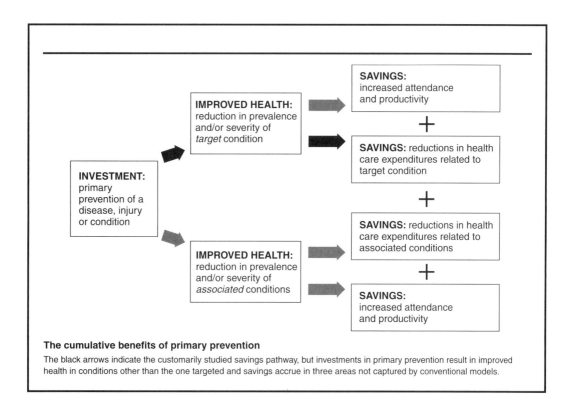

The cumulative benefits of primary prevention

The black arrows indicate the customarily studied savings pathway, but investments in primary prevention result in improved health in conditions other than the one targeted and savings accrue in three areas not captured by conventional models.

Figure 9-1 Multiplier Effects

Source: Prevention Institute and the California Endowment. (2007). *Reducing health care costs through prevention.* Available at http://www.preventioninstitute.org/documents/HE_HealthCareReformPolicyDraft_091507.pdf. Accessed December 18, 2007.

resulting prevalence of the condition, and the implications for health care expenditures. Today's public expenditure on prevention is an investment in future health and productivity. Preventing illness and injury reduces not only suffering but also costs and burdens on the health care system. Health outcomes can be improved not only through quality treatment but also by preventing poor health before it occurs by employing and expanding proven prevention efforts. Based on a review of published sources, Table 9-1 delineates a few examples of national prevention savings. The total accrued savings for every $18 invested in the selected prevention efforts is a total of $393.93 to $461.60 saved in health care costs, social services, and lost productivity. Given concerns about escalating health care costs, further building and disseminating the case for the cost effectiveness of prevention can help build more support for investment in it.

Table 9-1
Cost Savings through Prevention

Source: Prevention Institute, unpublished, 2007.

Every $ Invested in:	Produces Savings of:
Investments in workplace safety	$4–6 in reduced illnesses, injuries, and fatalities (U.S. Department of Labor)
Breastfeeding support by employers	$3 in reduced absenteeism and health care costs for mothers and babies and improved productivity (United States Breastfeeding Committee, 2002)
Lead abatement in public housing	$2 in reduced medical and special education costs and increased productivity (Brown, 2002)
Child safety seats	$32 in direct medical costs and other costs to society (Eichelberger, 2003)
High-quality preschool programs	$7 from averted crime, remedial services, and child welfare services (Schweinhart, Barnes, & Weikhart, 1993)
The measles-mumps-rubella vaccine	$16.34 in direct medical costs (Centers for Disease Control and Prevention, 1999)

*More current economic modeling was not available at the time of press but can be found at www.preventioninstitute.org.

Lessons from Prevention Successes: Changing Norms

Prevention has demonstrated success. Tobacco is one example. A generation ago virtually every public space was smoke filled and, despite the surgeon general's pronouncement that tobacco smoke was risky for health, the norm was to light up or accept others lighting up in public. Education campaigns about the danger of smoke, even secondhand smoke, had little impact and stop smoking clinics had marginal success.

> ### A Case Study of Smoking Restrictions
>
> In the early 1980s, two cities limited smoking in sections of restaurants and public spaces, and these laws in Berkley and San Francisco were initially dismissed as "fringe tactics" from out-of-the-mainstream communities. Then, a coalition formed to change the law in a more moderate county and its 18 different cities. Before long, the partnership between public health, the American Cancer Society, and the American Heart and Lung Associations became a model replicated in numerous spots across California and then throughout the United States. Organizations started voluntarily restricting smoking, something they previously would have been reluctant to do. Although the space regulated was limited (e.g., sections of public places, such as restaurants), these efforts signaled a new norm.

Norms are collective beliefs, assumptions, and standards (Berkowitz, 2003). These modest behavioral changes engendered and rapidly led to momentum for more. As the norms changed, the spaces where smoking was limited increased, support for tax increases on cigarettes surged, and smoking rates dropped (California Department of Health Services, 2006).

Similar stories can be told about most other prevention successes. Mass behavior change never occurs because of information alone. Norms change shaped by changes in policies and organizational practices generally function as the tipping factor that changes behavior. Each prevention success is different from another. But, in every case, it took leaders who believed something could and should change. It took courage taking on industry, lobbyists, and public opinion. It took moving from information to norms change through comprehensive approaches. It required overcoming obstacles so large they were described as insurmountable. In every single case, success was a product of focusing on changing the environment, which in turn influenced individual behaviors.

Trajectory of Health Disparities: A Framework for Understanding and Reducing Disparities

The frequency and severity of injury and illness is not inevitable. An analysis of the underlying causes of medical conditions reveals a trajectory by which poor health outcomes develop and worsen. The health disparities trajectory (see Figure 9-2) depicts elements that contribute to inequitable health, mental health, and safety outcomes in low-income communities and communities of color. First, some individuals are born into a society that neither treats people nor distributes opportunity equally, creating environments that put low-income communities and communities of color at risk for poorer health and safety outcomes. Second, these environments disproportionately produce exposures and behaviors that contribute to poor physical and mental health, resulting in the need for medical care. A lack of access to medical care and lower quality diagnosis and treatment leads to higher rates of sickness, disability, and mortality. The circles, decreasing in size, represent the relative contribution to increasing disparities. That is to say, the environment, with an effect on health directly and indirectly through shaping behaviors, significantly determines health status. The arrows, which increase in size and get darker in shading from left to right, reflect growing disparities and increasing poor health status. Factors at each of these levels—environment, exposures and behaviors, and medical care—shape poorer health and safety outcomes in low-income communities and communities of color and cumulatively contribute to the widening health gap. Understanding these pathways in greater detail clarifies what actions are needed to eliminate health disparities.

As depicted in Figures 9-2 and 9-3, the environment encompasses the social determinants of health (see "Clarification of Terms No. 1"), which includes **root factors** (racism, discrimination, poverty, and other forms of oppression) and the social, economic, and physical environment of a community.

Clarification of Terms No. 1: Social Determinants of Health

The *social determinants of health* encompass the multitude of social conditions in which we live that have an impact on health. Three broad categories of social determinants are social institutions, including cultural and religious institutions, economic systems, and political structures; surroundings, including neighborhoods, workplaces, towns, cities, and built environments; and social relationships, including position in social hierarchy, differential treatment of social groups, and social networks. These can potentially be altered by social and health policies and programs.

This includes, for example, the presence of toxic contamination, higher rates of joblessness, inadequate access to nutritious food and exercise, less effective transportation systems, and targeted marketing of unhealthy products.

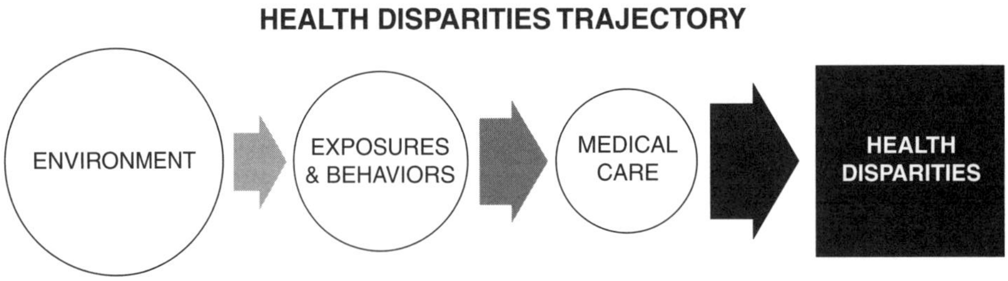

HEALTH DISPARITIES TRAJECTORY

Figure 9-2 Health Disparities Trajectory
Source: Courtesy of Rachel Davis and Larry Cohen, Prevention Institute.

EXPLANATION OF HEALTH DISPARITIES TRAJECTORY

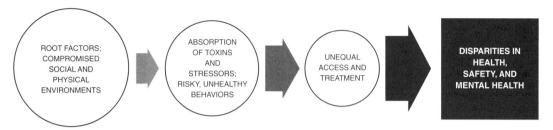

Figure 9-3 Explanation of Health Disparities Trajectory
Source: Courtesy of Rachel Davis and Larry Cohen, Prevention Institute.

These environments shape exposures and behaviors, which are the manifestation of the environment in the population and individuals. Exposures and behaviors in an unhealthy environment include breathing polluted or contaminated air and exposure to other toxins; experiencing stressors associated with root factors (e.g., poverty and racism) and with living in impoverished community environments; and practicing risky and unhealthy behaviors (e.g., poor eating and activity patterns, tobacco and alcohol use, and violence). These all contribute to the onset of illness, injury, and mental health problems. Illness, injury, and mental health problems prompt the need for medical care. Inequities in access to and quality of medical care are well documented (IOM, 2003) and contribute to even greater disparities. Although it is critical that medical care inequities be eliminated, at this point in the trajectory, there are already significant disparities in health status.

In order to significantly reduce disparities, intervention should not only occur to improve medical care but also occur as early in the trajectory as possible to ensure that people are not becoming sick or injured in the first place. This is the goal of primary prevention, which aims to remove the conditions in the environment that give rise to poor health and safety and to enhance the conditions that give rise to good physical health, mental health, and improved safety.

Take Two Steps Back to Reduce Disparities: From Medical Care to Environment

There are many illnesses and injuries that disproportionately affect people from low-income communities and communities of color (see Table 9-2). Many health problems interact, contributing to the excess burden of a disease in a population (Centers for Disease Control and Prevention [CDC], n.d.). They result from both largely genetic and external factors (McGinnis & Foege, 1993). The external factors can be modified, in contrast to inborn factors that cannot be altered, and account for nearly 50% of annual deaths—

Table 9-2

Disproportionate Onset
of Illness and Injury

- Asthma
- Cancer
- Cardiovascular disease
- Depression
- Diabetes
- Diseases of the heart, lungs, kidneys, bladder, and neurological system
- Hepatitis B
- HIV infection
- Injuries from violence
- Low birth weight and other problems at infancy
- Post-Traumatic Stress Disorder
- Sexually transmitted diseases
- Unintentional injuries

and the impaired quality of life that frequently precedes them (McGinnis & Foege, 1993).

The determinants of health and safety are multifaceted; the four forces that shape health are environment, lifestyles, heredity, and medical care services (Blum, 1981). Behavioral and lifestyle factors account for more than half of premature mortality, while environmental exposure to hazards accounts for 20% and health care for 10% (Adler & Newman, 2002). Similarly, research confirms that the explanations for disparities involve multiple factors. Because disparities may largely reflect a combination of socioeconomic differences, differences in health-related risk factors, environmental degradation, direct and indirect consequences of discrimination, and differences in access to health care (IOM, 2003), there have been calls for addressing the social and political context (Giles & Liburd, 2007) in order to reduce them.

One way to think about a prevention-oriented model for reducing health disparities is to think backwards from a given health problem or medical condition, such as diabetes, injury, or cancer, to the exposures and behaviors that might produce such a problem or condition. From that point, it can be traced further back to elements in the environment that underlie the exposures and behaviors. This is, in effect, taking two steps back. The first step back is from medical care, which most typically means access and treatment, to the exposures and behaviors that contributed to the need for medical care. For example, type 2 diabetes is an illness requiring treatment and taking a step back would be to the behaviors that led to the illness, such as unhealthy eating and a sedentary lifestyle, in order to prevent future occurrences of type 2 diabetes. The second step back is from these behaviors to the environment that shaped them. In this example, unhealthy eating and a sedentary lifestyle can be linked to the availability of healthy, affordable food and safe places to be active in the community.

For the most part, attention to addressing disparities has focused predominantly on issues related to medical care. Disparate health and treatment outcomes have been attributed to cultural and linguistic barriers; lack of stable relationships with primary care providers; financial incentives to limit services; financing and delivery fragmentation; and possible bias, prejudice, clinical uncertainty, and stereotyping (IOM, 2003). Ensuring that all individuals have access to quality medical care is one vital part of a comprehensive strategy to reduce health disparities. Quality health care means culturally competent, accessible health care for everyone. A quality health care system will provide preventive services and emergency response; diagnose, treat, and manage disease and injury; support rehabilitation; and reduce the severity and repeat occurrences of disease.

Taking two steps back is critical because, as important as quality medical care is, improving it is only part of the solution to reducing health disparities. Medical care and intervention play important restorative or ameliorating roles after disease occurs (Blum, 1981), but even by providing universal health care coverage to all citizens, patterns of disease and injury that follow the socioeconomic status (SES) gradient would still remain (Adler & Newman, 2002). While medical care is vital, there are three reasons why addressing access to and quality of medical care *alone* will not significantly reduce disparities:

- *Medical care is not the primary determinant of health.* Of the 30-year increase in life expectancy since the turn of the century, only about 5 years of this increase are attributed to medical care interventions. Even in countries with universal access to care, people with lower socioeconomic status have poorer health outcomes.
- *Medical care treats one person at a time.* By focusing on the individual and specific illnesses as they arise, medical treatment does not reduce the incidence or severity of disease among groups of people because others become afflicted even as others are cured (IOM, 2000).
- *Medical intervention often comes late.* Medical care is usually sought after people are sick. Today's most common chronic health problems, such as heart disease, diabetes, asthma, and HIV/AIDS, are never cured. Therefore, it is extremely important to prevent them from occurring in the first place.

Therefore, in order to address disparities, it is critical to not only improve the access to and quality of medical care for preventive services, screening, and treatment, it is also vital to address the reasons why people from low-income communities and communities of color become disproportionately ill and injured in the first place.

One Step Back: From Medical Care to Exposures and Behaviors

The first step back is from medical care to exposures and behaviors. Exposures and behaviors are those characteristics that capture the risks of poor health, safety, and mental health outcomes, such as exposure to environmental toxins, risky or unhealthy behaviors, and experiencing chronic stressors associated with racism or poverty or witnessing violence.

This first step back to exposures and behavior is explained in a study by McGinnis and Foege (1993). In an analysis of the contributing factors to fatal conditions in the United States, they identified a set of nine factors strongly linked to the major causes of death (see Table 9-3) which they labeled "actual causes of death" (see Clarification of Terms No. 2).

Clarification of Terms No. 2: Actual Causes of Death

For instance, when looking at the actual causes of death, if lung cancer is the medical condition, the cause can often be traced back to smoking. As McGinnis and Foege note, the origins of disease and injury are multifactorial in nature and may act independently or synergistically. For example, alcohol is a significant contributor to numerous unintentional and violent injuries, sexually transmitted diseases, cancers, and liver disease. According to the analysis, when external factors contribute to deaths, the deaths are by definition premature and are often preceded by impaired quality of life (McGinnis & Foege, 1993).

Seven of the actual causes are related to human behavioral choices, such as tobacco, diet and activity patterns, motor vehicles, firearms, and alcohol; however, many aspects of the environment shape behaviors. Far more than air, water, and soil, the environment is anything external to individuals, including community behavioral norms (Cheadle, Wagner, Koepsell, Kristal, & Patrick, 1992). For example, poor choices about diet and physical activity, which account for approximately one-third of premature deaths in

Table 9-3
The Relationship Between Leading Health Problems and Actual Causes of Death

Source: McGinnis, J.M., & Foege, W.H. (1993). Actual causes of death in the United States. *Journal of the American Medical Association*, 270, 2207–2213.

Actual Causes of Death	Leading Health Problems and Medical Conditions
Tobacco	cancer, cardiovascular disease, low birth weight and other problems at infancy, and burns
Diet and activity patterns	cardiovascular and heart disease, cancers, and diabetes
Alcohol	risk factor for injuries (motor vehicle, home, work, burns, and drowning) and cancer (Alcohol is associated with an increased risk of violence, which may include the use of firearms and increased risk-taking behaviors, which includes sexual behavior).
Microbial agents	pneumococcal pneumonia and other bacterial infections, hepatitis, HIV, and other viral infections
Toxic agents	cancer, cardiovascular disease, and diseases of the heart, lungs, kidneys, bladder, and neurological system
Firearms	homicide, suicide, and unintentional injury
Sexual behavior	sexually transmitted diseases, excess infant mortality rates, cervical cancer, Hepatitis B and HIV infection
Motor vehicles	injury and death to passengers and pedestrians
Illicit use of drugs	infant deaths, suicide, homicide, motor vehicle injury, HIV infection, pneumonia, hepatitis, and endocarditis

the United States, are not based just on personal preference or information about health risks. An individual will have a harder time changing his or her behavior if he or she lacks sufficient income to purchase food, is targeted for the marketing of unhealthy products, and does not have access to healthy foods. Similarly, it is much harder for people to be physically active when streets are unsafe and there are few gyms or parks. One analysis asserts that shifts have altered the environment to one that encourages sedentary occupations, high-calorie food consumption, and higher costs for physical activity (Mitka, 2003). The environment plays a particularly important role in low-income and minority communities, where limited household income and geographic isolation leave residents without access to many alternatives. A landmark study of the relationship between supermarket access and dietary quality found that African-Americans living in neighborhoods with a lower density of supermarkets were less likely to meet dietary recommendations for fruits and vegetables compared to neighborhoods where more markets were available (Morland, Wing, & Roux, 2002).

Despite the available evidence, prevention efforts focus on behavior change alone, such as through health education and counseling efforts, which ignore the larger environmental factors that can work against the educational message. Educational efforts will have greater impact if they are linked with efforts to change environmental conditions. Although lower income levels are associated with a higher prevalence of risky behaviors, such as tobacco use, physical inactivity, and high-fat diet, there is a risk of "blaming the victim" by viewing behaviors as simply lifestyle choices (Adler & Newman, 2002). Behavioral change is not only motivated by knowledge but also by a supportive social environment and access to facilitative services (McGinnis & Foege, 1993), support from other societal mechanisms (Blum, 1981), and an emphasis on setting up social conditions that promote health (Giles & Liburd, 2007). The evidence that the environment is far and away the major determinant of health has been marshaled time and time again (Blum, 1981). Behaviors are shaped and controlled by social, physical (Adler & Newman, 2002), and cultural (IOM, 2000) environments that are associated with socioeconomic status (Adler & Newman, 2002).

Beyond shaping behavior, the environment also directly affects health. The actual causes list includes specific environmental hazards—microbial and toxic agents. These can be described as symptoms of the environment. Environmental quality tends to be worse in areas in which the population is either low income or primarily people of color. Toxic sites are concentrated in areas where low-income and minority populations reside (Lee, 2002). Housing is more likely to be a source of lead, insect dust, and other harmful contaminants. Further, low-income people of color may have higher exposure to industrial hazards in their workplaces. The environment also affects health outcomes by producing higher stress levels, which can contribute to poorer mental health and health outcomes.

For example, children who hear gunshots may be more likely to experience asthmatic symptoms (Husain, 2002). Chronic stress may contribute to other poor health outcomes such as cardiovascular disease and some forms of cancers. The impact of social, economic, and political exclusion results in a "weathering," whereby health reflects cumulative experience of stress (due to factors such as discrimination, inadequate incomes, unsafe neighborhoods, lack of neighborhood services, and multiple health problems) rather than chronological or developmental age (Geronimus, 2001).

Given the overwhelming influence of the environment in producing symptoms of ill health—in the form of toxins, shaping risky and unhealthy behaviors, and stressors—altering environments is a critical strategy to reduce disparities. It may also be more cost effective to prevent at the community and environmental levels than at the individual level (IOM, 2000). Indeed, there has been a call for more resources to be directed at underlying determinants of illness and injury (McGinnis, Williams-Russo, & Knickman, 2002).

The Second Step Back: From Exposures and Behaviors to Environment

The second step back is from exposures and behaviors to environment. Many community leaders and health advocates intuitively understand that the environment is a primary determinant of health. Further, it is also a key determinant of health disparities. Focusing on the environment—the social determinants of health—remains an underutilized approach to reducing disparities and a tremendous opportunity to prevent illness and injury before their onset.

The environment represents both the root factors of illness and injury (racism, discrimination, poverty, economic **disparity**, and other forms of oppression) and the community conditions (physical, economic, social, and cultural) that reflect how the root factors play out at the community level. For the purposes of this analysis, *community* refers to a physical place—the geographic area that encompasses the places where people live, work, and socialize—although it can also refer to a group of people who identify around a particular characteristic or experience, such as immigration, faith, age, and sexual orientation. Place-based strategies, with an emphasis on community participation and building community capacity, are extremely promising. In order to fundamentally close the health gap, there is a need to focus on the community environment and the broader factors that shape place.

Working towards the elimination of social and economic inequalities per se is a critical aspect of efforts to reduce health disparities. The weight of racism, oppression, and economic disparity takes its toll on health. Socioeconomic status is a key underlying factor of health (Adler & Newman, 2002). Education, income, and occupation influence health, which includes exposure to damaging agents, the social environment, health care, behavior–lifestyle, and chronic stress. Efforts to eliminate disparities include building more understanding of root factors and their impact on health outcomes; using social determinant status indicators for measurement and change; improving socioeconomic status (e.g., earned income tax credit); and righting injustices, such as through affirmative action and reparations. The goals of such efforts are to reduce racism, poverty, and other forms of oppression; to establish a "level playing field"; and to reverse damages experienced from a history of bias, discrimination, and limited opportunities.

Further, understanding how these root factors play out at the community level contributes to a valuable understanding of why health disparities exist and what can be done to minimize the influence of root factors on health outcomes (see Table 9-4). Individual income alone has been shown to account for less than one-third of increased health risks among Blacks (Schultz, Parker, Israel, & Fisher, 2001). Segregation and other neighborhood and community factors make up the additional risk (Jackson, Anderson, Johnson, & Sorlie, 2000; Schultz et al., 2001).

Community conditions, largely influenced by the root factors, can be improved through a **community health** approach. A community health approach builds on strengths and assets within communities and advances community elements that have an impact on health, mental health, and safety. Knowing exactly which factors, how they interact, and examples of specific activities and approaches that can make a difference is key to making a difference. The community clusters and factors presented here are an important step in this process.[3]

The 13 community factors are organized into 3 interrelated clusters—equitable opportunity, people, and place (see Table 9-5)—and either directly influence health and safety outcomes via exposures (e.g., air, water, soil quality,

Table 9-4
Examples of How Root Factors Play Out at the Community Level

Source: Mikkelsen, L., Cohen, L., Bhattacharyya, K.,Valenzuela, I., Davis, R. & Gantz, T. (2002). *Eliminating health disparities: The role of primary prevention.* Oakland, CA: Prevention Institute.

People affected by health disparities more frequently live in environments with

- Toxic contamination and greater exposure to viral or microbial agents in the air, water, soil, homes, schools, and parks
- Inadequate neighborhood access to health-encouraging environments including affordable, nutritious food, places to play and exercise, effective transportation systems, and accurate, relevant health information
- Violence that limits the ability to move safely within a neighborhood, increases psychological stress, and impedes community development
- Joblessness, poverty, discrimination, institutional racism, and other stressors
- Underperforming schools
- Targeted marketing and excessive outlets for unhealthy products including cigarettes, alcohol, and fast food
- Community norms that do not support protective health behaviors

---

[3] The community factors are based on an iterative process conducted from July 2002 to March 2003. The process consisted of a scan of peer-reviewed literature and relevant reports and interviews with practitioners and academics as well as an internal analysis that included brainstorming, clustering of concepts and information, and a search for supporting evidence as the analysis progressed. Based on the findings of this scan and analysis, the authors identified a set of community factors that could be linked to health outcomes in the research and were ratified by a national expert panel (Davis, Cook, & Cohen, 2005).

Table 9-5
Community Factors
Affecting Health, Safety,
and Mental Health
Source: Prevention Institute. (2007a). *Good health
counts: A 21st century
approach to health and
community for California.*
Los Angeles: The California Endowment.

EQUITABLE OPPORTUNITY

1. Racial justice, characterized by policies and organizational practices that foster equitable opportunities and services for all; positive relations between people of different races and ethnic backgrounds

2. Jobs & local ownership, characterized by local ownership of assets, including homes and businesses; access to investment opportunities, job availability, the ability to make a living wage

3. Education, characterized by high quality and available education and literacy development across the lifespan

THE PEOPLE

1. Social networks & trust, characterized by strong social ties among persons and positions, built upon mutual obligations; opportunities to exchange information; the ability to enforce standards and administer sanctions

2. Community engagement & efficacy, characterized by local/indigenous leadership; involvement in community or social organizations; participation in the political process; willingness to intervene on behalf of the common good

3. Norms/acceptable behaviors & attitudes, characterized by regularities in behavior with which people generally conform; standards of behavior that foster disapproval of deviance; the way in which the environment tells people what is okay and not okay

THE PLACE

1. What's sold & how it's promoted, characterized by the availability and promotion of safe, healthy, affordable, culturally appropriate products and services (e.g. food, books and school supplies, sports equipment, arts and crafts supplies, and other recreational items); limited promotion and availability, or lack, of potentially harmful products and services (e.g. tobacco, firearms, alcohol, and other drugs)

2. Look, feel & safety, characterized by a well-maintained, appealing, clean, and culturally relevant visual and auditory environment; actual and perceived safety

3. Parks & open space, characterized by safe, clean, accessible parks; parks that appeal to interests and activities across the lifespan; green space; outdoor space that is accessible to the community; natural/open space that is preserved through the planning process

4. Getting around, characterized by availability of safe, reliable, accessible and affordable methods for moving people around, including public transit, walking, biking

5. Housing, characterized by availability of safe, affordable, available housing

6. Air, water & soil, characterized by safe and non-toxic water, soil, indoor and outdoor air, and building materials

7. Arts & culture, characterized by abundant opportunities within the community for cultural and artistic expression and participation and for cultural values to be expressed through the arts

stressors) or indirectly via behaviors that in turn affect health and safety outcomes (e.g., the availability of healthy food affects nutrition).

Equitable Opportunity

This cluster refers to the level and equitable distribution of opportunity and resources. Access and **equity** affect health in fundamental ways over a lifetime. The availability of jobs with living wages, absence of discrimination and racism, and quality education are all important. Underlying economic conditions play out through a variety of effects, and poverty is closely associated with poor health outcomes (Adler & Newman, 2002). Economic inequity, racism, and oppression can serve to maintain or widen gaps in socioeconomic status (Adler & Newman, 2002). Lower education levels are associated with a higher prevalence of health risk behaviors such as smoking, being overweight, and low physical activity levels (Lantz et al., 1998). High school graduation rates correlate closely with poor health outcomes (Adler & Newman, 2002).

A Case Study of Economic Development

Long-term poverty and lack of hope or opportunity can be devastating for individuals and communities. Being able to support oneself and one's family fosters self-sufficiency and dignity while reducing the stresses associated with poverty and being unemployed. When adults and youth cannot find appropriate employment, they are more likely to turn to crime and violence and associated illicit activities, such as selling drugs. Individuals and communities without resources are less likely to be able to develop strategic responses to health issues (for example, providing healthy food or eliminating lead from houses and soil). Establishing employment programs that link employees to their community fosters community ownership and connection and can result in positive changes for the neighborhood. Since the 1960s, government has invested in community development corporations designed to provide agile, strategic assistance to neighborhoods with few resources. The most effective community development corporations have been those that have brought together coalitions of community stakeholders. The community development corporations–led citizen involvement has consistently created better neighborhoods. In many cases, it also created a new cadre of energetic and skilled leaders, able to seize further opportunities to advance neighborhood interests (The Urban Institute, 2005).

Although economic development is rarely recognized as a key strategy to reduce disparities, well-designed economic development efforts, in fact, can address multiple community health issues simultaneously. Recognizing that residents of low-income communities in Philadelphia were experiencing high rates of diet-related chronic disease, the nonprofit Philadelphia Food Trust (PFT) launched an effort to bring supermarkets into low-income areas where access to fresh food and produce was poor. The PFT concluded that the number of supermarkets in the lowest income neighborhoods of Philadelphia was 156% fewer than in the highest income neighborhoods (Philadelphia Food Trust, n.d.).

(continues)

Leaders of the PFT-inspired Food Marketing Task Force, along with two state representatives, pushed for the development of the Pennsylvania Fresh Food Financing Initiative in the fall of 2004. To date, the Pennsylvania Fresh Food Financing Initiative has committed resources to 5 supermarket projects and has committed $6 million in grants and loans to leverage this investment. These 5 projects will result in the creation of 740 new jobs and represent $22,378,000 in total project costs. In addition, at the time of publication, there are over 20 projects in the financing pipeline, ranging from 6,000 square-foot corner stores to 60,000-square-foot full-service supermarkets (Philadelphia Food Trust, n.d.).

Applying a health lens to economic development is critical to ensuring that these efforts help close the health gap. This means ensuring that economic development efforts are designed to affect the 13 community factors. For example, in many communities, small corner stores are the primary food outlets. Many of these stores depend on alcohol sales to survive. Projects such as Literacy for Environmental Justice in San Francisco have worked to develop incentives and plans to help small stores transition to selling fresh food instead of junk food and liquor (Literacy for Environmental Justice, n.d.). The impact is not only in terms of increased availability of fresh food but also reduced availability of alcohol—a key factor in preventing violence, and increased support of local ownership.

People   This cluster refers to the relationships between people, the level of engagement, and norms, all of which influence health and outcomes. Strong social networks and connections correspond with significant increases in physical and mental health, academic achievement, and local economic development, as well as lower rates of homicide, suicide, and alcohol and drug abuse (Buka, 1999; Wandersman & Nation, 1998). For example, children have been found to be mentally and physically healthier in neighborhoods where adults talk to each other (Wilkenson, 1999). Social connections also contribute to a community's willingness to take action for the common good, which is associated with lower rates of violence (Sampson, Raudenbush, & Earls, 1997); improved food access (Pothukuchi, 2005); and anecdotally with such issues as school improvement, environmental quality, improved local services, local design and zoning decisions, and increasing economic opportunity. Changes that benefit the community are more likely to succeed and more likely to last when those who benefit are involved in the process (CDC, 1997); therefore, active participation by people in the community is important. Additionally, the behavioral norms within a community "may structure and influence health behaviors and one's motivation and ability to change those behaviors" (Emmons, 2000, p. 251). Norms contribute to many preventable social problems, such as substance abuse, tobacco use, levels of violence, and levels of physical activity. For example, traditional beliefs about manhood are associated with a variety of poor health behaviors, including drinking, drug use, and high-risk sexual activity (Eisler, 1995).

Place   This cluster refers to the physical environment in which people live, work, play, and go to school. Decisions about place, including look, feel, and safety; transportation; open space; product availability and promotion; and housing can influence physical activity, tobacco use, substance abuse, injury and violence, and environmental quality. For example, physical activity levels are influenced by conditions such as enjoyable scenery (Jackson, n.d.), the proximity of recreational facilities, street and neighborhood design (CDC, 2000), and transportation design (Hancock, 2000). A well-utilized public transit system contributes to improved environmental quality; lower motor vehicle crashes and pedestrian injury; less stress; decreased social isolation; increased access to economic opportunities, such as jobs (Hancock, 2000); increased access to needed services, such as health and mental health services (B. Helfer, personal communication, March 11, 2003); and access to food, because low-income households are less likely than more affluent households to have a car (Cotterill & Franklin, 1995). What is sold and how it is promoted also play a role. For example, for each supermarket in an African-American census tract, fruit and vegetable intake has been shown to increase by 32% (Morland et al., 2002). Further, the presence of alcohol distributors in a community is correlated with per capita consumption (Schmid, Pratt, & Howze, 1995). Poor housing contributes to health problems in communities of color (Schultz et al., 2001) and is associated with increased risk for injury and violence; exposure to toxins, molds, viruses, and pests (PolicyLink, 2002); and psychological stress (Geronimus, 2001).

A Case Study of the Built Environment

Over the past decade there has been a growing recognition of the critical ways in which physical structures and infrastructure, the *built environment*, impact the physical and mental health of community residents. The built environment is the manmade surroundings that provide the setting for human activity, from the largest-scale civic surroundings to the smallest personal place. Momentum for long-term sustainable change can be generated through increases in community efficacy built on improved cohesion and trust. Two tactics for transforming the built environment are emerging as important in reducing disparities. One is the building of campaigns to address existing deficits in the built environment in a community. The other is to create mechanisms for the assessment of the health implications of proposed investment that would alter existing infrastructure, such as new transit routes, new buildings, and changes to utility services. Both are necessary.

(continues)

An example of effective modification of the existing environment was carried out in Boyle Heights, a predominantly Latino neighborhood in Los Angeles. Neighborhood residents were concerned about the lack of open space and available walking paths. They partnered with the Latino Urban Forum to create a 1.5 mile walking–jogging path around the Evergreen Cemetery. Rates of physical activity increased, and the Evergreen Jogging Path has become a catalyst for further community improvement projects (Aboelata et al., 2004).

The Trajectory as a Tool to Reduce Disparities and Promote Health Equity

Eliminating persistent and growing health disparities requires a public health strategy that not only includes but also goes beyond treating afflicted individuals. The three trajectory elements—environment, exposures and behaviors, and medical care—correspond to public health classifications of primary, secondary, and tertiary prevention (see Prevention Trajectory), which are increasingly being referred to as universal, selective, and indicated. The environment affects the entire population and thus interventions at this point in the trajectory are *universal*; negative exposures and behaviors manifest in an at-risk population, and thus interventions will be more *selective*, focusing on those who have been exposed or are engaging in risky behaviors; and finally, medical care is *indicated* for those who are sick and injured.

The trajectory from environment to exposures and behaviors to medical care and the inequities at each point represents a continuum of why health disparities occur. Although intervention is necessary at each point in the trajectory in order to reduce disparities, implementing changes in the environment has the most potent capacity to positively affect the population's health and to reduce disparities, and the community clusters and factors provide a valuable framework for selecting strategies for action. Quality intervention at each point in the trajectory can synergistically improve health, safety, and mental health outcomes and foster health equity.

Strengthening environments and improving medical care are not only necessary elements in the strategy to reduce health disparities but are mutually supportive. High-quality, accessible health care contributes to improving community environments. Providing timely and effective diagnosis and treatment not only reduces demands on the medical system, it also better enables people to contribute to the community environment through such activities as work and civic participation. Further, an effective health care institution will provide preventive care and will be active in encouraging the kinds of community services and policies that keep people healthy. An effective health care institution can also improve the local economy by purchasing local products and employing local residents.

Positive behaviors and environments equally improve the success of treatment and disease management. Some specific examples include the following:

- Healthy eating and activity habits are not only critical for prevention but also for disease management, such as for diabetes, cardiovascular disease, HIV/AIDS, and cancer treatment.
- Improved air quality—indoors and outdoors—reduces asthma triggers.
- A reliable, affordable, and accessible transportation system transports people to screening and treatment appointments.
- Literacy improves the ability to read and understand prescription labels—both directions and warnings.
- Strong social networks are associated with people looking out for each other and taking care of each other during treatment and recovery.

A Tool for Evaluating and Changing Community Environments: THRIVE (Tool for Health and Resilience in Vulnerable Environments)

THRIVE is a community **resilience** assessment tool that helps communities bolster factors that will improve health and safety outcomes and reduce disparities. It provides a framework for community members, coalitions, public health practitioners, and local decision makers to identify factors associated with poor health outcomes in communities of color, to engage relevant stakeholders, and to take action to remedy the disparities. The tool is grounded in research and was developed with input from a national expert panel. It has demonstrated utility in urban, rural, and suburban settings. Within months of piloting, several communities had initiated farmers' markets and youth programs. At the community level, the THRIVE tool contributed to a broad vision about community health, confirmed the value of upstream approaches, challenged traditional thinking about health promotion, organized difficult concepts and enabled systematic planning, and proved to be a good tool for strategic planning at community and organizational levels.

THRIVE is not an end in itself; rather it is a tool that can be used as part of a community process to improve health. THRIVE can be used to inform all of the elements of a community planning process. For example, the information gleaned from the tool can be part of the needs assessment and identify priority areas for action. It can also serve as a framework for strategic planning, help identify which partners to engage in a coalition, and provide the context for community participation. It enables people to either start with specific health and safety concerns and to link these to community health factors or to start with community health factors. It then allows people to rate how well the community is doing on these, to prioritize factors, and, based on these priorities, to generate potential actions, examples of activities communities have undertaken to address the particular factors, and additional links and resources (Davis, Cook, & Cohen, 2005); for more information, visit the THRIVE website at http://www.preventioninstitute.org/thrive/index.php.

The Role of Public Health: A New Way of Doing Business

The analyses of community factors, trends, and directions that influence rates of disparities reveal the value of improving environments in order to close the health gap. This approach to improving health outcomes necessarily requires that the public health sector and health advocates approach health in a new way. It requires a new way of thinking and a new way of doing business. This is an approach that identifies a medical condition and asks, how do we treat this? It also requires understanding how the fundamental root causes of health disparities play out in the community in a way that affects health and injury and asking, who do we need to engage and what do we need to do in order to *prevent* people from getting sick and injured? Approaching health, and community, in this way requires a concerted focus on applying a health lens, comprehensive approaches, interdisciplinary collaboration, a resilience-based approach to working with communities, and evaluation and accountability.

Apply a Health and Health Disparities Lens

No one strategy will, in isolation, solve the disparities crisis. What has the most promise for reducing disparities is that efforts be promulgated with both a health lens and a focus on disparities. That is, efforts (e.g., planning and design, zoning, marketing, economic development) should be undertaken with attention not only to ensuring actions are designed to bolster community factors to improve health but also to ensuring actions are specifically designed to close the health gap. Public health has a key role to play in insisting that necessary players understand the health impact of their decisions and in working with them to ensure that they are contributing to, not compromising, good health.

Advance Comprehensive Approaches

It is important to understand that research is still examining which community factors may have greater influence; however, it is clear that no single strategy, program, or policy is the answer. Multiple changes are needed to shift community norms toward healthier behaviors. Based on experience with other public health issues, such as controlling tobacco or reducing impaired driving, a variety of changes help to build momentum and to gain traction and interest over time; incremental changes lead to others that ultimately change the overall dynamics.

To understand the necessary range of activities, practitioners have used the Spectrum of Prevention (Cohen & Swift, 1999), a tool that enables people and coalitions to develop a comprehensive plan while building on existing efforts. The spectrum (see Table 9-6) encourages movement beyond the educational or individual skill-building approach to address broader environmental and systems-level issues. When the six levels are used together, they produce a more effective strategy than would be possible by implementing an initiative or program in isolation. The spectrum has been used

Table 9-6
The Spectrum
of Prevention

Source: Cohen, L., & Swift,
S. (1999). The spectrum of
prevention: Developing a
comprehensive approach to
injury prevention. *Injury
Prevention*, 5, 203–207.

Levels of the Spectrum	Description
Strengthening individual knowledge and skills	Enhancing an individual's capability of preventing injury or illness
Promoting community education	Reaching groups of people with information and resources in order to promote health and safety
Educating providers	Informing providers who will transmit skills and knowledge to others
Fostering coalitions and networks	Bringing together groups and individuals for broader goals and greater impact
Changing organizational practices	Adopting regulations and norms to improve health and safety; creating new models
Influencing policy and legislation	Developing strategies to change laws and policies in order to influence outcomes in health, education and justice

to advance multiple efforts including, but not limited to, violence and injury prevention, physical activity and nutrition promotion, sustainability of mental health promotion, and lead prevention.

Efforts employing the spectrum as an organizing tool are most effective when they simultaneously take action at multiple levels while also create synergy between levels. Work at different levels can serve to build together toward change. Efforts at the top levels of the spectrum may have the greatest impact on broad population health and disparity reduction but will not be successful unless momentum has been built at the upper levels.

**Generate
Interdisciplinary
Approaches**

Improving community health cannot be achieved by any one organization or by addressing one individual at a time. Eliminating racial and ethnic health disparities and improving health outcomes requires participation from key public and private institutions working in partnership with communities.

Institutions, including banks, businesses, government, schools, health care, and community service groups, have a major influence on community environments. The decisions they make—such as whether to accommodate pedestrian and bicycle travel on city streets, where to locate supermarkets or alcohol outlets, or what efforts to take to reduce hazardous emissions—influence health behaviors and health outcomes. As employers, investors, and purchasers, each has an impact on the local economy. As providers of services, they influence what is and is not available to community residents. As prominent facilities within communities, they help establish norms for students, employees, and the general public. By providing activity breaks, creating welcoming stairwells, or ensuring healthy affordable food options, these facilities can create an atmosphere that supports healthy behavior. Schools are an important community resource and an excellent venue for reaching families. While meeting educational needs, they can both promote healthy behaviors and link students to services and support.

Engaging all communities in shaping solutions and taking action for change is critical. Communities need to be involved in identifying the health problems of greatest concern, examining the critical pathways to illness and injury, and working to alter these pathways. There are many strengths in communities of color upon which to anchor an effective strategy. Strong family ties and social networks, trust and respect among community members, and health-promoting traditions, such as active lifestyles or high fruit and vegetable diets, are all resilience factors that need support and enhancement for reducing health disparities.

Foster Community Resilience

Community resilience is the ability of a community to recover from and/or thrive despite the prevalence of risk factors. Prevention strategies have focused largely on reducing risk factors. Equally important is building upon and enhancing resilience in communities. Enhancing community resilience can have long-term, positive impacts on individual and community health.

Every community has strengths and sources of resilience. Building on a community's strength can contribute to needed change. In order to substantially reduce health disparities, a long-term plan that consistently builds momentum and involves community partners is required. Focusing on building community capacity and resilience has three important results: community members are brought into the process and feel a greater vested interest in successful change; community members can apply new skills to address health factors outside of the current initiative and are able to respond to advances and emerging practices (as opposed to being passive recipients); and community members gain skills and a sense of efficacy that can permeate many aspects of their lives and improve broad life outcomes.

Studies show that resilience factors can counteract the negative impact of risk factors (Bradley et al., 1994; Smith, Lizotte, Thornberry, & Krohn, 1995). For instance, while a high availability of firearms and alcohol within a community is a risk factor for violence, positive social norms can provide social controls that are protective against the use of weapons. One study demonstrates that the effects of protection on reducing problem behaviors become stronger as levels of risk exposure increase (Pollard, Hawkins, & Arthur, 1999). In effect, resilience factors moderated the negative effects of exposure to risk. Effective approaches need to include attention to both risk and resilience (Pollard et al., 1999; Smith et al., 1995). Addressing risk factors results in the absence of factors that threaten health and safety; however, it does not necessarily achieve the presence of conditions that support health.

Drive Evaluation and Accountability

Public health has an important contribution to make in regards to data and evaluation and using this capacity to measure progress and to establish benchmarks for accountability. Community indicator reports—published reports that use a carefully selected set of indicators to track the social, health, and economic conditions in a defined geographic area—are a valuable tool for this (Flores, Davis, & Culross, 2007; Prevention Institute, 2007a). The most comprehensive and valuable reports are able to monitor trends over time and offer some interpretation about the magnitude and direction of any changes. Simply making indicators available will not result in change. Effective indicator reports frame the information in a way that can lead to action; they identify relevant policies and steps that can be undertaken to improve the indicator. Reports and report cards also work best in a context of accountability (i.e., when the agencies or organizations responsible for acting on the information are clearly identified). Community indicator reports facilitate community improvement in a number of different ways. They may foster community engagement and collaboration, improve health care quality, identify agendas for public resource distribution, set baselines for government performance, monitor progress in government performance or community health and well-being, inform public policy development and advocate for specific policies, or do a combination of these. Some reports focus on improving community health through a particular sector, whereas others suggest multisector collaborations to achieve the desired outcome.

One of the most important considerations is a commitment to ongoing community input. Community input ensures that reports and the process of developing reports reflect local priorities and keep the meaning of indicators transparent and clearly understood by populations for whom the report is intended. The process of developing a community indicator report can facilitate dialogue on issues that matter, translate collaboration into a meaningful product, and allow communities to think through a vision for a healthy future. The process of taking an interest in and contributing to the improvement of the conditions for health in a community can also be valuable to a community's overall health. The process is what makes the difference; the report is a tool that results from the process.

CONCLUDING REMARKS

Of the 5% of health dollars spent on health promotion and disease prevention (McGinnis & Foege, 1993), relatively few resources are devoted to prevention initiatives that address the major influences, or underlying factors, that negatively impact health. Because these factors interact to cause a greater burden of disease among certain groups of people, it is critical that these factors be addressed to close the gap in health disparities. Successfully reducing these disparities requires a broad approach that pays attention to the environment instead of focusing on medical care alone. In many cases, decisions are made without awareness of their relationships to health outcomes. When communities and institutions make decisions more explicitly, they can improve health and reduce disparities. By examining the trends and analyzing these against what is known about how to reduce disparities, priorities for action will emerge. Public health leaders and practitioners have a significant role to play as major catalysts and players to move forward this approach.

Primary prevention, with an emphasis on changing the environment (root factors and the physical and social environment), is an emerging craft that shapes comprehensive solutions, thus achieving a broad impact. With its emphasis on a community orientation, multidisciplinary collaboration, and organizational and policy-level changes, this approach can significantly improve the health of individuals, families, and communities who are most impacted by poor health and premature death.

The opportunity to reduce health disparities is palpable. Communities and government agencies are grappling with the complex issue of health disparities. The seriousness of the consequences and the inadequacies of current approaches make a new way of working a requirement. In addition to improving the health of individuals and communities, the approach presented here provides a tremendous opportunity to equip communities with skills to proactively address other issues that affect them. For those most at risk, furthering the movement for an environmental and systematic approach to health will reduce morbidity and mortality, save money, and improve the quality of life.

Health disparities are in part the result of a long history of governmental and institutional policies and practices that have put minorities at a higher risk of illness and injury. Reversing the impact of these policies and practices requires a long-term commitment from public and private institutions to improve the environments in communities of color and low-income communities and should be a major goal of public health.

DISCUSSION QUESTIONS

1. Jack Geiger offered prescriptions for food and shoes at the community clinic he started in Mississippi. What are some other things medical facilities today could offer that would have a great impact on health?

2. Why does medical care alone have limited ability to impact health disparities?

3. Why is it important to look at the environment as well as behaviors when looking at how disparities in health are produced?

4. Why is prevention a necessary strategy to address health disparities?

5. Are there community elements that consistently show up as having an impact on multiple illnesses, injuries, conditions, or disparities?

6. Think about a two steps back approach to type 2 diabetes. What does that look like when you take a step back from the illness (diabetes) and medical care to exposures and behaviors and then take another step back to the social and physical environment?

REFERENCES

Aboelata, M. J., Mikkelsen, L., Cohen, L., Fernández, S., Silver, M., Fujie Parks, L., & DuLong, J. (Eds.). (2004). *The built environment and health: 11 profiles of neighborhood transformation.* Oakland, CA: Prevention Institute.

Adler, N. E., & Newman, K. (2002). Socioeconomic disparities in health: Pathways and policies. *Health Affairs, 21*(2), 60–76.

Berkowitz, A. D. (Ed.). (2003). *The social norms resource book.* Little Falls, NJ: PaperClip Communications.

Blum, H. L. (1981). Social perspective on risk reduction. *Family and Community Health, 3*(1), 41–50.

Bradley, R. H., Whiteside, L., Mundfrom, D. J., Casey, P. H., Kelleher, K. J., & Pope, S. K. (1994). Early indications of resilience and their relation to experiences in the home environments of low birthweight, premature children living in poverty. *Child Development, 65,* 346–360.

Brown, M. (2002). Costs and benefits of enforcing housing policies to prevent childhood lead poisoning. *Medical Decision Making, 22,* 482–492.

Buka, S. (1999). *Results from the project on human development in Chicago neighborhoods.* Presented at the 13th Annual California Conference on Childhood Injury Control, San Diego, CA.

California Department of Health Services, Tobacco Control Section. (2006). *California tobacco control update 2006.* Sacramento, CA: CDHS/TCS. Available at http://www.cdph.ca.gov/programs/tobacco/Documents/CTCPUpdate2006.pdf.

California HealthCare Foundation. (2005a). *Health care costs 101.* Available at http://www.chcf.org. Accessed February 2006.

California HealthCare Foundation. (2005b). *Health care costs 101: California addendum.* Available at http://www.chcf.org. Accessed February 2006.

Caplan, R., & Rodberg, L., (1994). *Rx: Federal support for community health: An innovative community-based approach to preventive health.* Available at http://www.context.org/ICLIB/IC39/Caplan.htm. Accessed July 25, 2006.

Center for Chronic Disease Prevention and Health Promotion. (n.d.) Syndemics Prevention Network. Available at http://www.cdc.gov/syndemics/. Accessed June 15, 2003.

Centers for Disease Control and Prevention, Public Health Practice Program Office. (1997). *Principles of community engagement.* Atlanta, GA: U.S. Department of Health and Human Services.

Centers for Disease Control and Prevention. (1999). *An ounce of prevention . . . What are the returns?* (2nd ed.). Atlanta, GA: U.S. Department of Health and Human Services.

Centers for Disease Control and Prevention. (2000). *Active community environments* (factsheet). Available at http://www.cdc.gov/nccdphp/dnpa/physical/health_professionals/active_environments/aces.htm. Accessed March 2009.

Cheadle, A., Wagner, E., Koepsell, T., Kristal, A., & Patrick, D. (1992). Environmental indicators: A tool for evaluating community-based health-promotion programs. *American Journal of Preventive Medicine, 8,* 345–350.

Chenoweth, D. (2005). *The economic costs of physical inactivity, obesity, and overweight in california adults: Health care workers' compensation, and lost productivity.* Topline Report, California Department of Health Services. Available at http://www.wellnesstaskforce.org/PDF/obese.pdf. Accessed January 2009.

Cohen, L., & Swift, S. (1999). The spectrum of prevention: Developing a comprehensive approach to injury prevention. *Injury Prevention, 5*, 203–207.

Colliver, V. (2007). Preventive health plan may prevent cost increases: Safeway program includes hot line, lifestyle advice. *San Francisco Chronicle.* Available at http://sfgate.com/cgi-bin/article.cgi?f=/c/a/2007/02/11/BUG02O20R81.DTL. Accessed March 2009.

Cotterill, R. W., & Franklin, A. W. (1995). *The urban grocery store gap.* Storrs, CT: Food Marketing Policy Center, University of Connecticut (Food Marketing Policy Issue Paper No. 8).

Davis, R., Cook, D., & Cohen, L. (2005). A community resilience approach to reducing ethnic and racial disparities in health. *American Journal of Public Health, 95*(12), 2168–2173.

Eichelberger, M. R. (2003). The vaccine that prevents "accidents." *SAFE KIDS Worldwide*, (September 22).

Eisler, R. M. (1995). The relationship between masculine gender role stress and men's health risk: The validation of construct. In R. F. Levant and W. S. Pollack (Eds.), *A new psychology of men* (p. 207–225). New York, NY: Basic Books.

Emmons, K. M. (2000). Health behaviors in a social context. In L. F. Berkman and I. Kawachi (Eds.). *Social epidemiology* (p. 251). New York, NY: Oxford University Press.

Farley, T., & Cohen, D. (2005). *Prescription for a healthy nation: A new approach to improving our lives by fixing our everyday world* (p. xi). Boston, MA: Beacon Press.

Flores, L. M., Davis, R., & Culross, P. (2007). Community health: A critical approach to addressing chronic diseases. *Preventing Chronic Disease, 4*(4). Available at http://www.cdc.gov/pcd/issues/2007/oct/07_0080.htm.

Geiger, H. J. (2005). The unsteady march. *Perspectives in Biology and Medicine,48*, 1–9.

Geronimus, A. (2001). Understanding and eliminating racial inequalities in women's health in the United States: The role of the weathering conceptual framework. *Journal of the American Medical Women's Association, 56*(4), 133–136.

Ghez, M. (2000). Getting the message out: Using the media to change social norms on abuse. In C. Renzetti, J. Edleson, and R. Bergen (Eds.), *Sourcebook on violence against women* (p. 419). Thousand Oaks, CA: Sage Publications.

Giles, W. H., & Liburd, L. (2007). Achieving health equity and social justice. In C. Cohen, V. Chavez, and S. Chehimi (Eds), *Prevention is primary: A renewed approach to community wellbeing* (p. 25–40). San Francisco, CA: Jossey Bass.

Hancock, T. (2000). Healthy communities must also be sustainability communities. *Public Health Reports, 115*(March/April & May/June),151–156.

House, J. S., & Williams, D. R. (2000). Understanding and reducing socioeconomic and racial/ethnic disparities in health. In B. Smedley and S. Syme (Eds.), *Promoting health: Intervention strategies from social and behavioral research* (p. 81–124). Washington, DC: National Academy Press.

Husain, A. (2002). Psychosocial stressors of asthma in inner-city school children. Poster presentation at *Putting the Public Back into Public Health: 130th APHA Annual Meeting*, (November). Philadelphia, PA.

Institute of Medicine. (2000). A social environmental approach to health and health interventions. In B. D. Smedley and S. L. Syme SL (Eds.), *Promoting health: Intervention strategies from social and behavioral research* (p. 15). Washington, DC: National Academy of Sciences.

Institute of Medicine. (2003). *Unequal treatment: Confronting racial and ethnic disparities in health care.* In B. Smedley, A. Stith, and A. Nelson A, (Eds.). Washington, DC: The National Academies Press.

Jackson, S. A., Anderson, R. T., Johnson, N .J., & Sorlie, P. D. (2000). The relations of residential segregation to all-cause mortality: A study in black and white. *American Journal of Public Health, 90*(4), 615–617.

Jackson, R. J. (n.d.) *Creating a healthy environment: The impact of the built environment on public health* (Centers for Disease Control and Prevention). Available at http://www.sprawlwatch.org. Accessed December 19, 2002.

Lantz, P.M., House, J.S., Lepkowski, J.M., Williams, D.R., Mero, R.P., & Chen, J. (1998). Socioeconomic factors, health behaviors, and mortality. *Journal of the American Medical Association, 279*(21),1703–1708.

Lee, C. (2002). Environmental justice: Building a unified vision of health and the environment. *Environmental Health Perspectives, 110*(Suppl. 2), 141–144.

Literacy for Environmental Justice. (n.d.). Available at http://www.lejyouth.org. Accessed August 12, 2006.

McGinnis, J.M., & Foege, W.H. (1993). Actual causes of death in the United States. *Journal of the American Medical Association, 270,* 2207–2213.

McGinnis, M., Williams-Russo, P., & Knickman, J .R. (2002). The case for more policy attention to health promotion. *Health Affairs, 21*(2), 78–93.

Mikkelsen, L., Cohen, L., Bhattacharyya, K., Valenzuela, I., Davis, R., & Gantz, T. (2002). *Eliminating health disparities: The role of primary prevention.* Oakland, CA: Prevention Institute.

Minority Health and Health Disparities Research and Education Act. (2000). United States Public Law, *106-525,* 2498.

Mitka, M. (2003). Economist takes aim at "big fat" U.S. lifestyle. *Journal of the American Medical Association, 289,* 33–34.

Morland, K., Wing, S., & Roux, A. D. (2002). The contextual effect of the local food environment on residents' diets: The atherosclerosis risk in communities study. *American Journal of Public Health, 92*(11),1761–1768.

National Institutes of Health. (2002). *NIH's strategic research plan and budget to reduce and ultimately eliminate health disparities* (Vol. I). Available at http://ncmhd.nih.gov/our_programs/strategic/pubs/Volumel_031003EDrev.pdf. Accessed June 26, 2008.

Philadelphia Food Trust. (n.d.) Supermarket campaign. Available at http://www.thefoodtrust.org/php/programs/super.market.campaign.php. Accessed August 12, 2006.

PolicyLink. (2002). *Reducing health disparities through a focus on communities.* Oakland, CA: Author.

Pollard, J. A., Hawkins, J. D., & Arthur, M. W. (1999). Risk and protection: Are both necessary to understand diverse behavioral outcomes in adolescence? *Social Work Research, 23*(3), 145–158.

Pothukuchi, K. (2005). Attracting supermarkets to inner-city neighborhoods: Economic development outside the box. *Economic Development Quarterly, 19,* 232–244.

Prevention Institute. (2007a). *Good health counts: A 21st century approach to health and community for California.* Los Angeles, CA: The California Endowment.

Prevention Institute. (2007b). Dr. Jack Geiger in key elements of prevention efforts. In C. Cohen, V. Chavez, and S. Chehimi (Eds.), *Prevention is primary: A renewed approach to community wellbeing* (p. 100-101). San Francisco, CA: Jossey Bass.

Prevention Institute and the California Endowment. (2007). *Reducing health care costs through prevention*. Available at http://www.preventioninstitute.org/documents/HE_HealthCareReformPolicyDraft_091507.pdf. Accessed December 18, 2007.

Sampson, R. J., Raudenbush, S. W., & Earls, F. (1997). Neighborhoods and violent crime: A multilevel study of collective efficacy. *The American Association for the Advancement of Science, 277*(5328:15), 918–924.

Schmid, T. L., Pratt, M., & Howze, E. (1995). Policy as intervention: Environmental and policy approaches to the prevention of cardiovascular disease. *American Journal of Public Health, 85*(9), 1207–1211.

Schultz, A., Parker, E., Israel, B., & Fisher, T. (2001). Social context, stressors, and disparities in women's health. *Journal of American Medical Women's Association, 56*(4), 143–149.

Schweinhart, L. J., Barnes, H. V., & Weikart, D. P. (1993). Significant benefits: The high/scope perry preschool study through age 27. *Monographs of the High/Scope Educational Research Foundation, 10*.

Shiell, A., & McIntosh, K. (2006). Some economics of health promotion: What we know, don't know and need to know before spending to promote public health. *Harvard Health Policy Review, 7*, 21–31.

Smith, C., Lizotte, A. J., Thornberry, T. P., & Krohn, M. D. (1995). Resilient youth: Identifying factors that prevent high-risk youth from engaging in delinquency and drug use. In J. Hagan (Ed.), *Delinquency and disrepute in the life course: Contextual and dynamic analyses* (p. 217–247). Greenwich, CT: JAI Press.

The Urban Institute. (2005). *The impact of community development corporations on urban neighborhoods*. Washington, DC: Metropolitan Housing and Communities Policy Center.

Wandersman, A., & Nation, M. (1998). Urban neighborhoods and mental health: Psychological contributions to understanding toxicity, resilience, and interventions. *American Psychologist, 43*, 647–656.

Wilkenson, R. (1999). Income inequality, social cohesion, and health: Clarifying the theory—a reply to Muntaner and Lynch. *International Journal of Health Services, 29*, 525–545.

U.S. Department of Labor, Occupational Safety and Health Administration. (n.d.) *Safety pays*. Available at http://www.osha.gov/dcsp/smallbusiness/safetypays/index.html. Accessed March 2009.

United States Breastfeeding Committee. (2002). *Workplace breastfeeding support* [issue paper]. Raleigh, NC: United States Breastfeeding Committee.

10
CHAPTER

The truth® Campaign: Using Countermarketing to Reduce Youth Smoking

Jane A. Allen, MA
Donna Vallone, PhD, MPH
Ellen Vargyas, JD
Cheryl G. Healton, DrPH
American Legacy Foundation

OBJECTIVES

After reading this chapter, you should

- Understand the evidence base for using countermarketing to prevent and reduce tobacco use
- Understand the importance of branding in developing an effective public health campaign
- Understand how a variety of evaluation tools can be combined to develop a clear assessment of a countermarketing campaign
- Understand key barriers to effective countermarketing, particularly the tobacco industry

KEY TERMS

Brand
Countermarketing
Sensation seeking

Tobacco industry
truth® campaign
Youth smoking

Introduction to the truth® Campaign

The **truth® campaign** is a branded, national smoking prevention campaign designed to reach at-risk youth, ages 12 to17 years, primarily through edgy television advertisements with an antitobacco-industry theme (Farrelly et al.,

2002a; Farrelly, Davis, Haviland, Messeri & Healton, 2005). Young adults, ages 18 to 24 years, compose an important secondary audience.

The truth® campaign features fast-paced, hard-edged ads that present facts about the addictiveness of smoking, the number of deaths and amount of disease attributed to smoking, the ingredients in cigarettes, and the marketing practices of the tobacco industry. Market research experts have long asserted that the "just say no" approach to public health messaging is counterproductive (McKenna, Gutierrez & McCall, 2000; Reputation Management, 1998). For this reason, truth® campaign ads do not tell youth what to do or what not to do. They do not preach, and they are not disrespectful of smokers. Rather, the ads convey factual information and encourage young people to make up their own minds about smoking and the **tobacco industry**. The campaign features youth spokespersons with personal characteristics often associated with smoking, such as rebelliousness, independence, and risk taking. The truth® campaign co-opts these stereotypical social images to change norms about not smoking (Evans, Price, & Blahut, 2005).

The television component of the truth® campaign is supplemented by radio ads, a robust and growing presence on the Internet, and an annual, grass roots "truth® tour." The truth® tour is a summer bus tour that brings "crew members" to cities across the nation and provides an opportunity for youth to encounter the campaign in a dynamic setting. American Legacy Foundation launched the truth® campaign in 2000; it was and still is the only national **youth smoking** prevention campaign in the United States not sponsored by the tobacco industry.

Evidence for the Effectiveness of Countermarketing Campaigns

Countermarketing is a mass-media communication strategy that has been used by public health organizations in recent years to counter tobacco industry advertising and promotion and other protobacco media influences, such as smoking imagery in movies (Centers for Disease Control and Prevention [CDC], 2003). There is excellent evidence from state, national, and international studies that tobacco countermarketing campaigns are an effective way to reduce youth smoking prevalence (CDC 2003; National Cancer Institute, 2008). As a result, countermarketing is one of the CDC's recommended "best practices" for tobacco control (CDC, 2007). Effective countermarketing campaigns are those that focus youth attention on the business practices of the tobacco industry, have "edgy" youth spokespersons, and have good visibility among the intended audience (Flay, 1987; Goldman & Glantz, 1998; Hornik, 2002; McKenna et al., 2000; Warner, 2001; Siegel, 1998). The impact of a countermarketing campaign can be enhanced by the presence of other antitobacco influences, such as high state cigarette taxes, smoke-free policies, and school or community-based prevention and cessation programs (CDC, 2007; Hersey et al., 2005).

Three state and two national countermarketing campaigns can be considered model programs because they have been rigorously evaluated and found to be associated with reduced youth smoking rates. These programs include the campaigns of Florida, California, Massachusetts, and the 1967–1971 U.S. campaign that took place under the Fairness Doctrine. The final model program is American Legacy Foundation's national truth® campaign.

Florida
The Florida truth campaign focused entirely on youth, with media as one component of a comprehensive campaign. The media was considered intensive and novel; an antitobacco industry approach was used as a primary message strategy. A variety of studies demonstrated that the campaign reduced smoking, reduced the risk of initiation, and reduced the likelihood of progressing to established smoking. Nearly all youth in Florida (92% of 12- to 17-year-olds) could accurately describe one of the campaign advertisements in the year after the campaign launched (Zucker et al., 2000). From 1998 to 2000, smoking prevalence declined significantly among students in Florida, from 18.5% to 11.1% among middle school students and from 27.4% to 22.6% among high school students (Bauer, Johnson, Hopkins, & Brooks, 2000). A longitudinal study showed that exposure to the campaign lowered the risk of smoking initiation and, among current smokers, the likelihood of progressing to established smoking (Sly, Hopkins, Trapido & Ray, 2001). Moreover, the campaign had a dose-response effect; higher levels of campaign exposure were associated with lower likelihood of smoking initiation and progression to established smoking (Sly et al., 2001; Sly, Trapido & Ray, 2002).

California
The California Tobacco Control Program is a comprehensive program primarily focused on adults; however, it is designed so that youth are also exposed to campaign media. An anti-industry approach is among several message strategies employed. Most published studies focus on the campaign's positive impact on adult smoking rates, per capita consumption, and cessation (Fichtenberg & Glantz, 2000); however, there is evidence that the campaign also reduced youth smoking rates and increased the proportion of youth who report never having smoked. Among youth aged 12 to 17 years, the proportion who had never smoked increased from 1990 to 1999. Respondents were more likely to be "never smokers" if they were 12 years or younger in 1990, when most program components were put in place (Chen, Li, Unger, Liu, & Johnson, 2003). Although adolescent smoking increased from 1993 to 1996, this trend began to change in 1996. From 1996 to 1999 the proportion of youth reporting established smoking declined from 9.9% to 8.0% (Gilpin et al., 2001). The California Department of Public Health reports declines in youth smoking from 1996 to 2002 (California Department of Health Services Tobacco Control Section, 2004).

The national truth® campaign may have been a factor in the decline in youth smoking during this period.

Massachusetts   The Massachusetts antismoking media campaign consisted of television, radio, and billboard advertising, designed to reach youth and adults. Campaign advertisements focused largely on tobacco industry practices and the health effects of tobacco use. The media campaign was considered emotionally arousing, was fairly intense (costing $8 per capita over 4 years), and took place in the context of newly established state taxes on cigarettes (L. Biener, personal communication, 2006; Siegel & Biener, 2000). A large proportion of youth (71%) reported exposure to the television component of the media campaign. A longitudinal study showed that 12- and 13-year-old youth who were exposed to the campaign in 1993 were 50% less likely to progress to established smoking over the next 4 years. These youth were also less likely to have an inflated perception of peer smoking rates—a perception associated with an increased likelihood of smoking (Siegel & Biener, 2000).

The Fairness Doctrine Campaign   From 1967 through 1971, the Federal Communication Commission (FCC) Fairness Doctrine required broadcasters to show approximately 1 public service antitobacco ad for every 3 tobacco ads they aired (U.S. Department of Health and Human Services [DHHS], 1989). Although the advertisements were not designed specifically for youth and represented a variety of messages, during the period of the campaign, per capita cigarette sales decreased by 7%, youth smoking decreased by 3%, and youth who reported watching more television during this period were found to be less likely to smoke (DHHS, 1989; Lewit, Coate & Grossman, 1981). Another study concluded that smoking rates among adults would have been significantly higher from 1964 to 1978 had it not been for the campaign (Warner & Murt, 1982). These ads went off the air when Congress prohibited all broadcast media advertising of cigarettes. Studies reported a notable increase in smoking rates shortly thereafter (Warner, 1986).

The Development of the truth® Campaign

The Master Settlement Agreement   In 1998, 46 state attorneys general and other state officials and all of the major tobacco companies signed the Master Settlement Agreement (MSA) to resolve the states' legal claims against the tobacco companies. The MSA prohibits the marketing of cigarettes and other tobacco products to youth; prohibits the use of cartoon characters, such as Joe Camel, in tobacco advertising; eliminates tobacco industry sponsorship of sporting events and restricts the number and type of other events the industry can sponsor; eliminates all outdoor advertising, such as billboards and transit ads; bans free samples for youth; and bans all industry-branded merchandise (Office of Attorney General, 1998). The MSA also altered tobacco industry corporate practice. It restricted lobbying; dissolved the Tobacco Institute, the Council for Tobacco

Research, and the Center for Indoor Air Research; and prohibited companies from entering agreements with one another to limit or suppress tobacco-related research. The MSA made internal industry documents public. Finally, the MSA provided a substantial amount of money to the signing states and to a national foundation (to be created). The states were awarded $206 billion as a result of the settlement (Office of Attorney General, 1998). It was expected, although not required, that at least some of this money would be used to fund smoking prevention and cessation programs, thereby reducing the financial and human cost of tobacco to states. Although some states did implement programs to reduce smoking rates, particularly in the period immediately following the settlement, most states have used their MSA funds for other purposes (Campaign for Tobacco Free Kids, 2006).

The Establishment of the American Legacy Foundation

The MSA provided $150 million over 10 years for the establishment of a national foundation and another $1.45 billion to the foundation from 2000 through 2003 for the purpose of educating the public about the dangers of tobacco use (Office of Attorney General, 1998). The purpose of the national foundation was to "support (1) the study of and programs to reduce youth tobacco products usage and youth substance abuse in the states and (2) the study of and educational programs to prevent disease associated with the use of tobacco products in the states" (Office of Attorney General, 1998, p. 25). The foundation was later named the American Legacy Foundation.

Key Elements of the truth® Campaign

The truth® campaign was based in substantial part on the now defunct Florida truth campaign, which effectively reduced rates of youth tobacco use in Florida (Bauer et al., 2000). Both the Florida truth campaign and Legacy's national truth® campaign have intellectual roots in the work of a panel of youth marketing experts convened in 1996 by the Columbia School of Public Health and funded by the CDC (Columbia Marketing Panel, 1996; McKenna et al., 2000). The Columbia expert panel identified three critical elements for a successful youth tobacco prevention media campaign. First, noting teens' extreme brand-consciousness and the pervasiveness of tobacco brands, it called for the creation of a teen-focused non-smoking—or "counter" tobacco—brand. Second, it recognized that a teen-focused campaign must talk to teens in their own voice and not talk down to them. Third, the panel recommended that the counter brand highlight the actions of the tobacco industry in marketing cigarettes, including its failures to be truthful about cigarettes' addictiveness and health effects (Columbia Marketing Panel, 1996; McKenna et al., 2000). These became key elements of Legacy's national truth® campaign.

The truth® Campaign is Grounded in Behavior Change Theory and Media Research

Effective campaigns are based on behavior change theory. They have a clearly defined target audience and feature messages that are designed to influence knowledge, beliefs, social norms, and attitudes that are statistically associated with the behavior the campaign seeks to change (Fishbein, 1967; Flay & Burton, 1990; Rosenstock, Strecher, & Becker, 1988). Some theoretical models assert that self-efficacy is strongly linked to successful change for certain behaviors (Bandura, 1986; Rosenstock et al., 1988). Behavior change theories posit that shifts in knowledge, beliefs, and self-efficacy precede changes in attitudes and behavior (Bandura, 1986; Fishbein, 1967; Rosenstock et al., 1988). Messages should be pretested, with particular attention paid to the possible differential effectiveness of campaign messages by race–ethnicity and socioeconomic status (Niederdeppe, Fiore, Baker & Smith, 2008; Vallone, Allen, Clayton, & Xiao, 2007). The truth® campaign was developed, implemented, and evaluated in conjunction with this evidence base. For example, one of the first tests of campaign effectiveness was whether campaign exposure was associated with statistically significant change in specific beliefs and attitudes that were linked with intention not to smoke in the coming year (Farrelly et al., 2002a).

Message delivery is as important as message development. Advertisements should be novel or provocative to gain and hold the attention of the audience (Flay, 1987; Hornik, 2002). The intensity and duration of the campaign must be sufficient for it to generate substantial exposure within the target audience, though optimal levels of exposure have not been identified (Flay, 1987; Flay & Burton, 1990; Hornik, 2002). Recent research shows that the effects of media exposure can be short lived, suggesting that campaign effectiveness can be increased by airing ads at regular intervals (Wakefield et al., 2008). Insufficient exposure is one possible reason that some promising, evidence-based campaigns have been unable to demonstrate behavior change (Hornik, 2002).

Comprehensive campaigns that include a media component—and media campaigns that operate in a context of other tobacco control initiatives—have shown greater or longer lasting effects as compared with media-only campaigns (National Cancer Institute, 2008). This is likely because comprehensive campaigns activate or encourage a "complex process of change in social norms" that supports individual efforts to quit (Hornik, 2002, p. 16). However, research shows that tobacco industry marketing, including industry-sponsored antismoking advertisements, can undercut the effectiveness of public health campaigns (Farrelly et al., 2002a; National Cancer Institute, 2008; Wakefield et al., 2006).

truth® is a Brand   One of the greatest strengths of truth® is that it has been positioned as a **brand** (Evans, Wasserman, Bertoletti, & Martino, 2002; Evans et al., 2004; Evans, Price & Blahut, 2005). Brands are often used as a means of self-expression, and youth are particularly sensitive to the messages they convey to peers through their brand choices. The tobacco industry has some of the most well-known brands in the world; one study of tobacco brand awareness among youth showed that, among 8th grade students, 95% recognized Joe Camel and 55% recognized the Marlboro Man (as cited in Evans et al., 2005). The truth® campaign was designed to compete directly with tobacco industry brands; in essence, truth® was designed to "take market share from the tobacco industry" (Evans, Wasserman, Bertoletti, & Martino, 2002, p.17). The truth® campaign looked to popular teen brands such as Nike and Mountain Dew as examples of how to effectively reach youth. Studies of the effectiveness of the truth® brand show that it generated a high level of brand equity among the target audience and that "internalizing" the brand was associated with greater reductions in smoking uptake than was simple campaign exposure (Evans et al., 2002; Evans et al., 2005). In other words, truth® campaign ads should be effective when experienced as discrete units, but they are more powerful when the viewer places them in the context of the larger body of messages and images that constitute the truth® brand.

The truth® Audience   The truth® campaign has always been designed to reach and influence those youth at greatest risk of smoking. In the earliest years of the campaign, advertisements were pretested with youth who were "open to smoking"—youth who had never smoked but who would not rule out trying a cigarette sometime in the next year or if a friend offered them one. More recently, campaign designers (and evaluators) have made use of a trait called "sensation seeking" to efficiently develop and deliver truth® advertisements. **Sensation seeking** is measured using one of several scales, an example of which is the Brief Sensation Seeking Scale IV (BSSS-4), which consists of four questions: I would like to explore strange places; I like to do frightening things; I like new and exciting experiences, even if I have to break the rules; and I prefer friends who are exciting and unpredictable (Stephenson, Hoyle, Palmgreen & Slater, 2003).

Sensation seeking has been linked repeatedly to a variety of youth risk behaviors, including cigarette smoking (Martin et al., 2002; Slater, 2003; Zuckerman, Ball & Black, 1990). A number of studies demonstrate that sensation seeking can be used to segment the audience in an effort to more effectively produce and deliver public health messages that will resonate with those at greatest risk (Palmgreen et al., 1991; Palmgreen et al., 1995; Palmgreen, Donohew, Lorch, Hoyle, & Stephenson, 2001). For example, campaign messages and advertising executions can be tested within focus groups composed of individuals who score high on a sensation-seeking scale to help ensure that these communication vehicles resonate with this target population. Those most at risk, high sensation seekers, have been found to respond to messages that are high in "message sensation value"—"the degree to which a message elicits sensory, affective, and arousal responses" (Palmgreen, Stephenson, Everett, Baseheart & Francies, 2002, p. 404). To more effectively reach the target audience, advertising executions can be placed within the context of television programming found to be popular with high sensation-seeking youth. Thus, media buys that embed high-sensation value messages in high-sensation value programming have the best chance of reaching populations segmented on this psychographic variable. The designers of the truth® campaign have capitalized on this emerging body of research to increase the reach and impact of the truth® campaign.

A word of caution: a recent study based on Legacy Media Tracking Survey (LMTS) data suggests that the BSSS-4 is less reliable and valid for

African-American youth than other youth (Vallone, Allen, Clayton, & Xiao, 2007). Furthermore, African-American youth who are open to smoking or have experimented with cigarettes have statistically significantly lower mean sensation-seeking scores than their White and Hispanic counterparts (Vallone, Allen, Clayton, & Xiao, 2007). Taken together, these findings suggest that the BSSS-4 performs less than optimally among African-American youth, particularly those at greatest risk of progressing to established smoking. For this reason, the American Legacy Foundation and others who use sensation seeking as a segmenting variable must be cautious in placing too great a degree of confidence in the ability of this measure to determine whether campaigns are reaching and influencing the desired target audience. While we await further research to identify a sensation-seeking measure that functions equally well across race–ethnicity, sensation seeking should be considered a useful, but not perfect, campaign development and evaluation tool.

Evaluation Tools

The LMTS and Legacy Media Tracking Online (LMTO)

The LMTS is a nationally representative, random-digit-dial (RDD), cross-sectional telephone survey of youth and young adults ages 12 to 24 years. It was developed to track awareness of, and receptivity to, Legacy's truth® campaign. It also measures tobacco-related beliefs, attitudes and behaviors, sensation seeking, openness to smoking among youth who are not current smokers, exposure to secondhand smoke, and exposure to pro and anti-tobacco influences in the home, the school, and the mass media. Eight waves of LMTS data (including a baseline wave) were collected from December 1999 through January 2004. African-American, Hispanic, and Asian youth were oversampled in each survey wave to ensure that sample sizes would be large enough to produce accurate estimates for these populations. Response rates ranged from 60% in 2001 to 30% in 2004 (Vallone, Allen & Xiao, in press). The decline in response rates over time reflects a pattern that has been observed throughout the field in recent years, possibly because of the increase in the numbers of sales and survey calls (Curtin, Presser, & Singer, 2005). Legacy has used the LMTS over the years as a tool to assess audience exposure to the truth® campaign, with particular focus on how exposure is influenced by changes in the media purchasing plan, and to assess audience reactions to groups of ads with a unified theme and style. In this way, the LMTS has enabled Legacy to capitalize on successful media strategies and to minimize those that appear to be less robust.

In 2005, in response to declining telephone response rates and the cost of telephone survey data collection, Legacy shifted to an online media tracking survey called Legacy Media Tracking Online (LMTO) (Wunderink, et al., 2007). There were drawbacks and benefits to the move to an online survey. Perhaps the greatest drawback was that the change in the method of survey administration meant that data collected prior to 2005 could not be directly compared with data collected afterward. For example, LMTS data had often been used to determine how well a new group of ads resonated with youth relative to earlier, successful ads. Because Legacy's analysis of the data suggested that the mode of survey administration influenced the magnitude of youth responses to a certain degree, comparing an ad flight from 2006 (collected using LMTO) with one from 2002 (collected using LMTS) would be potentially misleading. A second drawback was that LMTO data was not considered rigorous enough for publication in a peer-reviewed journal, because it was based on a convenience sample rather than one that had been randomly drawn. These drawbacks were offset by several important benefits, the most important being that online data collection was substantially less expensive than telephone data collection. As a result, Legacy could have surveys in the field more frequently than it would have had it continued to use phone surveys, particularly as Foundation funds were in decline. Although the new data collections were not comparable to those collected using the LMTS, they were comparable to one another, and they appropriately fulfilled the primary goal of Legacy's media tracking—monitoring youth exposure and reactions to the truth® campaign. The LMTO has been used, as was the LMTS, to assess the ongoing health of the campaign. Eight waves of LMTO data have been collected to date.

Biochemical Validation Study

Legacy conducted a biochemical validation study to assess whether the truth® campaign could have created a social context that elevated social desirability response bias on surveys, as measured by an increase in underreporting of smoking (Messeri et al., 2007). This could give rise to data that falsely suggests a campaign-induced decline in youth smoking, or it could exaggerate campaign effects. Data was obtained from a national sample of 5,511 students from 48 high schools that were matched to schools sampled for the 2002 National Youth Tobacco Survey (NYTS) (Messeri et al., 2007). Self-reported smoking was compared with biochemical indicators of smoking, measured using saliva cotinine. The study showed the overall rate of underreporting was 1.3%, and the level of truth® exposure was not related to underreporting (Messeri et al., 2007). This study suggests that the truth® campaign was not an important cause of social desirability responses on surveys among high school students and that, in general, underreporting smoking is not a major source of error in school-based surveys.

Outcomes

Awareness of and Receptivity to the Campaign

A 2002 study based on LMTS data showed that in the first 9 months of the campaign, 75% of all 12- to 17-year-olds nationwide could accurately describe at least 1 truth® ad (Farrelly et al., 2002a). This finding was based on a conservative measure of awareness called *confirmed awareness*. Confirmed awareness is documented in the following way. The interviewer first asks the respondent if they are aware of any of the truth® campaign ads. If the respondent reports general truth® awareness, the interviewer then describes the beginning of a truth® ad currently or recently on the air. The youth is then asked to describe the end of the ad in his or her own words. The interviewer, who has been trained by viewing videos of the ads in question, then determines whether the youth has accurately described the ad. This measure of confirmed awareness ensures that youth do not provide false awareness responses to the interviewers.

The same 2002 study showed that during the first 9 months of the campaign, truth® influenced key youth attitudes toward tobacco in the expected direction and was associated with lower intention to smoke, though this latter finding was marginally statistically significant at $p = 0.09$ (Farrelly et al., 2002a). Change in relevant attitudes, and to an even greater degree, change in intention to behave in a particular way are excellent predictors of actual behavior change down the line. Furthermore, a second study published the same year showed that truth® was equally appealing across race–ethnicity (Farrelly et al., 2002b). For these reasons, in the first year of the campaign, Legacy was optimistic that truth® would prove to be effective at the national level and that it would influence behavior of at-risk youth regardless of race-ethnicity.

A more recent study indicates that, from 2000-2004, females had lower levels of confirmed awareness of the truth® campaign as compared with males, and youth who lived in lower education zip codes were less likely to have confirmed campaign awareness as compared with those in higher education zip codes (Vallone, Allen & Xiao, in press). These findings suggest that the effectiveness of the truth® campaign may be enhanced by developing strategies to increase campaign awareness among females and youth from lower education zip codes.

Changing Smoking Behavior

One study to date has explored the effect of the campaign by race/ethnicity (Cowell, Farrelly, Chou & Vallone, 2009). That study showed that while exposure to the truth® campaign was statistically significantly associated with intention not to smoke in the future among youth who had never smoked (OR = 2.02, p = 0.001), the results were more robust among African American youth (OR = 5.39, p = 0.001) as compared with white (OR = 1.76, p = 0.062) or Hispanic youth (OR = 2.00, p = 0.064) (Cowell, Farrelly, Chou & Vallone, 2009). Among youth who had tried smoking, but were not current smokers, the association was strong and statistically significant among youth overall (OR = 5.70, p = 0.000) and across all racial ethnic groups: African American (OR = 6.11, p = 0.002); white (OR = 6.53, p = 0.000); Hispanic (OR = 5.83, p = 0.000) (Cowell, Farrelly, Chou & Vallone, 2009).

A 2005 study used Monitoring the Future (MTF) and media delivery data (gross ratings points, or GRPs) to demonstrate a dose-response relationship between campaign exposure and smoking prevalence among youth in grades 8 through 12, so that youth with greater exposure to the campaign were less likely to be current smokers (Farrelly et al., 2005). The study concluded that the truth® campaign was responsible for an estimated 22% of the nation-wide decline in youth smoking from 1999 to 2002 (Farrelly et al., 2005). A more recent, longitudinal study, based on data collected during annual interviews with a cohort of youth from 1997 through 2004, indicated that exposure to the truth® campaign was associated with a decreased risk of smoking initiation (relative risk = 0.80, p = 0.001). Based on these results, the authors estimate that 450,000 youth were prevented from smoking between 2000 and 2004 as a result of the truth® campaign (Farrelly, Nonnemaker, Davis, Hussin, 2009).

Cost Effectiveness A cost-effectiveness study indicates that the truth® campaign was economically efficient (Holtgrave, Wunderink, Vallone & Healton, 2009). Using methods established by the U.S. Panel on Cost-effectiveness in Health and Medicine, the authors estimate that the campaign recovered its costs, and saved between $1.9 billion and $5.4 billion in medical costs for society (Holtgrave, Wunderink, Vallone & Healton, 2009). An additional analysis uses a conservative method that takes into account the argument that individuals who never smoke or who quit smoking live longer than smokers, and thus incur additional medical costs due to their longer lifespan; in this analysis the authors estimate that the cost per Quality Adjusted Life Year (QALY) saved is $4,302 (Holtgrave, Wunderink, Vallone & Healton, 2009).

Barriers to Effective Countermarketing

The Tobacco Industry

Litigation

The tobacco industry has sought to end or obstruct effective countermarketing campaigns, including through litigation. Lorillard Tobacco Company (with the support of the other major tobacco manufacturers) attempted to shut down the American Legacy Foundation through litigation, based on the claim that the truth® campaign "vilified" and "personally attacked" them, which was in violation of the MSA (Vargyas, 2007). In 2006, almost exactly 5 years after the Foundation's dispute with Lorillard began, the Delaware Supreme Court unanimously held that none of the Foundation's advertisements violated the MSA (*Lorillard Tobacco Company v. American Legacy Foundation*, 903 A.2d 728 [Del Supr. 2006]). Nevertheless, the long legal battle significantly burdened the Foundation, consuming financial and human resources that could have been otherwise spent on the public health mission of the organization. In another unsuccessful but lengthy legal attack on a successful countermarketing campaign (*R.J. Reynolds v. Shewry*), Lorillard and R.J. Reynolds challenged the California antitobacco advertisements on a number of grounds.

Industry-Sponsored Youth Smoking Prevention Campaigns

The tobacco industry has sponsored several national youth smoking prevention campaigns, the most prominent examples of which are Philip Morris' Think. Don't Smoke and Talk. They'll Listen. Think. Don't Smoke featured a "just say no" type message for youth, while Talk. They'll Listen was ostensibly targeted to parents. The same 2002 study that showed a marginally statistically significant association between truth® campaign exposure and lower likelihood of intending to smoke within the next year also showed that exposure to Think. Don't Smoke was associated with a *greater* likelihood of intending to smoke within the next year ($p = 0.05$; Farrelly, et al., 2002a). Shortly after the publication of this study, and a public call from American Legacy Foundation for them to take the ads off the air, Philip Morris ended the ad campaign.

Striking evidence that tobacco industry-sponsored media campaigns are ineffective or counterproductive also comes from a recent study that looked at the effects of tobacco industry–sponsored youth prevention campaigns on over 100,000 youth (Wakefield et al., 2006). The study showed a dose-response relationship between campaign exposure and tobacco-related attitudes, so the greater number of industry-sponsored ads a youth saw the more likely they were to have lower perceived harm of smoking (odds ratio = 0.93), stronger approval of smoking (odds ratio = 1.11), stronger intentions to smoke in the future (odds ratio = 1.12), and stronger likelihood of having smoked in the past 30 days (odds ratio = 1.12; Wakefield et al., 2006). These findings suggest that industry-sponsored campaigns may have no effect or a counterproductive effect on youth tobacco use.

The Lorillard campaign, Tobacco is Wacko! If You're a Teen, never had the media weight to reach even a small segment of U.S. youth (Allen & Xiao, 2009), but if it had, it is likely that it also would have had a counterproductive effect on youth smoking. The campaign slogan Tobacco is Wacko! If You're a Teen suggests that smoking is only unwise for teens but that it might be appropriate for adults. This particular message may well increase the appeal of smoking among young people who want to emulate adult behavior. Indeed, now public Lorillard documents show that internal concerns had been voiced about the slogan, particularly the "if you're a teen" language, but, as explained by the company's general counsel, Lorillard's president had made it clear that Lorillard "made the decision based on legitimate business concerns and we [Lorillard] must stick by it" (V. Lindsey, e-mail to Ronald Milstein, Lorillard Tobacco Company (Bates No.: 97011359), 2000; R. Milstein, e-mail to Victor Lindsley, Lorillard Tobacco Company (Bates No. 99282955, 2000).

New Products that Appeal to Youth

Despite the MSA's prohibition of marketing to youth, the tobacco industry routinely brings new tobacco products to the market, many of them designed and/or marketed to appeal to young smokers. For example, in 1999, R.J. Reynolds Tobacco Company began heavily promoting Camel Exotic

Blends—flavored cigarettes packaged in colorful tins of a distinctive size and shape. These Camel cigarettes were offered in seasonal, limited-time-only flavors such as Twista Lime and Kauai Kolada during the summer and Warm Winter Toffee and Winter MochaMint in the winter. In 2004, Brown and Williamson Tobacco Company launched a line of their popular cigarette brand, Kool, in flavored varieties called Mocha Taboo, Caribbean Chill, Midnight Berry, and Mintrigue.

There was substantial public health concern about the appeal of these cigarettes to youth who have never smoked or to those who are light and/or intermittent smokers. Flavors sweetened the taste of tobacco, making these cigarettes easier for younger smokers to tolerate, and they were sold in bright, striking packaging. Internal tobacco company documents strongly suggest that flavored cigarettes were designed to appeal primarily to young adults (Carpenter, Wayne, Pauly, Koh, & Connolly, 2005; Lewis & Wackowski, 2006; Wunderink et al., 2007). This is of particular concern because 18- to 24-year-olds, who are of legal age and not protected by the MSA, serve as role models for youth.

In addition to the flavored cigarettes, in 2004, Brown and Williamson sponsored a hip-hop oriented Kool Mixx campaign, targeted at urban youth. Most recently, R.J. Reynolds launched a new brand, Camel No. 9, with significant appeal to young girls and women. Not only does the brand name evoke the famous Chanel No. 5 perfume but it is packaged in a distinctive black box with a hot pink or teal green (for menthol) camel logo and edging and has been promoted with a line of branded items that include rubber bracelets, sequined cell phone jewelry, lip gloss, compact mirrors, and novelty purses, all of which appeal to a young audience. The brand has been heavily advertised in women's fashion magazines.

The state attorneys general have been active in enforcing the MSA provisions against youth targeting. They filed actions and reached settlements under which flavored cigarettes were taken off the market and Brown and Williamson stopped the Kool Mixx campaign. However, at the time this chapter went to press, no formal action had been taken with regard to Camel No. 9.

Smoking in the Movies and on TV

There is a growing body of literature on the prevalence of tobacco use in movies and the association between exposure to tobacco use in movies and youth smoking (National Cancer Institute, 2008; Sargent, 2005). Recent research indicates that images of tobacco use in movies are common, including in youth-rated movies, and that youth are exposed to and recall these tobacco images (Charlesworth & Glantz, 2005; Dalton et al., 2002; Goldstein, Sobel, & Newman, 1999; Mekemson et al., 2004; CDC, 2005; Sargent, Worth, & Tanski, 2006; Thompson & Yokota, 2001). Images of smoking in televised movie trailers are also common (Healton et al., 2006).

A number of studies have documented the relationship between exposure to movie stars' use of tobacco in films and youth smoking initiation or susceptibility to tobacco use (Distefan, Gilpin, Sargent, & Pierce, 1999; Distefan, Pierce, & Gilpin, 2004; Pechmann & Shih, 1999; Tickle, Sargent, Dalton,

Beach, & Heatherton, 2001). Pechmann and Shih demonstrated that 9th grade nonsmokers who watched a movie in which the lead characters smoke were more likely to report intentions to smoke in the future, compared with their peers who watched the same movie from which the smoking images had been removed (Pechmann & Shih, 1999). This study showed that seeing an antitobacco ad prior to viewing the movie eradicated this association. A 1999 survey of more than 6,000 youth by Distefan, Gilpin, Sargent, and Pierce found tobacco use of favorite movie stars to be associated with youth smoking status (Distefan et al., 1999). A longitudinal study expanding on this research demonstrated that, among girls who did not smoke at baseline, having a favorite movie star who smoked in 1996 doubled the risk of smoking by 1999 (Distefan et al., 2004.)

Frequency of exposure to tobacco use in movies also plays a role in susceptibility to smoking. Sargent et al. demonstrate a positive, dose-response association between exposure to tobacco use in movies and susceptibility to smoking (2002). A longitudinal follow-up of these students more than a year later indicated that 17% of those in the highest quartile of exposure had begun smoking, compared with 3% of those in the lowest. Multivariate analysis indicated that 52% of these initiations were a result of having seen tobacco use in movies (Dalton et al., 2003). A recent national cross-sectional study confirmed these results (Sargent et al., 2005).

Major public health organizations in the United States and worldwide have called upon the film industry to take 4 steps to reduce the impact of these images on youth smoking: (1) certify that no one involved with the production received anything of value from anyone in exchange for using or displaying tobacco; (2) require that strong antismoking ads be aired prior to movies that depict tobacco use; (3) stop identifying specific tobacco brands; and (4) rate movies that include smoking "R" (National Cancer Institute, 2008). Recently, 41 state attorneys general called upon the heads of all film industry studios to pair classic truth® campaign ads with any DVD or downloaded movie that includes smoking imagery.

Weakness in the Master Settlement Agreement

Although the MSA imposes restrictions on marketing tobacco to youth, the tobacco companies have continued to reach youth through new communication channels, such as the Internet, purported smoking prevention campaigns, and new products such as flavored cigarettes. The attorneys general have taken action to enforce the MSA, but as one inappropriate practice is addressed, others emerge.

The Future of truth®

Decline of Funding for the American Legacy Foundation and truth®

A major weakness of the MSA is a "sunset clause" specifying that after 2003 the participating tobacco companies are obligated to contribute to the Foundation's public education fund only in years in which their collective industry market share represents 99.05% of the U.S. tobacco market. The MSA public education funds are the major source of funding for the Foundation and have supported the truth® campaign and most of its other activities. The failure to reach this extremely high market share threshold has resulted in markedly reduced funding available for truth® in the coming years (Vargyas, 2007). At least one state level study suggests that defunding successful tobacco use prevention campaigns may signal a rise in pro-tobacco beliefs and attitudes, and an increase in youth intention to smoke. (Sly et al., 2005).

truth® or Consequences

In 2000, 70% of the truth® media purchase was on network television; in 2007, 70% was on cable television. This shift from network to cable TV was prompted by changes in the media environment, such as the increase in the number of television channels available and the associated splintering of the audience, and by an internal analysis showing that Legacy could reach the vast majority of the truth® audience more cost effectively through cable television. Overall, the new media strategy has worked well for Legacy and the truth® campaign; however, because of uneven nationwide cable penetration, a segment of the truth® target audience was receiving less campaign exposure than their peers. These youth tended to live in more rural areas, which already placed them at higher risk for smoking (Johnston, O'Malley, Bachman, & Schulenberg, 2007). Legacy was concerned that these youth especially were being underserved by the truth® campaign. As a result, Legacy applied for and received funding from the CDC to implement a program called truth® or consequences. The truth® or consequences campaign involves purchase of local network airtime for truth® in 41 designated media markets across the United States. The media campaign is supplemented by a grants program to develop and implement local programs for open-to-smoking youth.

CONCLUDING REMARKS

The truth® campaign is an evidence-based, countermarketing campaign that has been demonstrated to prevent smoking initiation among at-risk youth. The success of the campaign is attributed largely to three key characteristics: (1) its peer-to-peer message strategy; (2) the use of branding; and (3) its antitobacco industry theme. Campaign evaluation studies have been rigorous and ongoing and have been published in the peer-reviewed literature. Results of these analyses have been used to ensure awareness and receptivity to the campaign's message among the target audience, and thus, to increase the efficacy of the campaign.

Despite the campaign's success, there remain substantial barriers to the successful implementation of this youth smoking prevention initiative. We urge the public health community to continue to develop and implement strong countermarketing campaigns regardless of threats from the tobacco industry or other entities; to continue to fund and conduct research related to the impact of youth exposure to pro- and antitobacco media messages; and to work to effect policy change to enhance and complement countermarketing efforts. An effective countermarketing campaign should be considered the centerpiece of any comprehensive effort to reduce youth smoking in the United States as recommended by the CDC and the IOM (CDC, 2007; IOM, 2007).

DISCUSSION QUESTIONS

1. How strong is the evidence in support of using countermarketing to reduce youth tobacco use?
2. What strategies did the truth® campaign use to effect behavior change?
3. How and why did evaluators combine research tools to assess the truth® campaign?
4. What are the barriers to effective tobacco countermarketing?

REFERENCES

Allen, J & Xiao, H. (2009). Legacy Media Tracking Data. Unpublished raw data.

Bandura, A. (1986). *Social foundations of thought and action: A social cognitive theory.* Englewood Cliffs, NJ: Prentice Hall.

Bauer, U. E., Johnson, T. M., Hopkins, R. S., & Brooks, R. G. (2000). Changes in youth cigarette use and intentions following implementation of a tobacco control program: Findings from the Florida Youth Tobacco Survey, 1998-2000. *Journal of the American Medical Association, 284*(6), 723–728.

Biener, L. (2000). Adult and youth response to the Massachusetts anti-tobacco television campaign. *Journal of Public Health Management and Practice, 6*(3), 40–44.

California Department of Health Services Tobacco Control Section Update. (2004). Available at http://www.dhs.ca.gov/tobacco/documents/pubs/2004TCSupdate.pdf. Accessed December 13, 2007.

Campaign for Tobacco Free Kids. (2007). *A broken promise to our children: The 1998 state tobacco settlement seven years later.* Washington, DC: Campaign for Tobacco Free Kids.

Carpenter, C. M., Wayne, G. F., Pauly, J. L., Koh, H. K., & Connolly, G. N. (2005). New cigarette brands with flavors that appeal to youth: Tobacco marketing strategies. *Health Affairs, 24*(6), 1601–1610.

Centers for Disease Control and Prevention. (2003). *Designing and implementing an effective tobacco counter-marketing campaign.* Atlanta, GA: CDC, National Center for Chronic Disease Prevention and Health Promotion, Office on Smoking and Health.

Centers for Disease Control and Prevention. (2005). Tobacco use, access, and exposure to tobacco in media among middle and high school students–United States, 2004. *Morbidity and Mortality Weekly Report, 54*(12), 297–301.

Centers for Disease Control and Prevention. (2007). *Best practices for comprehensive tobacco control programs—2007.* Atlanta, GA: CDC, National Center for Chronic Disease Prevention and Health Promotion, Office on Smoking and Health.

Charlesworth, A., & Glantz, S. A. (2005). Smoking in the movies increases adolescent smoking: A review. *Pediatrics, 116*(6), 1516–1528.

Chen, X., Li, G., Unger, J. B., Liu, X., & Johnson, C. A. (2003). Secular trends in adolescent never smoking from 1990 to 1999 in California: An age-period-cohort analysis. *American Journal of Public Health, 93*(12), 2099–2104.

Columbia Marketing Panel. (1996). *Tobacco counter-marketing strategy recommendations* [draft report].

Cowell, A. J., Farrelly, M. C., Chou, R. & Vallone, D. M. (2009). Assessing the impact of the national 'truth' antismoking campaign on beliefs, attitudes, and intent to smoke by race/ethnicity. *Ethnicity and Health, 14*(1), 75–91.

Curtin, R., Presser, S., & Singer, E. (2005). Changes in telephone survey nonresponse over the past quarter century. *Public Opinion Quarterly, 69,* 87–98.

Dalton, M. A., Sargent, J. D., Beach, M. L., Titus-Ernstoff, L., Gibson, J., Ahrens, M. B., Tickle, J., & Heatherton, T. F. (2003). Effect of viewing smoking in movies on adolescent smoking initiation: A cohort study. *Lancet, 362*(9380), 281–285.

Dalton, M. A., Tickle, J. J., Sargent, J. D., Beach, M. L., Ahrens, M. B., & Heatherton, T. F. (2002). The incidence and context of tobacco use in popular movies from 1988 to 1997. *Preventive Medicine, 34,* 516–523.

Distefan, J. M., Gilpin, E. A., Sargent, J. D., & Pierce, J. P. (1999). Do movie stars encourage adolescents to start smoking? Evidence from California. *Preventive Medicine, 28,* 1–11.

Distefan, J. M., Pierce, J. P., & Gilpin, E. A. (2004). Do favorite movie stars influence adolescent smoking initiation? *American Journal of Public Health, 94*(7), 1239–1244.

Evans, W. D., Wasserman, J., Bertoletti, E., & Martino, S. (2002). Branding behavior: The strategy behind the truth campaign. *Social Marketing Quarterly, 8*(3), 17–29.

Evans, W. D., Price, S., Blahut, S., Hersey, J., Niederdeppe, J., & Ray, S. (2004). Social imagery, tobacco dependence and the truth campaign. *Journal of Health Communication, 9,* 425–441.

Evans, W. D., Price, S., & Blahut, S. (2005). Evaluating the truth brand. *Journal of Health Communication, 10,* 181–192.

Farrelly, M.C., Nonnemaker, J., Davis, K.C. & Hussin, A. (2009). The influence of the national truth® campaign on smoking initiation. *American Journal of Preventive Medicine,* Feb 9. [Epub ahead of print].

Farrelly, M. C., Healton, C. G., Davis, K. C., Messeri, P., Hersey, J. C., & Haviland, M. L. (2002a). Getting to the truth: Evaluating national tobacco countermarketing campaigns. *American Journal of Public Health, 92*(6), 901–907.

Farrelly, M. C., Davis, K. C., Yarsevich, J., Haviland, M. L., Hersey, J. C., Girlando, M. E., & Healton, C. G. (2002b). *Getting to the truth: Assessing youths' reactions to the truth® and "Think. Don't Smoke" tobacco counter-marketing campaigns* [First Look Report 9]. Washington, DC: American Legacy Foundation.

Farrelly, M. C., Davis, K. C., Haviland, M. L., Messeri, P., & Healton, C. G. (2005). Evidence of a dose-response relationship between "truth" antismoking ads and youth smoking prevalence. *American Journal of Public Health, 95*(3), 425–431.

Fichtenberg, C. M., & Glantz, S. A. (2000). Association of the California Tobacco Control Program with declines in cigarette consumption and mortality from heart disease. *New England Journal of Medicine, 343*(24), 1772-1777.

Fishbein M. (1967). A consideration of beliefs and their role in attitude measurement. In M Fishbein (Ed.), *Readings in attitude theory and measurement* (p. 257–266). New York, NY: Wiley.

Flay, B. R. (1987). Mass media and smoking cessation: A critical review. *American Journal of Public Health, 77*(2), 153–160.

Flay, B. R., & Burton, D. (1990). Effective mass media communication strategies or health campaigns. In C. Atkin and L. Wallack (Eds.), *Mass communication and public health: Complexities and Conflicts* (p. 129–146). Newbury Park, CA: Sage.

Gilpin, F. A., Fmery, S. L., Farkas, A. J., Distefan, J. M., White, M. M., & Pierce, J. P. (2001). *The California Tobacco Control Program: A Decade of Progress, Results from the California Tobacco Surveys, 1990-1998.* La Jolla, CA: University of California, San Diego.

Goldman, L. K., & Glantz, S. A. (1998). Evaluation of antismoking advertising campaigns. *Journal of the American Medical Association, 279*(10), 772–777.

Goldstein, A. O., Sobel, R. A., & Newman, G. R. (1999). Tobacco and alcohol use in G-rated children's animated movies. *Journal of the American Medical Association, 28*(12), 1131–1136.

Healton, C. G., Watson-Stryker, E. S., Allen, J. A., Vallone, D. M., Messeri, P. A., Graham, P. R., Stewart, A. M., Dobbins, M. D., & Glantz, S. A. (2006). Televised movie trailers: Undermining restrictions on advertising tobacco to youth. *Archives of Pediatric and Adolescent Medicine, 160*(9), 885–888.

Hersey, J. C., Niederdeppe, J., Ng, S. W., Mowery, P., Farrelly, M., & Messeri, P. (2005). How state counter-industry campaigns help prime perceptions of tobacco industry practices to promote reductions in youth smoking. *Tobacco Control, 14*(6), 377–383.

Holtgrave, D.R., Wunderink, K.A., Vallone, D.M. & Healton, C.G. (2009). Cost-Utility Analysis of the National truth® Campaign to Prevent Youth Smoking. *American Journal of Preventive Medicine*, Feb 9. [Epub ahead of print]

Hornik, R. (Ed.). (2002). *Public health communication: Evidence for behavior change.* London, NJ: Lawrence Erlbaum Associates, Publishers.

Institute of Medicine. (2007). *Ending the tobacco problem: A blueprint for the nation.* Washington, DC: The National Academies Press.

Johnston, L. D., O'Malley, P. M., Bachman, J. G., & Schulenberg, J. E. (2007). *Monitoring the Future national survey results on drug use, 1975-2006: Volume I, Secondary school students* (NIH Publication No. 07-6205). Bethesda, MD: National Institute on Drug Abuse.

Lewis, M. J., & Wackowski, O. (2006). Dealing with an innovative industry: A look at flavored cigarettes promoted by mainstream brands. *American Journal of Public Health, 96*(2), 244–251.

Lewit, E. M., Coate, D., & Grossman, M. (1981). The effects of government regulation on teenage smoking. *Journal of Law and Economics, 24*(3), 545–569.

Lorillard Tobacco Company v. American Legacy Foundation, 903 A.2d 728 (Del Supr. 2006).

Martin, C. A., Kelly, T. H., Rayens, M. K., Brogli, B. R., Brenzel, A., Smith, W. J., & Omar, H. A. (2002). Sensation seeking, puberty, and nicotine, alcohol, and marijuana use in adolescence. *Journal of the American Academy of Child and Adolescent Psychiatry, 41*, 1495–1502.

McKenna, J., Gutierrez, K., & McCall, K. (2000). Strategies for an effective youth counter-marketing program: Recommendations from commercial marketing experts. *Journal of Public Health Management and Practice, 6*(3), 7–13.

Mekemson, C., Glik, D., Titus, K., Myerson, A., Shaivitz, A., Ang, A., & Mitchell, S. (2004). Tobacco use in popular movies during the past decade. *Tobacco Control*, *13*(4), 400–402.

Messeri, P. A., Allen, J. A., Mowery, P. D., Healton, C. G., Haviland, M. L., Gable, J. M., & Pedrazzani, S. D. (2007). Do tobacco countermarketing campaigns increase adolescent under-reporting of smoking? *Addictive Behavior*, *32*(7), 1532–1536.

National Cancer Institute. (2008). *The role of the media in promoting and reducing tobacco use* (Tobacco Control Monograph No. 19; NIH Pub No. 07-6242). Bethesda, MD: U.S. Department of Health and Human Services, National Institutes of Health, National Cancer Institute.

Niederdeppe, J., Fiore, M. C., Baker, T. B., & Smith, S. S. (2008). Smoking-cessation media campaigns and their effectiveness among socioeconomically advantaged and disadvantaged populations. *Am J Public Health*, *98*(5), 916–924.

Office of Attorney General, California Department. (1998). *Master Settlement Agreement*. Available at http://ag.ca.gov/tobacco/pdf/1msa.pdf. Accessed December 13, 2007.

Palmgreen, P., Donohew, L., Lorch, E. P., Hoyle, R. H., & Stephenson, M. T. (2001). Television campaigns and adolescent marijuana use: Tests of sensation seeking targeting. *American Journal of Public Health*, *91*, 292–296.

Palmgreen, P., Donohew, L., Lorch, E. P., Rogus, M., Helm, D., & Grant, N. (1991). Sensation seeking, message sensation value, and drug use as mediators of PSA effectiveness. *Health Communication*, *3*, 217–227.

Palmgreen, P., Lorch, E. P., Donohew, L., Harrington, N. G., D'Silva, M., & Helm, D. (1995) Reaching at-risk populations in a mass media drug abuse prevention campaign: Sensation seeking as a target variable. *Drugs and Society*, *8*, 27–45.

Palmgreen, P., Stephenson, M. T., Everett, M. W., Baseheart, J. R., & Francies, R. (2002). Perceived message sensation value (PMSV) and the dimensions and validation of a PMSV scale. *Health Communication*, *14*, 403–428.

Pechmann, C., & Shih, C. (1999). Smoking scenes in movies and antismoking advertisements before movies: Effects on youth. *Journal of Marketing*, *63*, 1–13.

Reputation Management. (1998). Why Just Say No Won't Do. *Reputation Management*, 26–40.

R.J. Reynolds Tobacco Company; Lorillard Tobacco Company; R. J. Reynolds Smoke Shop, Inc. v. Sandra Shewry, Director of the California Department of Health Services; Dileep G. Bal, Acting Chief of the Tobacco Control Section of the California Department of Health Services; State of California. United States District Court, Eastern District of California. September 28, 2004.

Rosenstock, I. M., Strecher, V. J., & Becker, M. H. (1988). Social learning theory and the Health Belief Model. *Health Education Quarterly*, *15*(2), 175–183.

Sargent, J. D. (2005). Smoking in movies: impact on adolescent smoking. *Adolescent Medicine Clinics*, *16*(2), 345–370.

Sargent, J. D., Beach, M. L., Adachi-Mejia, A. M., Gibson, J. J., Titus-Ernstoff, L. T., Carusi, C. P., Swain, S. D. Heatherton, T. F., & Dalton, M. A. (2005). Exposure to movie smoking: Its relation to smoking initiation among U.S. adolescents. *Pediatrics*, *116*(5), 1183–1191.

Sargent, J. D., Dalton, M. A., Beach, M. L., Mott, L. A., Tickle, J. J., Ahrens, M. B., & Heatherton, T. F. (2002). Viewing tobacco use in movies. Does it shape attitudes that mediate adolescent smoking? *American Journal of Preventive Medicine*, *22*(3), 137–145.

Sargent, J., Worth, K., & Tanski, S. (2006). *Legacy First Look Report 16. Trends in top box office movie tobacco use 1996-2004.* Washington, DC: American Legacy Foundation.

Siegel, M. (1998). Mass media antismoking campaigns: A powerful tool for health promotion. *Annals of Internal Medicine, 129*(2), 128–132.

Siegel, M., & Biener, L. (2000). The impact of an antismoking media campaign on progression to established smoking: results of a longitudinal youth study. *American Journal of Public Health, 90*(3), 380–386.

Slater, M. D. (2003). Sensation-seeking as a moderator of the effects of peer influences, consistency with personal aspirations, and perceived harm on marijuana and cigarette use among younger adolescents. *Substance Use and Misuse, 38*, 865–880.

Sly, D. F., Arheart, K., Dietz, N., Trapido, E. J., Nelson, D., Rodriguez, R., McKenna, J., & Lee, D. (2005). The outcome consequences of defunding the Minnesota youth tobacco-use prevention program. *Preventive Medicine, 41*(2), 503–510.

Sly, D. F., Hopkins, R. S., Trapido, E., & Ray, S. (2001). Influence of a counteradvertising media campaign on initiation of smoking: The Florida "truth" campaign. *American Journal of Public Health, 91*(2), 233–238.

Sly, D. F., Trapido, E., & Ray, S. (2002). Evidence of the dose effects of an antitobacco counteradvertising campaign. *Preventive Medicine, 35*, 511–518.

Stephenson, M. T., Hoyle, R. H., Palmgreen, P., & Slater, M. D. (2003). Brief measures of sensation seeking for screening and large-scale surveys. *Drug and Alcohol Dependence, 72*, 279–286.

Thompson, K. M., & Yokota, F. (2001). Depiction of alcohol, tobacco, and other substances in G-rated animated feature movies. *Pediatrics, 107*(6), 1369–1374.

Tickle, J. J., Sargent, J. D., Dalton, M. A., Beach, M. L., & Heatherton, T. F. (2001). Favorite movie stars, their tobacco use in contemporary movies, and its association with adolescent smoking. *Tobacco Control, 10*(10), 16–22.

U.S. Department of Health and Human Services. (1989). *Reducing the health consequences of smoking: 25 years of progress. A report of the Surgeon General* [DHHS Publication No. 89-8411] Washington, DC: U.S. Department of Health and Human Services, Public Health Service, Centers for Disease Control, Center for Chronic Disease Prevention and Health Promotion, Office on Smoking and Health.

Vallone, D., Allen, J. A. & Xiao, H. Is Socioeconomic status associated with awareness of and receptivity to the truth® campaign? In press at *Drug and Alcohol Dependence.*

Vallone, D., Allen, J. A., Clayton, R. R., & Xiao, H. (2007). How reliable and valid is the brief sensation seeking scale (BSSS-4) for youth of various racial/ethnic groups? *Addiction, 102*(2S), 71–78.

Vargyas, E. (2007). Opposition to effective social marketing: Lorillard Tobacco Company's failed attempt to shut down the American Legacy Foundation. *Cases in Public Health Communication and Marketing.* Available at http://www.gwumc.edu/sphhs/departments/pch/phcm/casesjournal/index.cfm. Accessed December 13, 2007.

Wakefield, M., Terry-McElrath, Y., Emery, S., Saffer, H., Chaloupka, F. J., Szczypka, G., Flay, B., O'Malley, P. M., & Johnston, L. D. (2006). Effect of televised, tobacco company-funded smoking prevention advertising on youth smoking-related beliefs, intentions, and behavior. *American Journal of Public Health, 96*(12), 2154–2160.

Wakefield, M. A., Durkin, S., Spittal, M. J., Siahpush, M., Scollo, M., Simpson, J. A., Chapman, S., White, V., & Hill, D. (2008). Impact of tobacco control policies and mass media campaigns on monthly adult smoking prevalence. *American Journal of Public Health, 12,* 1443-1450.

Warner, K. E. (1986). Selling health: A media campaign against tobacco. *Journal of Public Health Policy, 7*(4), 434–439.

Warner, K. F. (2001). Related tobacco control policy: From action to evidence and back again. *American Journal of Preventive Medicine, 20*(2S), 2–5.

Warner, K. E., & Murt, H. A. (1982). Impact of the antismoking campaign on smoking prevalence: A cohort analysis. *Journal of Public Health Policy, 3*(4), 374–390.

Wunderink, K., Allen, J. A., Xiao, H., Duke, J., Green, M., & Vallone D. (2007). *American Legacy First Look Report 17. Cigarette preferences among youth: Results from the 2006 Legacy Media Tracking Online (LMTO).* Washington, DC: American Legacy Foundation.

Zucker, D., Hopkins, R. S., Sly, D. F., Urich, J., Kershaw, J. M., & Solari, S. (2000). Florida's "truth" campaign: A counter-marketing, anti-tobacco media campaign. *Journal of Public Health Management and Practice, 6*(3), 1–6.

Zuckerman, M., Ball, S., & Black, J. (1990). Influences of sensation seeking, gender, risk appraisal, and situational motivation on smoking. *Addictive Behavior, 5,* 209–220.

Case Study of a Data Informed Response to Youth Gun Violence: Pennsylvania Injury Reporting and Intervention System (PIRIS)

Michelle R. Henry, BA
Robert D. Ketterlinus, PhD

OBJECTIVES

After reading this chapter, you should

- Understand the value of a multisystem collaborative violence prevention effort for young people
- Understand the link between injury surveillance and reporting and individual-level intervention
- Be able to define uses of data collected from program participants

KEY TERMS

Case management	Management information system
Firearm-related injury	Multisystem intervention
Injury surveillance	Violence intervention

Introduction

Gunshot wounds are a leading cause of death in the United States, accounting for 11,624 homicides; 16,750 suicides; and 235 unintentionally inflicted shooting deaths in 2004 (Centers for Disease Control [CDC], 2004). In urban areas, homicides comprise the majority of firearm-related death, and young people—youth between the ages of 15 and 24 years—are at greatest risk. Firearm-related homicide is the second most common cause of death among Americans of this age group, second only to deaths from motor vehicle accidents (CDC, 2004).

Firearm injuries are costly. In 2000, the total lifetime cost of firearm injuries for 15- to 24-year-olds in the United States was more than $12 billion. For Pennsylvanians age 15 to 24 years, firearm injuries were the 2nd leading cause of death and the 6th leading cause of injury hospitalization in 2004. The total hospitalization charges for firearm injuries in this age group were about $61.6 million (CDC, 2004).

In March 2005, Pennsylvania Governor Edward G. Rendell established the Commission to Address Gun Violence to recommend changes that emphasize prevention, community focus, and collaboration to reduce gun violence. An extensive report included a recommendation to develop and implement a hospital-based **injury surveillance** system that is actively connected to social service and intervention providers (Commonwealth of Pennsylvania, 2005a). In response to this, the Pennsylvania Department of Health created a unique pilot project called the Pennsylvania Injury Reporting and Intervention System (PIRIS) to address gun violence among 15- to 24-year-olds in Philadelphia. (Commonwealth of Pennsylvania, 2005b). The goal of PIRIS is to reduce the risk of recurring violence among young victims of gunshots and their peers by connecting gunshot victims and their families with needed social services that might be beneficial to their recovery, health, and overall well-being.

PIRIS was designed to improve the well-being of the participants and their families by addressing medical, economic, and mental health needs, as well as by helping participants resume daily activities. Support provided by the program helps young people continue to make a healthy transition to adulthood (work and education) and helps participants, caregivers, and families avoid some of the catastrophic impacts of these injuries (economic and psychosocial).

PIRIS is currently being implemented at 3 Philadelphia hospital trauma centers: Albert Einstein Medical Center; the Hospital of the University of Pennsylvania; and Temple University Hospital. In 2005, together these hospitals treated 39% of **firearm-related injuries** among persons ages 15 to 24 years in the commonwealth (Pennsylvania Trauma Systems Foundation, 2005). With the goal of providing immediate intervention when a firearm victim is admitted to one of these trauma centers, the hospital emergency room and/or trauma social workers introduce the PIRIS project to all gunshot victims between the ages of 15 and 24 years of age who are admitted to the hospital, and upon written permission from the patient and/or his or her legal guardian, the social workers make a referral to Public Health Management Corporation's (PHMC) PIRIS case management intervention staff.

PIRIS Components

There are four main components to PIRIS: case management services, community level **violence intervention**, a quality and improvement assessment of the case management component, and comprehensive injury surveillance. Enrollment in the **case management** component of PIRIS provides the participant with a variety of information and referral services, including assistance with health insurance, education, job training, counseling, family needs, legal issues, parenting, and recreational activities. Intervention services are also provided to the families of the participants. PIRIS aims to help the participants and their family members to recognize the conditions that may have contributed to their exposure to violence and to develop individual plans to help prevent further violence.

In addition to serving participants and their families, the PIRIS program addresses violence on a community level. The Philadelphia Anti-Drug/Anti-Violence Network (PAAN) is a PIRIS partner charged with providing community outreach services specifically targeted to communities or neighborhoods where the shootings took place and where the participants live. PAAN is given data on the incident locations from PHMC PIRIS intervention staff and organizes community rallies and special events aimed to bring together community members, government, and other stakeholders to address the violence that is taking place in their communities. Activities that take place during these rallies include information sharing on available services, resources, and job opportunities, as well as identifying community problems that need to be addressed, such as lighting on the street and the need for police presence.

PHMC researchers lead the quality and improvement assessment component of PIRIS, collecting and analyzing extensive PIRIS basic client and service data as well as results from several assessment survey instruments used to monitor and report on the impact of the case management services, to refine the PIRIS project, and to make recommendations for future anti-violence interventions.

PIRIS also contains a comprehensive injury surveillance component. This larger data collection effort is spearheaded by the Firearm Injury Center at Penn, the Center for Clinical Epidemiology and Biostatistics, and the Pennsylvania Trauma System Foundation. This effort is designed to enhance the state's ability to replicate PIRIS throughout the commonwealth and helps to identify individual and system outcomes that are used to evaluate the effectiveness of PIRIS interventions and the value of the data collection system.

Figures 11-1 and 11-2 further illustrate the PIRIS **multisystem intervention** approach and how PIRIS partners collaborate to provide data and coordinate services to PIRIS participants. Table 11-1 provides a comprehensive list of all PIRIS collaborative partners.

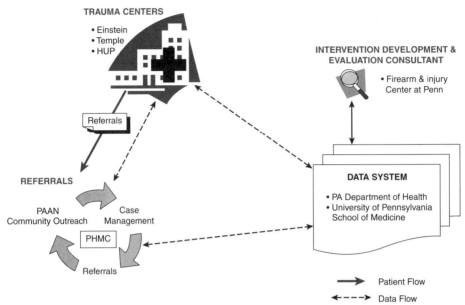

Figure 11-1 PIRIS Structure and Operations
Source: Pennsylvania Department of Health.

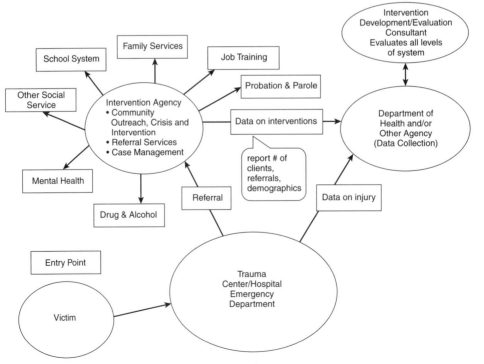

Figure 11-2 The PIRIS Multi-Intervention System Approach
Source: Pennsylvania Department of Health.

Table 11-1 PIRIS Collaborative Partners *Source:* Pennsylvania Department of Health.	Pennsylvania Department of Health (PA DOH)
	Philadelphia Department of Public Health (PDPH)
	Public Health Management Corporation (PHMC)
	Albert Einstein Medical Center (AEMC)
	Temple University Hospital (TUH)
	Hospital of the University of Pennsylvania (HUP)
	Firearm & Injury Center at Penn (FICAP), University of Pennsylvania
	Pennsylvania Trauma Systems Foundation (PTSF)
	Center for Clinical Epidemiology and Biostatistics (CCEB), University of Pennsylvania
	Philadelphia Anti-Drug / Anti-Violence Network (PAAN)

About the PIRIS Case Study

This case study examines the development and ongoing quality and improvement assessment of this public health approach and the unique collaboration of PIRIS partners to address the repercussions of gun violence among 15- to 24-year-olds. In the next sections, we provide brief descriptions of the two main PIRIS components—the PIRIS Reporting System and PIRIS Intervention—including a discussion of data collected and how data is used to inform program implementation and improvement.

Description of PIRIS Reporting System

Description of the System

Establishing a gunshot injury data system to identify youth who have been shot and to collect individual-level information on each victim helps (1) determine the incidence of gunshot injury among this population, (2) describe characteristics of the victims, and (3) recruit patients into the PIRIS intervention.

The way the PIRIS surveillance data system works is that each trauma center in the state has an individual serving full time as the trauma registrar, who, on a daily basis, enters the medical charts of new patients who are treated at their center for traumatic injuries. Through an agreement with the Pennsylvania Trauma Systems Foundation, these in-hospital data are integrated into the PIRIS data system. Although entered daily, the data are accessed for the purposes of PIRIS on a periodic basis, rather than daily. This process is typical of how surveillance systems are designed, because they are generally used to produce information that is analyzed for epidemiologic research conducted retrospectively.

The intervention component of PIRIS, however, identifies patients in real time so that they can be contacted in person and recruited as intervention participants.[1] This recruitment effort is being conducted by staff members in each trauma center, as described in the following section.

The PIRIS surveillance data system is supplemented by links to another existing data source: the Weapons Related Injury Surveillance System (WRISS). WRISS was initiated in 2002 and is overseen by the Philadelphia Police Department, toward the goal of identifying and collecting information on each shooting that occurs in Philadelphia (Ahlman, L., Kurtz, E., and Flint, A., 2007). The WRISS data was made available to the PIRIS project by the Philadelphia Adult Probation and Parole Department.

Description of PIRIS Intervention, Data Collected, and Use of Data

Description of the Intervention

PIRIS-participating hospital trauma center staff (typically a social worker) identifies youth eligible for the PIRIS intervention—15- to 24-year-old gunshot victims who are admitted to the hospital and who are not in police custody. The program identifies only those who are admitted to the hospital; patients who are seen and released from the emergency department are not included in either the data system or recruitment into interventions.

Hospital social workers approach potential PIRIS clients once they have been admitted and stabilized. The social worker explains the program to the youth and his or her parents, if appropriate, and asks if they would like to talk to a PHMC case manager about the program. If the youth and his or her parents agree, the social worker faxes a referral form to PHMC that includes youth and parent contact information. A PHMC case manager contacts the youth to schedule a time to meet and to explain more about the program. If the youth agrees to participate in the program, the case manager schedules a home visit with the youth and his or her parents. During the home visit, the case manager gathers more information about the youth and family and conducts an initial needs assessment. The case manager then creates a service plan that includes information about and referrals to agencies that can help the youth and his or her parents obtain services addressing their needs, including obtaining health insurance, education, job

---

[1] Each PIRIS participant has an electronic record created, maintained, and stored in the PIRIS database. Only PIRIS employees have access to the participant data, and individual paper records are kept in locked files. PIRIS case management staff and other authorized program partners have access to participant records. At the time of enrollment, participants or their authorized representative, sign Consent to Participate and Share Information forms, granting permission to share their personal information gathered throughout the intervention with other PIRIS partners. This authorization form expires in 1 year from the date of signature and must be renewed each year if the participant is still active in the program.

training, transportation, counseling, legal assistance, parenting support, recreational activities, and other services. The needs assessment and service plan are updated periodically as needed.

Data Collected

Assessment is an ongoing process that the case manager begins early in the relationship with the PIRIS participant and re-evaluates on a regular basis. Information gathered throughout the case management process includes, but is not limited to, age, gender, ethnicity, household composition, health history, employment history, educational level, legal issues, relationship issues, history of child abuse, substance abuse issues, mental health history, financial status, and parenting issues, if applicable. In addition, the case manager and participant jointly identify problems and associated goals to work on throughout the participant's tenure in the program. The assessment process aims to answer the following questions:

- What kind of life experiences has the participant had prior to the gunshot incident and enrollment in the PIRIS intervention?
- What is going on now for the participant?
- What is the most important or immediate issue at this time?
- Where would the participant like to be?
- What resources, talents, or experiences can he or she use to make the desired changes?
- What steps does he or she need to take to make the changes?

Information gathered from the assessment is documented into PIRIS's **management information system** (MIS). Because the assessment is an ongoing process throughout the participant's tenure in the program, the database is updated as the participant's status is altered, goals change, or new resources are acquired. Furthermore, while the participant is in the program, the case manager enters participant needs assessments and service plans into the MIS, records the status of each goal identified by the participant (e.g., goal achieved, in progress, not achieved), and documents the reason that the participant is discharged from the program (length of participation is also recorded in the MIS). The MIS is also used to record the service referrals and services received, as well as the type and number of contacts between case managers and participants and family members.

Initial Case Management Assessment

The initial case management assessment is guided by three primary case management assessment tools: the Global Appraisal of Individuals Needs—Quick (GAIN-Q); a risk assessment; and a case record face sheet.

The GAIN-Q instrument is a widely used evidence-based biopsychosocial assessment used to identify various life problems among adolescents and adults in the general population (Dennis & Kaminer, 2006; Titus & Dennis, 2003). The GAIN-Q is administered by the PIRIS case manager within 30 days of the initial home visit and helps the case manager identify a variety of problems that the gunshot victim may have experienced prior to his or her enrollment in the program, including low educational and employment status, sources of stress, involvement in violence (as a victim and perpetrator), physical and mental health, and legal and substance abuse related problems.

The GAIN-Q intake assessment asks participants to reflect on their personal experiences over their lifetime, during the past year (12 months), during the past 90 days, and at the current time. By asking questions that refer to these different time periods, case managers can assess lifetime risk factors and experiences, determine current case management and social service needs, and monitor progress towards achieving case management goals. In addition, research and evaluation staff, using primarily questions pertaining to the past 90 days and at the current time, can similarly monitor participant progress during PIRIS participation and postdischarge. The GAIN-Q takes approximately 15 minutes to administer, and participants receive a $20 payment for each completed GAIN-Q assessment to reimburse them for their time.

While the participant is still in the program, the case manager administers a follow-up version of the GAIN-Q, called the GAIN-Q Monitoring instrument (GAIN-QM), every 3 months in order to track changes in participant's problems. After the participant is discharged from the program, PHMC research staff continues to administer the GAIN-QM up until 1 year after program discharge.

The risk assessment tool was originally created to predict participants who are most difficult to engage in the program, to predict which participants are least likely to achieve their goals, and to identify participants who would most benefit from intensive supportive services soon after they enroll in the program. After a brief pilot period, the risk assessment tool was revised with a shift in perspective and purpose so that the emphasis is less on predicting success and is instead on ensuring that case managers use the assessment data they collect about a participant's personal history to make appropriate referrals to needed social services.

The case record face sheet is used by case managers to document and ensure systematic collection of participant demographic and contact information; current involvement with the criminal justice system, social service system, and other antiviolence programs; circumstances of the gunshot incident that led the youth to PIRIS eligibility; housing conditions and needs; and social support (e.g., living with others, involvement in a religious community).

Case Management Quality and Improvement Assessment

PHMC researchers employ several assessment and survey instruments to assess the case management component of PIRIS. The assessment tools used include the GAIN-Q assessment, the GAIN-QM assessment, a GAIN Supplemental Assessment, and a case management Client Satisfaction Survey. The newly revised risk assessment was implemented as part of the case management intake process in September 2008 as another instrument used to measure case management effectiveness. This tool will be used primarily as a mechanism for determining whether appropriate referrals were made to social service agencies during the case management process.

As noted earlier, the GAIN-Q is a full biopsychosocial evaluation tool for clinical assessment (diagnosis, individualized treatment planning) and program evaluation. The GAIN-QM is a tool for monitoring how individuals respond to treatment and services during and/or after program participation. The GAIN-QM contains a subset of questions from the GAIN-Q intake assessment, so it is possible to evaluate an individual's progress using both survey instruments.

The GAIN-QM is administered to PIRIS participants every 90 days postintake throughout the duration of program participation and at 6 and 12 months postdischarge. The GAIN-QM is administered by PIRIS case management staff while the participant is enrolled in the program and then by PHMC research staff postdischarge. PIRIS participants receive a cash incentive each time they complete the GAIN-Q and GAIN-QM surveys.

The GAIN Supplemental Assessment is administered to former PIRIS participants at 6 and 12 months postdischarge by PHMC research staff. The supplemental survey assesses postprogram progress towards specific individual goals established during case management and monitors education, employment, and health status as well as recurrence of violence. Participants receive a cash incentive each time they complete the GAIN Supplemental Assessment.

The Client Satisfaction Survey asks former PIRIS participants to reflect on their experiences about case management assistance with specific needs, case management adherence to protocol and appropriate behavior, and communication with case managers. This survey is administered by PHMC research staff within 30 days after discharge from the program. Participants receive a $10 cash incentive for completing the survey.

A summary of intervention-related data currently collected and used to inform program implementation and program improvement is presented in Table 11-2. All data is entered into the MIS for access by PIRIS case management, research, and administrative staff.

Use of Data to Inform Program Implementation and Improvement

PHMC's research team utilizes a general framework for assessment of the PIRIS intervention and use of data for program implementation and improvement. PHMC's PIRIS intervention team, including case management and research staff, engages in five phases of a continuous inquiry and learning process using data described in the previous section.

Framework for Selection and Use of PIRIS Intervention Data to Inform Program Implementation and Improvement

- Phase 1: Planning and preparing to conduct a program evaluation
- Phase 2: Collecting and documenting data
- Phase 3: Analyzing and interpreting the data
- Phase 4: Sharing results with stakeholders
- Phase 5: Action planning and final report

Source: Camino, Zeldin, Mook, and O'Connor, 2004.

Instrument	Key Measures	When Administered	Who Administers
GAIN-Q	Demographics, lifetime experiences, sources of stress, physical health, emotional and behavioral health, substance use, service utilization	Intake, every 3 months during PIRIS enrollment	PIRIS case managers
GAIN-QM	Subset of GAIN-Q questions pertaining to experiences and service utilization in the past 90 days	Every 90 days postintake throughout the duration of program participation and at 6 and 12 months postdischarge	PIRIS case managers and PHMC research staff
GAIN Supplement	Post-program progress toward goals established during case management (e.g., education, employment, and health goals), recurrence of violence	Six and 12 months postdischarge	PHMC research staff
Risk Assessment	Service referrals	Intake	PIRIS case managers
Case Record Sheet	Demographic and contact information, service system involvement, circumstances of the gunshot incident, housing conditions and needs, social support	Intake	PIRIS case managers
Client Satisfaction Survey	Satisfaction with case management services	Within 30 days after discharge	PHMC research staff
Case Management Data	Needs, goals, goal attainment, service referrals, services received, time in program, number of case management contacts, reasons for discharge7	Ongoing data collection and assessment	PIRIS case managers

Table 11-2
PIRIS Intervention Data and Data Sources
Source: Pennsylvania Department of Health.

For the purposes of the PIRIS project, Phase 4 (sharing the results with the group) involves sharing results with the intervention staff during intervention team meetings and sharing results with the PIRIS partners (as shown in Table 11-1) at quarterly PIRIS project meetings. Furthermore, the report mentioned in Phase 5 (action planning and finalizing the report) includes both informal reports for the intervention team and formal progress reports to the PIRIS funder and other partners.

The following examples illustrate how PIRIS intervention data have been used to inform program implementation and improvement.

Example 1: Use of Data to Inform Program Implementation and Improvement

PIRIS data is used to improve program processes and to target, improve, and expand the many components of the intervention. Examining data on total number of gunshot wound patients, along with the numbers of eligible and recruited participants, helped improve hospital and case management data collection and recruitment processes. Using this data to project additional patient load has helped guide plans to expand the system. Data from the pilot project also contributes to plans for other trauma centers to assure that those plans use the most effective and efficient ways of targeting postdischarge services to young gunshot wound patients.

All partners are provided with feedback from the PIRIS data system. This has helped each institution document the importance of providing follow-up care to young gunshot patients and to increase their focus on preventing future injury. Data also are used to identify ways that other service systems can be improved, based on challenges that are documented by case managers as they work with participants and their families. Data relevant to optimal operation of PIRIS components, as well as information on best practices targeted to participant characteristics, are shared with all PIRIS partners and an advisory group of public health and community experts. Problems and opportunities are then identified, and specific actions are proposed in response. This represents an important part of an ongoing, continuous quality assessment and improvement process for PIRIS components and the PIRIS system as a whole.

Example 2: Types and Number of Participant Goals

An analysis of the first 103 completed GAIN-Q intake assessment surveys completed by newly enrolled PIRIS participants[2] found that 80 participants (80.0%) responded that they want help with family, school, work, health, emotional, behavioral, alcohol, drug, or legal problems. When asked to describe more specifically with what they wanted help, PIRIS participants said that they needed help with finding a job; graduating from school or earning a GED; obtaining, maintaining, or managing health insurance; emotional well-being; recovering from physical injuries sustained in the gun-related incident that brought them to PIRIS; housing; loans; substance abuse; paying bills; transportation; clothing; food; and legal issues. These responses are reflected in the goals that are set for the participant as part of the intensive case management provided by PIRIS.

Analysis of the case management service plans (recorded in the PIRIS MIS) for the first 44 participants discharged from PIRIS showed that out of 12

---

[2] More than 100 GAIN-Q intake assessments were completed with newly enrolled PIRIS participants from May 2006 through July 2008 ($n = 103$).

different categories of goals,[3] participants identified the greatest number of goals in the areas of health (133 goals made), education (80 goals), and employment problems and needs (92 goals). Together, these goals accounted for over one-half (52.6%) of the 580 goals made by this PIRIS cohort.

These findings reflected the case managers' anecdotal reports regarding participants' goals and helped reinforce the case managers' efforts to allocate more of their time seeking new sources of health, education, and employment services. The identification of these goals illustrates the need for post-discharge services that help young gunshot wound victims stay, or get back on track from health transitions to becoming productive adults.

Given the traumatic nature of the gunshot violence experienced by PIRIS participants, the PIRIS intervention team expected that youth would identify mental health services as a goal, and given the age range of the participants, it was anticipated that substance abuse services might also be a fairly common goal. However, findings from the first 44 discharged PIRIS participants show just 5% of goals set (4.8%, $n = 28$) as pertaining to behavioral health (substance abuse and mental health) services. This percentage seems quite low given anecdotal reports from case managers that a large majority of PIRIS participants smoke marijuana on almost a daily basis. (Case managers report that participants generally do not view their drug use as a problem.)

In contrast to the goals set, GAIN-Q intake assessment data for the first 103 participants enrolled in PIRIS reveal that PIRIS participants experienced a wide range of personal stresses during the 12 months prior to the gunshot incident that led to PIRIS enrollment. For instance, some participants reported deaths of a family member or close friend (30.7%, $n = 31$), both in gun violence related incidents and in accidents, and several reported that they witnessed these fatal events. In addition, two-thirds (63.4%, or 64 individuals) reported that during the past 12 months, they were attacked with a weapon, beaten, sexually abused, or emotionally abused.[4] One in 4 PIRIS participants reported symptoms of depression; 25 (25.0%) reported feeling very trapped, lonely, sad, blue, depressed, or hopeless about the future. In addition, 45% of PIRIS participants ($n = 45$) reported using alcohol, marijuana, cocaine, heroin, or other substances during the 12 months prior to the gunshot incident. These findings suggest the need for different approaches to screening and assessing mental health and substance abuse service needs for participating youth, perhaps resolving issues of stigma or institutional barriers to appropriate interventions.

These data corroborated case managers' intuition of "hidden" behavioral problems and, in turn, have stimulated case managers to address the

---

[3] The 12 categories of PIRIS participant goals include children, education, employment, finances, health (physical and mental), housing, legal, parenting education, program participation, relationships, sexual health, and substance abuse.

[4] From the data, we do not know if participants were referencing the gun-related incident that led to their PIRIS enrollment.

apparent disconnect among some participants about problems that can result from this type of illegal drug use. For example, case managers discovered that some participants are not aware that some employers require a drug test as part of the hiring process and/or administer random drug tests. Case managers talk to youth about possible problems they may face if they continue to use drugs in these types of situations and discuss options for helping them become drug free, including referrals to appropriate behavioral health services.

Case managers have also observed that those participants having behavioral health problems (identified through reports by significant others or from other sources) have not admitted that they may have an alcohol or drug problem or have not sought help with their drug–alcohol problems by the third month in the program; it is unlikely that they will seek help with their problems as part of PIRIS. Therefore, an important lesson learned is that additional efforts and resources should be focused on identifying behavioral health problems as early after a participant is enrolled in the program as possible, preferably within the first month or two.

Example 3: Explaining Differences in Goal Attainment

There is no predetermined length of stay in the PIRIS program. There are two types of discharges: (1) participant initiated and (2) program initiated. An ideal discharge planning process is program initiated, whereby both the participant and the case manager feel that most or all case management goals have been met, and the participant is no longer in need of the intensive case management services provided through PIRIS. A participant-initiated discharge is one that takes place before the case manager deems it as being an appropriate time to initiate the discharge process. For example, if the participant states that he or she is no longer interested in receiving PIRIS services or moves out of the service area, a discharge letter is mailed to the participant. Other participant-initiated discharges similarly result from a case manager being unable to continue engaging with the participant (e.g., missed visits, unreturned phone calls) or as a result of a participant encountering legal issues that impede engagement (incarceration, arrest, or bench warrant).

The decision to discharge a PIRIS participant is made after the case management team reviews feedback given by the participant, his or her service plan, and status of his or her goals, as well as other relevant information obtained from probation officers, teachers, and other professionals working with the PIRIS participant and his or her family. Based on this review, the case management supervisor enters a discharge reason code in the PIRIS MIS. In this section, reasons for discharge are categorized as "case management completed" (e.g., goals and needs have been met) or "unable to continue engagement" (e.g., extenuating legal circumstances, such as incarceration, whereabouts unknown, or lack of contact with case management staff).

A recent analysis of MIS data about the first 44 participants discharged from PIRIS found that in state fiscal year 2008 (July 1, 2007, to June 30,

2008), 2 out of 3 PIRIS participants (65.9%) were discharged because they were unable to continue engagement (Table 11-3).

The intervention team was interested in learning about differences between these two groups and how to use this information to increase the number of participants who achieved their goals. The research team, using the GAIN-Q and GAIN-QM data housed in the MIS, found that the groups did not differ by gender, age, race, or probation status at enrollment, and there were no statistical differences in the number of goals identified by the two groups.

Length of Stay in PIRIS

Findings from previous analyses conducted and shared with case management staff showed that the longer a participant stays in the program, the more likely the participant will achieve his or her goals. Consequently, the case management team goal is to keep participants engaged for as long as possible. On average, participants discharged in state fiscal year 2008 had stayed in the program for approximately 5.7 months. Not surprisingly, there was noticeable difference in length of stay in PIRIS depending on the reason for discharge; those who were discharged because they had completed case management were in the program an average of 4 months longer than those who were unable to continue engagement (Table 11-4).

Goals Met

On the whole, PIRIS participants who completed case management developed and met a greater number of goals than did those discharged from PIRIS because they were unable to continue engagement. Overall, two-thirds of former PIRIS participants had met all or most of their goals by the time they were discharged. However, individuals who were discharged because they were unable to continue engagement had met far fewer goals than those who had completed case management (Table 11-5).

Tables 11-6 and 11-7 highlight progress made in selected goal areas among individuals discharged because they had completed case management and

Table 11-3
Reasons for Discharge from PIRIS, Fiscal Year 2008 (*n* = 44)
Source: PHMC PIRIS MIS.

Reason for Discharge	***n* (%)**
Case management completed	15 (34.1%)
Unable to continue engagement	29 (65.9%)

Table 11-4
Length of Stay in PIRIS by Reason for Discharge, Fiscal Year 2008 (*n* = 44)
Source: PHMC PIRIS MIS.

	Reason for Discharge	
	Case management completed (*n* = 15)	**Unable to continue engagement (*n* = 29)**
Average number of months (days)	8.5 (261 days)	4.1 (123 days)
Range in days	92–715	14–502

Table 11-5
Comparison of Goals
Met by Reasons for
Discharge from PIRIS,
Fiscal Year 2008 ($n = 44$)
Source: PHMC PIRIS MIS.

	All or Most Goals Met	Some or Few Goals Met	No Goals Met	Total
Case management completed	15 (100.0%)	0 (0.0%)	0 (0.0%)	15
Lack of engagement	13 (44.8%)	12 (41.4%)	4 (29.0%)	29
Total	28 (63.6%)	12 (27.3%)	4 (9.0%)	44

Table 11-6
Selected Goals and
Status of Discharged
PIRIS Participants
Who Completed Case
Management, Fiscal
Year 2008 ($n = 15$)
Source: PHMC PIRIS MIS.

	Goal Status n (%)				
Goal Area	Met	In Progress	Unmet	Discontinued	Total Goals Set
Employment	54 (81.8%)	5 (7.6%)	2 (3.0%)	5 (7.6%)	66
Education	45 (80.4%)	6 (10.7%)	1 (1.7%)	4 (7.1%)	56
Health	36 (85.7%)	2 (4.8%)	3 (7.1%)	1 (2.4%)	42
Financial	25 (71.4%)	0 (0.0%)	4 (11.4%)	6 (17.1%)	35
Legal	19 (86.4%)	0 (0.0%)	1 (4.5%)	2 (9.1%)	22
Relationships	10 (47.6%)	0 (0.0%)	4 (19.0%)	7 (33.3%)	21
Housing	15 (93.8%)	1 (6.3%)	0 (0.0%)	0 (0.0%)	16
Mental–Emotional health	11 (84.6%)	0 (0.0%)	1 (7.7%)	1 (7.7%)	13
Parenting education	8 (72.7%)	1 (9.1%)	0 (0.0%)	2 (18.2%)	11
Children	9 (100.0%)	0 (0.0%)	0 (0.0%)	0 (0.0%)	9
Substance abuse	2 (66.7%)	0 (0.0%)	0 (0.0%)	1 (33.3%)	3
Total	**234 (79.6%)**	**15 (5.1%)**	**16 (5.4%)**	**29 (9.9%)**	**294**

Table 11-7
Selected Goals and Sta-
tus Discharged PIRIS
Participants Unable to
Continue Engagement,
Fiscal Year 2008 ($n = 29$)
Source: PHMC PIRIS MIS.

	Goal Status n (%)				
Goal Area	Met	In Progress	Unmet	Discontinued	Total Goals Set
Employment	16 (61.5%)	3 (11.5%)	3 (11.5%)	4 (15.4%)	26
Education	12 (50.0%)	1 (4.2%)	5 (20.8%)	6 (25.0%)	24
Health	60 (78.9%)	1 (1.3%)	15 (19.7%)	0 (0.0%)	76
Financial	13 (46.4%)	1 (3.6%)	11 (39.3%)	3 (10.7%)	28
Legal	33 (91.7%)	0 (0.0%)	2 (5.6%)	1 (2.8%)	36
Relationships	4 (28.6%)	0 (0.0%)	5 (35.7%)	5 (35.7%)	14
Housing	18 (54.5%)	2 (6.1%)	7 (21.2%)	6 (18.2%)	33
Mental–Emotional health	0 (0.0%)	0 (0.0%)	1 (50.0%)	1 (50.0%)	2
Children	3 (100.0%)	0 (0.0%)	0 (0.0%)	0 (0.0%)	3
Parenting education	2 (66.7%)	0 (0.0%)	0 (0.0%)	1 (33.3%)	3
Substance abuse	6 (60.0%)	0 (0.0%)	4 (40.0%)	0 (0.0%)	10
Total	**167 (65.5%)**	**8 (3.1%)**	**53 (20.8%)**	**279 (10.6%)**	**255**

those unable to continue engagement, respectively. These analyses found that the individuals who completed case management set more employment and education goals, and individuals discharged because they were unable to continue engagement set more health and legal goals. More specifically,

- participants who were discharged because they completed case management set two and one-half times as many employment goals (66 vs. 26 goals set) and more than twice as many education goals (56 vs. 24 goals set) as did the group discharged for inability to continue engagement; and
- participants discharged because they were unable to continue engagement had set twice as many health goals (76 vs. 35 goals set) and 40% more legal goals (36 vs. 21 goals set) as did the group discharged because they had completed case management.

As noted earlier, the number and percentage of goals met were highest among participants discharged because they had completed case management. However, more legal goals were developed and met among participants discharged for inability to continue engagement than among participants discharged because they completed case management.

Findings regarding goals set and goal status at discharge again highlight the importance of extending participation in PIRIS so that immediate needs can first be addressed (e.g., health issues) and so that more complex and long-term goals, such as education and employment obtainment, can then be addressed.

Example 4: Addressing Program Strengths and Weaknesses Through Client Satisfaction

Retrospective Client Satisfaction Survey

Between April 2006 and February 8, 2008, 94 PIRIS participants were discharged from the program. As of June 30, 2008, efforts to contact all past participants had been initiated, and PIRIS interviewers had successfully completed satisfaction surveys with 35 of the 91 retrospective participants (38.5%) deemed eligible for this study. One individual declined to be interviewed and 2 former participants are unreachable because they have moved for personal or legal protection reasons. Results presented in this section are preliminary findings, as the retrospective survey is currently in process.

Locating Participants

PHMC research staff has devised a multipronged approach to facilitate location of individuals for participation solicitation: (1) phone calls are made to the most up-to-date phone numbers available in the MIS, as provided by case management; (2) home visits are conducted when phone contact is either not feasible (no working number) or is unsuccessful; and (3) prison records are checked to determine if inability to contact a former PIRIS participant is due to his or her incarceration. At the time of follow-up, six former PIRIS participants were incarcerated; of these, three have successfully completed satisfaction surveys.

Interviewers typically attempt 1 to 10 contacts before locating a participant and determining whether or not that individual will participate in the follow-up. Future analyses will examine the locating process to assess types (phone, home visit, prison visit) and number of contacts made to document the best way to reach this hard-to-find population. This information will be useful to interviewers and case managers in maintaining contact with this hard-to-reach population.

Preliminary Results

The Client Satisfaction Survey asks about case management assistance with specific needs, case management adherence to protocol and appropriate behavior, and communication with case managers. Selected results of the first 35 satisfaction surveys completed by PIRIS participants are discussed below.

Overall, former PIRIS participants reported satisfaction with case management services, with the vast majority (96.9%, $n = 33$) reporting that their case manager was helpful overall. Satisfaction with case management helpfulness in meeting specific needs was particularly high in the areas of assistance with maintaining family relationships (92.9%, $n = 26$); assistance with involvement in positive leisure-time activities (89.6%, $n = 26$); assistance with obtaining, maintaining, and/or resolving problems with benefits (86.2%, $n = 25$); and assistance with obtaining and using community resources, such as transportation and social agencies (82.8%, $n = 24$).

All but two former participants responded positively to questions regarding case management adherence to protocol and appropriate behavior. For example, the majority of participants agreed that case managers appropriately introduced themselves at intake, returned phone calls promptly, were available when needed, listened carefully, involved the participant's family, and seemed to understand the participant's unique needs. Feedback regarding specific or negative experiences, such as a case manager being unreachable due to a disconnected phone line, is immediately reported to case management staff and is readily addressed for improved service provision.

Finally, participants were given the opportunity to respond to an open-ended question regarding what they perceive to be their biggest accomplishments during PIRIS participation and/or ways in which the PIRIS case management program helped achieve their biggest accomplishments. Participants reported that PIRIS involvement in case management helped improve relationships and social skills, increase self-confidence and respect, access health benefits, get back into school, make appointments on time, and overcome fears.

- "My communication with my family was my biggest accomplishment."
- "The case manager would have us talk together and work out our issues, and me and my mother never worked out our problems; we just got into a lot of fights."

- "She [case manager] helped me to understand that I can go places and not think I will be shot again."
- "Biggest progress was to help me physically, mentally, and to get me back in working condition and ready to go for a job."

Two individuals from this cohort indicated that case management could be improved by ensuring that all previously scheduled meetings with clients are cancelled and rescheduled in a timely fashion and that case managers could increase efforts to help find employment.

- "Case manager no shows, reschedule after the fact."
- "I wish they would have helped me get a job and keep me off the street."

Assessing the Client Satisfaction Survey Going Forward

The Client Satisfaction Survey has been revised for implementation July 1, 2008, to include further opportunity for qualitative feedback. The Client Satisfaction Survey was revised to include further opportunity for qualitative feedback, and was implemented July 1, 2008. The additions to the survey should yield rich information regarding specific aspects of programming that PIRIS participants appreciated or would have like to have seen improved. This feedback will be shared with the case management staff on a quarterly basis at a minimum and more frequently as specific issues are identified through the survey. Future analyses will also explore factors that may impact satisfaction, such as demographics and situational factors such as incarceration.

PIRIS as a Pilot System

The pilot phase of PIRIS was designed around a continuous process of data-driven quality assessment and improvement. This allowed the system to work with existing resources and within the standard operations of each participating institution. This was done to assure that the system would be seen as corresponding with the goals and abilities of each institution, thereby adding value and improving chances for sustainability. Flexibility and ongoing participation of all partners in data-informed improvements have provided a wealth of data for taking this program to scale.

CONCLUDING REMARKS

Gun violence is prevalent across the nation and is a public health issue because it affects a large population, results in premature death and disability, and can be prevented. Longer-term assessment must be maintained to determine the impact of violence interventions, such as PIRIS, on the participant and society and the cost savings to the health care system and society related to the prevention of firearm injuries and hospitalizations.

The ongoing assessment of injury surveillance and individual level client information integration will add to the current understanding of evidence-based programming to prevent youth violence, as well as increase the success of replication of this program across the state.

DISCUSSION QUESTIONS

1. What are some benefits to having a hospital-based injury surveillance system that is actively connected to social service and intervention providers?
2. Name two ways in which client level data can be used to improve a case management program.
3. How do participants discharged from PIRIS, because they have completed case management, differ from those who self-initiate discharge?
4. Describe a multi-pronged approach to follow-up with a difficult-to-engage group of individuals.

REFERENCES

Ahlman, L., Kurtz, E., & Flint, A. (2007). *Weapons related injury surveillance system (WRISS) report, Philadelphia, PA 2002–2006.* Available at http://fjd.phila.gov/pdf/criminal-reports/WRISS-REPORT-2002-2006.pdf.

Camino, L., Zeldin, S., Mook, C., & O'Connor, C. (2004). *Youth and adult leaders for program excellence: A practical guide for program assessment and action planning.* Madison, WI: University of Wisconsin–Extension.

Centers for Disease Control and Prevention. (2004). *WISQARS fatal injuries: Mortality reports. 2004 data.* Available at http://webappa.cdc.gov/sasweb/ncipc/mortrate.html. Accessed December 13, 2007.

Commonwealth of Pennsylvania. (2005a). *Governor Rendell Forms Commission to Curb Gun Violence in Pennsylvania.* Available at http://www.state.pa.us/papower/cwp/view.asp?A=11&Q=441815&tx=1.

Commonwealth of Pennsylvania. (2005b). *Commission on Gun Violence Issues Report to Governor Rendell.* Available at http://www.state.pa.us/papower/cwp/view.asp?Q=443005&A=11.

Dennis, M. L., & Kaminer, Y. (2006). Introduction to special issue on advances in the assessment and treatment of adolescent substance use disorders. *American Journal on Addictions, 15,* 1–3.

Pennsylvania Trauma Systems Foundation. (2005). *Pennsylvania Trauma Outcome Study.* Pennsylvania Trauma Systems Foundation Annual Report (p. 10). Mechanicsburg, PA: Pennsylvania Trauma Systems Foundation.

Titus, J. C., & Dennis, M. L. (2003). *GAIN-Q: Global appraisal of individual needs—quick administration and scoring manual (version 2).* Bloomington, IL: Chestnut Health Systems.

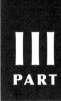

III
PART

Competencies Required for the Development of Successful Health Promotion Programs

Leadership in Health Promotion Programs

Bernard J. Healey, PhD
Robert S. Zimmerman Jr., MPH

OBJECTIVES

After reading this chapter, you should

- Understand the need for leadership skills in the development of health promotion programs
- Be aware of the need to develop power in order to lead others toward greater goal achievement
- Understand the role that needs to be played by the followers in the development of health promotion programs
- Be aware of the need for the use of communication skills in acquiring resources to continue and expand health promotion programs
- Be capable of understanding the need for leadership development in those who are responsible for the development and evaluation of health promotion programs

KEY TERMS

Charisma	Leadership
Culture	Traits
Influence	Transformational leadership

Introduction

Over the last 20 years, it has become evident that in order to reduce health care costs more must be done to keep people healthy. The promotion of healthy behaviors and the expansion of health promotion programs have become very popular with foundations, corporations, and various levels of government. These programs have shown to be an effective and efficient way of improving the population's health and reducing the costs associated with the development of expensive chronic diseases.

McKenzie, Neiger, and Thackeray (2009) argue that health educators need to be able to plan, implement, and evaluate health promotion efforts. These processes are very involved and require a great deal of preparation and training in order to be successful. This is going to require a change in the way in which these programs are developed and shared with stakeholders in the new program. Health promotion efforts will have to become a team effort with an emphasis on working together and encouraging innovation. There is clearly a strong element of **leadership** in every aspect of program development and implementation of the health promotion program.

Health promotion programs also require formal and informal leaders in order to be successful in achieving their goals and to ensure the continued funding for program continuation and expansion. In fact, leadership skills may very well be the missing ingredient from health promotion programs that fail. This leadership needs to be found in all of the stakeholders responsible for the success of the health promotion program from conception to final results.

Health promotion programs require strong leadership in order to accomplish their objectives and to obtain additional funds in order to expand. The health care delivery system in this country is in trouble not just because costs continue to rise but also because the system is not doing a very good job of preventing illness. Never have these problems been so numerous and so very difficult to solve. These problems can only be solved by strong leadership.

Sanders and Walters (2008) argue that an organization's vision is only as good as its leaders. Turnock (2009) points out that leadership development programs encourage envisioning the future and working with others to deal with future opportunities and threats. The health promotion specialist needs to develop these leadership skills in order to develop and implement health programs for their community.

Leaders need to create a **culture** in an organization where they are really the key sources for motivating new tasks and to accept changes as the opportunity for growth. Smircich and Morgan (2006) argue that leadership situations consist of an obligation and right of the leader to structure the new world, including the leader's vision for others. In other words, the leader needs to gain the ability to control the behavior of followers, allowing them to see and believe in the vision of the formal leader.

Leadership in health promotion programs must be looked at as a never-ending process. The vision has to include the education of all Americans from the many dangers of their own high-risk health behaviors. There is a need for strong, consistent, visible leadership that is essential to send a message of support to all Americans.

Evolution of Leadership

There is nothing new about the concept of leadership because it has been around since the beginning of civilization. Every society and generation has had leaders who arose to the demands of the time. These individuals have had the unique ability to mobilize the energy of their followers to attain important goals. These leaders were capable of sustainability in their effort to achieve their goals. They were capable of convincing followers that the goals being professed by the leader are the same as those who are following the leader. It was very evident that all leaders had the ability to **influence** large numbers of individuals toward the achievement of common goals. This ability is the reason behind some individuals achieving greatness and others not being as successful in implementing their vision.

Leadership is an attempt to gain influence over individuals that have the capability of helping to achieve common goals. There are many well known people—some good and some bad—that fit this definition of leadership: Gandhi, Hitler, Stalin, Lincoln, Kennedy, bin Laden, and Washington all fit this definition of leadership. They gained this influence or power from their charismatic way of articulating their goals. Although we do not agree with some of their goals, we cannot dismiss the fact that they were all capable of influencing others toward goals.

According to Western (2008), leadership must extend beyond the person and become more concerned about the challenge. By doing this, the leader is able to rally followers around a cause or a vision rather than around the leader. This allows us the ability to observe how individuals facing a challenge look for leadership or assume the responsibility of leadership themselves to face the particular challenge. This notion would help to explain how so many diverse leaders were successful at what they did despite the fact that they all had different skills. Perhaps rather than observing the leader, more attention should be paid to the particular challenge that forced leadership to come forth.

The world of work has been moving away from a bureaucratic design to more of a decentralized design, where the emphasis has changed from rules and regulations to results and to adding value to the product or service being delivered by the organization. This change in organizational structure is requiring a different type of leader with a different type of power to influence followers. The bureaucratic organization relied on legitimate power and control over rewards and punishments, which were largely a reflection of the organization and not the leader. The new world of work requires a leader with personal power that involves expertise and **charisma.** These leaders take their power with them when they leave an organization, which allows them to take risks in the way they and their followers go about developing and implementing new services.

Leadership Traits

Some of the older theories of leadership asserted that leadership qualities were inherited. From these theories developed the belief that several traits were responsible for one's ability to lead. Pierce and Newstrom (2006) define a *trait* as a general characteristic that could include individual motives, capacities, or patterns of behaviors. There are many who believe that these and other general traits may be the reason why he or she is a good leader.

Traits do matter in leadership, but they are not enough to define a good leader. Because traits cannot be taught, it makes very little sense to include trait theory in the development of leaders in health promotion. If certain traits are required to be a leader, then the old adage "he or she is a born leader" would seem to be true. There is no question that being gifted in speech or exuding self-confidence does not hurt your leadership capabilities. But it takes more than a trait to assist leaders in health promotion programs to influence followers toward goal accomplishment.

Many individuals in health promotion programs are pushed into leadership positions without any leadership training or development to help them with their enormous task. This has led many researchers to believe that certain traits of individuals are responsible for their leadership capabilities. Novick, Morrow, and Mays (2008) argue that having a certain trait, like being tall, does not in itself guarantee success as a leader.

There is no question that leaders are very different from other people. That difference may be a trait, the situation faced by the individual, exposure to a leadership training program, or a combination of all of these conditions. It is very important for leaders to be exposed to all of the leadership theories in order to understand the importance of leadership and to learn how to grow as a leader in order to handle the near impossible task facing the public health departments in the future. It helps for those placed in leadership positions in public health to learn how to lead.

Leadership Styles in Public Health

The style of the leader or the way he or she behaves is of great importance when dealing with participants that are purchasing a service. Health promotion is a service industry that, for the most part, communicates information to individuals regarding their health. This type of industry requires an administrator with a people-oriented leadership style. Novick et al. (2008) argue that most leaders in health services are pushed into their position with no leadership training. This is a critical piece of information because the success or failure of health promotion programs is directly related to the program director's ability to articulate a vision for the new promotion effort.

Northouse (2007) argues that leaders generally exhibit two kinds of behaviors: task behaviors and relationship behaviors. The leader of health promotion programs needs to understand that a combination of these behaviors may be required to accomplish public health goals.

The health promotion team is responsible for accomplishing the goals, while the leader is responsible for giving the team what it requires for goal accomplishment. Quite often the task behavior style may facilitate the goal accomplishment. The relationship style comes into play by helping the team members feel good and supported in what it is they are trying to achieve.

Manning and Curtis (2007) discuss the concept of a motive to lead. They argue that there are three motives to lead that include a desire for achievement, power or ability to influence others, and affiliation interpreted as an interest in helping others. There is no question that most people seek a career in public health because of a desire to help other people.

According to Kouzes and Posner (1995), every leader seeks challenge, exploits change, and understands the great risk that is present as a result of his or her actions. By definition, managers are not expected to go beyond the planned outcome. Leaders, on the other hand, allow the vision and not the planned outcome to determine the results of their activities.

Leadership is a small component of the entire process of public health management but one of the most important components, especially to organizations that supply services. Novick et al. (2008) point out that those responsible for the management of public health programs may not offer leadership to those programs because of lack of training or experience.

Table 12-1 shows many of the essential skills and competencies necessary to lead community health agencies in the twenty-first century. Because the majority of current and future public health problems will not be resolved by one agency, many of the skills listed in Table 12-1 are an absolute requirement for leaders who need to reach out to the community to solve problems. These skills, if developed and practiced by the health promotion leader, will make it easier to develop strong collaboration among government agencies, businesses, and the community.

The style of the leader is conditioned by the way the leader behaves. This behavior or style is especially visible in the leader's interaction with the employees of the organization or group where the leader practices his or her leadership skills in the accomplishment of goals. Northouse (2007) argues that this style seems to break down to one focusing on either task behavior or relationship behavior. This classification is supported by the majority of research that has been published on the leader's behavior. The task-oriented behavior by the leader works very well in some situations but fails in others. The relationship behavior has the same problem depending on the situation. There seems to be solid agreement among most researchers that the situation is the controlling variable that determines which leadership style works best with goal achievement by the leader.

It seems obvious that the way a leader behaves affects the employee's response to the leader and, ultimately, the performance of these followers. There were several studies of leadership theory conducted over the last 30 years that keep focusing on two major behaviors of leaders: task or work centered and employee centered or consideration behavior. Again, the type of behavior that worked best for the leader depended on the situation faced by the leader.

The motivation of both the leader and followers was also important in determining the leader and, ultimately, the behavior of the followers. A bureaucratic leader who is afraid of risk will not be effective in the achievement of health promotion goals in the twenty-first century. It will not take long for bureaucratic leader behavior to destroy the thick culture of health promotion workers.

Table 12-1
Leadership Skills

- Self-awareness
- Creating sustainable vision and translating that to a mission
- Decision making
- Problem solving
- Creative thinking
- Strategic thinking
- System thinking
- Entrepreneurial ability
- Building trust
- Working effectively in social systems
- Self-confidence
- Learning from experience
- Continuous quality improvement (CQI)
- Risk taking
- Priority setting
- Maintaining credibility
- Teaching
- Building teams within the institution
- Marketing
- Building relationships
- Communicating
- Persuasion
- Creating partnerships–fostering collaboration
- Developing others
- Building internal capacity
- Negotiation
- Delegating
- Creating organizational slack
- Forming teams and coalitions
- Management techniques
- Sensitivity
- Building infrastructure (e.g., improvement of information system capabilities)

Source: Novick, L. F., Morrow, C. B., & Mays, G. P. (2008). *Public health administration principles for population-based management* (2nd ed.). Sudbury, MA: Jones and Bartlett Publishers.

Once this culture is destroyed, it will take years to repair the damage. There is new research supporting the use of a transformational style of leadership in health-related departments.

Transformational Leadership and Public Health

Northouse (2007) points out that the **transformational leadership** style does not provide assumptions about how a leader should act; rather this style deals with the provision of a way to think about leading. The emphasis with this style is clearly on inspiration and innovation in the way the organization does business.

Tichy (1997) argues that a transformational leadership style encourages the leader to become involved not only in organizational goals but in the transformation of his or her followers into leaders themselves. This implies that the major role of a transformational leader is to positively energize those around the leader. This style allows the leader to create motivated followers that surround him or her, grasping for the energy provided by the leader and directed toward goal accomplishment.

This synergy allows the impossible not only to become possible but to become the norm for the organization. This is exactly the leadership style that is needed to provide direction through the ambiguity that confronts health promotion efforts in the United States today.

Novick et al. (2008) believe that transformational leadership requires true empowerment of all team members to accomplish predetermined goals for their program. Doing the right thing for the health of the people entails risk even from the very people that the leader is attempting to help.

Table 12-2 shows a comparison of the skills found in the transformational leader. Northouse (2007) points out that transformational leaders have the unique ability to get all team members more interested in the current project or organizational goal to be achieved rather than the member's own self interest. This type of leader should be communicating the goals of health promotion to all of the various constituencies that have the resources and support to make health promotion programs succeed. People are attracted to these leaders because they are able to explain their cause in such a way that supporters understand and want to be part of the movement to better health for all.

Leadership Development in Health Promotion Programs

Mays, Miller, and Halverson (2000) argue that the demand for professional development, especially leadership training, has grown in response to a multitude of external forces. These forces include the need for collaboration among many community agencies trying to make their communities healthier while also dealing with the ever-expanding emerging infections and the threat of bioterrorism.

In order to accomplish health promotion goals, leadership rather than management in health promotion is required. The Institute of Medicine (IOM, 2002) recognized the need for leadership training in the executive summary of its recent report titled *The Future of Public's Health in the 21st Century*. In this report, the IOM recommends that Congress increase funding for public health training, especially leadership training, for state and local health department's directors. The CDC also has responded with programs like the Public Health Leadership Institute and the National Public Health Leadership Development Network offering leadership development and training to public health professionals throughout the country. This

Table 12-2
Transactional vs. Trans-
formational Leadership:
Differences Between
Managing and Leading

	Transactional Leadership or Management Skills	**Transformational Leadership or Leadership Skills**
Performance:	Considered by leadership writers to produce ordinary performance	Considered by leadership writers to produce extraordinary performance
Goal:	To maintain the status quo by playing within the rules	To change the status quo by changing the rules
Goals arise out of:	Necessity, are reactive, and respond to ideas. They are deeply imbedded in the organization's history and culture	Desires; they are active, shaping ideas; may be a departure from organization's history and culture
Emphasis:	Rationality and control, limits choices, focuses on solving problems	Innovation, creativity to develop fresh approaches to long-standing problems, and open issues to new options
Attitudes towards goals:	Impersonal, if not passive attitudes	Personal and active attitude
Incentives:	Based on exchange of needs (i.e., "tit for tat")	Based on the greater good
Locus of reward:	Maximize personal benefits	Optimize systemic benefits
Requires:	Persistence, tough-mindedness, hard work, intelligence, analytical ability, tolerance, and goodwill	Genius and heroism
View work as:	Enabling processes, ideas, and people to establish strategies and make decisions	Creative, energizing, and emerging
Tactics employed:	Negotiate and bargain, use of rewards, punishment, and other forms of coercion	Inspire followers, create shared vision, motivate
	Strive to convert win–lose into win–win situations as part of the process of reconciling differences among people and maintaining balances of power	Strive to create new situations and new directions without regard to reconciling groups or power

Source: Novick, L. F., Morrow, C. B., & Mays, G. P. (2008). *Public health administration principles for population-based management* (2nd ed.). Sudbury, MA: Jones and Bartlett Publishers.

recommendation would certainly apply to those individuals leading health promotion programs.

Leadership skills are usually not part of the curriculum in schools of public health. According to the *The Nation's Health*, "getting an MPH [Masters of Public Health] does not necessarily confer on you the realities of practicing public health, just as medical schools do not necessarily train doctors to handle money or management issues," (Bailey, Stephanie Coursey, MD, MHSA, Chief of Centers for Disease Control and Prevention's Office of Public Health Practice, August 2007, p. 25).

It is uncommon to find leadership skills addressed in educational programs for those pursuing a career in public health or health promotion. The IOM (2002) points out that the MPH is the degree earned by many individual workers in public health and health promotion, especially those that remain in public health long enough to become program managers. A large number of individuals are found in leadership positions in public health and health promotion with academic preparation in areas other than public health and health education. Despite the academic certification of the public health leader, it is very rare to find individuals with strong leadership training credentials.

A very small part of the current workforce in health promotion receives training in public health before they begin their career. The average public health workers usually receive on-the-job training in a specific area of public health like epidemiology, public health nursing, laboratory science, and health education. Even if they have a degree or certification in the specific discipline where they are employed, there is probably no chance that they received training in leadership or communication skills while attaining their formal education.

The Nation's Health offered an excellent article in its August 2007 edition of "Leadership Institutes Help Public Health Workers Advance Careers." This article highlighted the value of public health workers attending one of the many public health institutes that offer professional development opportunities to public health practitioners across the United States. This would also apply to those working in health promotion programs.

Geoffrey Downie, MPA, program manager of the Mid-American Regional Public Health Institute, said that all institutes "share the belief that system thinking is a key component to effective leadership and that community health will improve if the public health infrastructure is sustained and supported." Joyce R Gaufin, executive director of the Great Basin Public Health Leadership Institute in Salt Lake City, commented about those who completed leadership training: "One of the most important individual benefits of participation is an increased sense of confidence about their own abilities and the actions they take as a leader" (*The Nation's Health*, 2007). These leadership training programs are usually a 1-year commitment, and the training is provided by expert faculty from leading schools of public health, business programs, and the private sector. Funding for these programs come from a variety of sources including CDC, state and local health agencies, and public health foundations.

These efforts at providing leadership training opportunities to those engaged in community health must be continued and expanded if we are serious about improving the public health of our nation. Kate Wright, director of the National Public Health Leadership Development Network, comments in the August 2007 edition of *The Nation's Health* that, "the need for leadership in public health is well documented, and many would agree that at no time in the nation's history has the need been greater" (p. 25).

There is a great deal of discussion about standardization by the various organizations that are providing leadership training programs to those working in community health programs. There is a need for best practices in leadership to be developed and shared with leaders and followers in all community health agencies throughout the country. In order to develop successful health promotion initiatives, the programs must be led by competent individuals with the necessary skills to make the programs succeed.

Leadership Skills

Leadership and Power

In order to be able to lead any group or organization, the leader needs to have a power base. Leadership involves the ability of an individual to influence others to accomplish a predetermined goal. Northouse (2007) argues that in order to influence individuals, a power relationship must exist between the leader and the followers. Because goal achievement requires change, the use of some form of power is required to make change happen.

Northouse (2007) points out that there are usually two major types of power found in individuals, which are derived from the position or are found in the individual. They are position and personal power. Lussier and Achua (2004) argue that perception of power may be the key ingredient in developing the ability to influence others.

Because many health promotion agencies are government sponsored, their structure is usually bureaucratic. A bureaucratic organization relies heavily on position power to achieve the goals of the organization. This type of power is derived from the top management or chief executive of the government entity and flows from the top of the organization downward. Lussier and Achua (2004) argue that position power involves legitimate, coercive, and reward power, which is owned by the organization and not the leader. This type of power can be taken away from the individual if mistakes are made. Therefore, bureaucratic leaders are always at risk of losing their position power if they anger those above them in the organization chart.

Risk is part of making change happen, and if one's career is placed at risk every time change is required, the bureaucratic leader is less inclined to be part of the change process. This has always been a recognized impediment to making rapid change happen. Unfortunately, health promotion leaders are well aware of the implied risk in their action when dealing with public health issues. There is always the chance that being part of the change process and in achieving their objectives, which often affects many people, they will anger some politically powerful individuals. The end result of this type of confrontation can result in the public health leader having to relinquish his or her position of power.

Lussier and Achua (2004) also discuss the personal type of power that can be found in leaders. Personal power comes forth from the leader and is owned by the leader. When individuals leave an organization, they take their personal power with them. Northouse (2007) argues that personal power is the ability to influence individuals because of being liked and respected by followers for their expertise. The two types of personal power usually found in leadership research are charisma and expertise found in a leader.

Lussier and Achua (2004) point out that charisma, or referent power, consists of certain traits found in an individual that are appealing to followers. This type of power results from relationships with others and usually involves friendship or loyalty between the leader and the follower. This type of power can be developed through education and training programs. It is interesting to note that personal power can quite often be found in followers who are not in any type of leadership position.

The transformational leadership style relies more on the personal power of the leader than it does on position power. The transformational process requires the leader to be considered a competent role model by his or her followers. These leaders have a vision of the future, and everything that they do is part of the road map to the attainment of that vision. One way to make faster progress in making the vision a reality is to get followers to buy into the vision through the use of the personal power of the leader.

Healthy People 2010 is a vision for population health that requires transformational leadership to achieve all of the objectives for the health of Americans. Novick et al. (2008) argues that in order to accomplish large goals that impact the public like those put forth in Healthy People 2010, the public health leaders require collaboration with others in the political landscape. This is where the transformational leadership style can serve the public health leader. The leader must also consider the enormous risk present in achieving these lofty goals.

Ability to Empower Staff in Health Promotion Programs

Health promotion leaders need to learn how to develop their staff and share the power of the agency with all of the staff involved in serving the public. Health promotion programs in this country are most dependent on their greatest resource, which is their workforce. These dedicated individuals come from a wide range of professions, educational backgrounds, and motivations for pursuing a career in public health. These are the followers that need to be energized toward accomplishment of health promotion goals by the leader.

These followers, because of their diverse training experience and their thick professional culture, cannot be managed for very long in a bureaucratic organization. They are different in that they need to be empowered both for personal growth and also for the accomplishment of organizational goals. They cannot be managed; they must be led and truly empowered by the leader, or they lose their motivation to perform.

According to Pierce and Newstrom (2006), it is very important to understand the role of the follower if one is ever to truly understand the process of leadership. The traits that make up the followers must be understood if we are to understand the receptivity of followers to certain types of leadership style. If the leader is ever going to be successful in his or her attempt at gaining the support of followers, a great deal of attention needs to be paid to followers' needs, perceptions, and expectations. The vast majority of followers in public health have longer tenure in their positions than the leader. They also have been through the change in management in the past. They are conditioned by what happened and did not happen with the previous leaders.

Empowerment becomes the ability of the leader to share power with followers in order to develop their own personal power. Position power is absent from this definition of empowerment by choice. One never really owns position power because the risk of loss of this type of power is always present. Every time position power is used to influence or lead, there is always the risk of loss associated with that action. The tendency for those with position power is to not take chances for fear of losing the power and damaging their career. To those that only have position power, change becomes the enemy and is therefore resisted.

Leaders who fear change tend to avoid empowering their followers because this empowerment increases the chances of loss of the leader's position of power. Health promotion programs have been the victim of many administrators who fit the category of not empowering their followers. Fortunately for the American public, some leaders with personal power and the ability to empower followers have been part of the history of health promotion efforts. Even with short tenure, they have been able to achieve lofty accomplishments in the promotion of good health.

Ability to Communicate

Novick et al. (2008) argue that the most important skills required for a leader in the twenty-first century are communication skills. Lussier and Achua (2004) also point out that the use of communication skills are required to present the mission statement, and goals of the program are essential to getting all stakeholders to become supportive of the leader's vision.

Northouse (2007) discusses the concept of emergent leadership where followers believe that the leader has gained influence over the group through his or her communication skills. Lussier and Achua (2004) argue that communication is actually a major part of the leadership strategy. There is a very strong relationship between communication skills and the effective performance of a leader. Communication tools are essential to leadership development and goal attainment in health promotion programs.

The IOM (2002) argues that health promotion leaders must be able to communicate internally and externally in order to distribute vital health information to their staff, other agencies, the media, and the community. They must also be able to gather information from the public about disease occurrence and to distribute health information concerning public health problems rapidly to the public.

The IOM (2002) argues that communication skills, along with an appreciation of the value of technology, can make health promotion a very effective tool in the epidemic of chronic diseases faced in this country. The IOM also recommends that all partners within the health promotion system make communication skills a critical core competency of their program. The IOM went on to recommend the expansion of vital information systems that are able to rapidly disseminate health-related information to those who need to know. The health promotion leader must understand and embrace the value of communication skills in the world of public health in the twenty-first century.

Conflict Management   The attainment of the goals of health promotion efforts in the twenty-first century will require the leader to deal with conflict and to learn how to manage that conflict. Conflict management is a skill that must be developed by the health promotion leader. Bureaucratic organizations usually see conflict as bad, and these organizations attempt to suppress conflict with a heavy reliance on rules and regulations that prevent conflict from ever developing. This also reduces the chances for creativity and innovation in the development and implementation of health promotion programs.

In the new world of health promotion, conflict needs to be seen as normal and even energizing and should actually be supported by the program leadership. Manning and Curtis (2007) argue that conflicting goals and personalities are expected when dealing with people in a healthy vibrant organization. The leader needs to be aware that change is the breeding ground for conflict and that part of the leader's role as change agent is dealing with this conflict. The leader in health promotion efforts must be aware that what he or she is attempting to do to improve the health of the community is going to cause conflict among some segments of the population. Health promotion programs are telling people that they must change behaviors that they would rather not change. Health promotion programs deal with sensitive issues like safe sex that, by their very nature, breed some conflict. This makes conflict management a very important skill that must be learned not only by the leader but also by the followers in health promotion efforts.

Conflict needs to be managed, and the leader needs to realize that the success of the health promotion agency may depend on how well the conflict is handled by the organization. Lussier and Achua (2004) argue that conflict management may take up to 20% of a leader's time and a great deal of his or her energy. The way that conflict is handled, especially in the area of health promotion programs, may be one of the most important skills required of a public health leader.

Conflict cannot and should not be avoided by the leader. Lussier and Achua (2004) point out that conflict resolution can build collaboration throughout the organization and sometimes the community. Collaboration is what is needed to make health promotion departments stronger and able to achieve greater goals as they move through the health problems they face in the twenty-first century.

Leaders as Change Agent

In order to improve and perhaps save our health care delivery system in the United States, profound change in operation must occur. Kotter (1995) argues that managers are usually engrossed with complexity, while leaders devote their time to change.

The pace of change has accelerated in recent years, and nowhere is the change process happening at a faster pace than in the service sector of our economy. Health promotion programs offer services; they are faced with dramatic change, and they too are caught up in the accelerated process of change. The leader of these programs must be capable of responding to change in terms of facing a new crisis and new responsibilities on a daily basis.

At no time will there ever be a greater demand for strong leadership than when dramatic change becomes present in the way business is done. Pierce and Newstrom (2006) discuss the need for leaders to have the ability to frame reality for their followers. This framing or structuring of the future must be done in a meaningful way for members of the organization to accept change and work to achieve it.

Lussier and Achua (2004) point out that leaders today must learn to manage change rather than to simply react to it. In fact, leaders must be able to exploit change for the opportunities that it can open for their organization. Change can also bring threats that the organization needs to be aware of and develop a proactive response in order to continue its growth. Change has frequently been the enemy of those in leadership positions in public health because they fear loss of the position of power.

Lussier and Achua (2004) point out that the leader and followers need to develop a concept of change as more of a process than a product. This would entail acceptance by the entire organization that environmental change is the catalyst needed to transform the organization to meet the vision espoused by the leader and accepted by his or her followers. It can then become a continuous process of quality improvement and growth for health promotion programs.

Stadler (2007) points out that one of the prerequisites for managing for the long term is to be conservative about change. This author advocates the exploitation of change while not advocating radical change without appropriate planning. In other words, the leader needs to first prepare the organization for opportunities that present themselves through change but to do so without considering the secondary effects of the action.

Culture Development

Culture is a combination of learned beliefs, values, rules, and symbols that are common to groups of people. The members of an organization very often take the culture for granted and usually are unaware of how important it is to their desire to remain or to not remain with this particular organization. The organizational culture is, in reality, the values that tend to rule the decision-making process of group members. This culture that is encouraged for all members to absorb becomes the one thing that always remains standard in the workplace. It is the way things are done on a daily basis in this particular workplace. It is what can make this a special place to work.

Sanders (2008) points out that a sustainable thick culture requires the leader to place the highest level of importance on people. This is so very important when the leader is responsible for the delivery of services. Many managers erroneously believe that they are responsible for building the culture of the organization. In reality, the culture is developed, nurtured, and thickened by the workers found throughout the organization. In fact, culture may very well be developed as a reaction to poor management and poor employee relations. These work groups have their own way of accomplishing goals of the organization, and in reality, this worker unity becomes the culture that determines the way things are done in the workplace. The best the manager can do is to try to accomplish goals by working with the existing culture. This is especially true of those who work in public health. These employees enjoy a unique bond that draws them to health education and convinces them that this is where they want to spend their career. It is nothing less than a feeling of family unity.

Those responsible for health promotion programs must understand and respect the value of the organization's culture. If the leader avoids dealing with the culture, transforming the organization to react to the changing environment becomes virtually impossible. The transformational leader, in order to be successful with public health employees, must become part of their culture or positive change will not happen. I have witnessed so many failed attempts by public health leaders to make change happen and then to fail in their quest because of the rigid culture of their employees. The culture actually works against them in their effort to produce change.

CONCLUDING REMARKS

There are two absolutely true statements about health promotion programs in the United States. These programs have a long list of unbelievable accomplishments with very limited resources. Through leadership, so much more can be accomplished.

It is one thing for health promotion agencies to develop the vision of a healthy America, but it is going to take sustained leadership to accomplish all of the goals outlined in *Healthy People 2010*. It is also going to take the collaboration among government, public health agencies, businesses, insurance companies, and the community to deal with the epidemic of chronic diseases that is growing in our country. Health promotion agencies have to provide the leadership to develop and nurture the partnerships that can make health goals achievable.

Those assigned leadership responsibilities have to receive leadership training and have to be given the opportunity to practice what they learn from the training programs. They cannot practice these skills in bureaucratic agencies where the leader is conditioned to fear change and to be fearful of taking risks to achieve the large goals of health promotion in America. They cannot work in agencies where their tenure is short and becomes shorter if they anger those in power by embracing change. They have to grow in their important positions, not hide from their responsibilities.

DISCUSSION QUESTIONS

1. What role does leadership play in the development of successful health promotion programs?
2. Explain the transformational leadership style and relate it to the development of health promotion programs.
3. Why is conflict management so very important in health promotion efforts?
4. What is the role of power in the development and implementation of community health promotion programs?

REFERENCES

Institute on Medicine Committee on Assuring the Health of the Public in the 21st Century. (2002).*The future of the public's health in the 21st century.* Washington, DC: National Academies Press.

Kotter, J. P. (1995). Leading change: Why transformation efforts fail. *Harvard Business Review*, (March–April), 59–67.

Kouzes, J. M., & Posner, B. Z. (1995). *The leadership challenge how to keep getting extraordinary things done in organizations.* San Francisco, CA: Jossey-Bass Publishers.

Lussier, R. N., & Achua, C. F. (2004). *Leadership theory application skill development* (2nd ed.). Mason, OH: Thomson South Western.

Manning, G., & Curtis, K. (2007). *The art of leadership* (2nd ed.). Boston, MA: McGraw Hill Irwin.

Mays, G. P., Miller, C. A., & Halverson, P. K. (2000). *Local public health practice: Trends & models.* Washington DC: American Public Health Association.

McKenzie, J. F., Neiger, B. L., & Thackeray, R. (2009). *Planning, implementing and evaluating health promotion programs: A primer* (5th ed.). San Francisco, CA: Pearson Education Inc.

Northouse, P. G. (2007). *Leadership theory and practice* (4th ed.). Thousand Oaks, CA: Sage Publications.

Novick, L. F., Morrow, C. B., & Mays, G. P. (2008). *Public health administration principles for population-based management* (2nd ed.). Sudbury, MA: Jones and Bartlett Publishers.

Pierce, J. L., & Newstrom, J. W. (2006). *Leaders and the leadership process readings, self-assessments, and applications* (4th ed.). Boston, MA: McGraw Hill Irwin.

Sanders, D. J. (2008). *Built to serve*. New York, NY: McGraw Hill Publishers.

Sanders, D. J., & Walters, G. (2008). *Equipped to lead: Managing people, process, partners, and performance*. New York, NY: McGraw Hill Publishers.

Smircich, L., & Morgan, G. (2006). *Leadership: The management of meaning*. Boston, MA: McGraw Hill Irwin.

Stadler, C. (2007). The four principles of enduring success. *Harvard Business Review*, (July–August 2007), 62–72.

The Nation's Health. (2007). Leadership institutes help public health workers advance careers. (August).

Tichy, N. M. (1997). *The leadership engine how winning companies build leaders at every level*. New York: Harper Collins Publisher.

Turnock, B. J. (2009). *Public health: What it is and how it works* (4th ed.). Sudbury, MA: Jones and Bartlett Publishers.

Western, S. (2008). *Leadership: A critical text*. Los Angeles, CA: Sage Publications.

Continuous Quality Improvement in Health Promotion Programs

Andrew Lanza, MSW

OBJECTIVES

After reading this chapter, you should

- Know the elements of a continuous quality improvement (CQI) model and how to apply these elements to health promotion programs
- Understand how a CQI model can complement or serve as an overlay for well-established methods of conducting health promotion
- Be familiar with key concepts associated with health promotion and how specific initiatives illustrate these concepts
- Be able to expand upon current understanding of health promotion and best practices

KEY TERMS

Continuous quality improvement
Deming Cycle
Geodemographic segmentation

Levels of prevention
PRIZM
Target segmentation

Introduction

Public health is the science and art of disease prevention, prolonging life, and promoting health and well-being through organized community effort for the sanitation of the environment, the control of communicable infections, the organization of medical and nursing services for the early diagnosis and prevention of disease, the education of the individual in personal health and the development of the social machinery to assure everyone a standard of living adequate for the maintenance or improvement of health (Winslow, 1920, p. 2183).

Previous chapters have described many of the essential ingredients of health promotion in the twenty-first century. Data gathering—through epidemiology and assessment, community engagement and planning, determination of goals and objectives, implementation and program evaluation—is considered some of the key aspects of health promotion. These methods have been well described and illustrated in other parts of this text. This chapter will review some of these and will provide evidence and information that will assist the public health student and professional in planning and implementing programs more logically. By applying the principles of a quality improvement process, as introduced by W. Edwards Deming decades ago, the public health professional can become more skilled in health promotion.

Increasingly, the health promotion field is challenged to do more, often with fewer resources. The measuring stick of success will undoubtedly be raised from informing and raising awareness to inspiring and facilitating action to promote and sustain healthy behaviors. The current stakes are too high to focus exclusively on individual responsibility, decision support, and behavior change. We must expand that focus to the "development of the social machinery to assure everyone a standard of living adequate for the maintenance or improvement of health," a vision for the field of public health that was articulated almost a century ago and continues to be relevant today (Winslow, 1920, p. 2183).

Our first working premise is that developing and sustaining best practices in health promotion may in fact be derived from peripheral areas rather than the health promotion field itself. This process can be seen when innovations are carried over or adapted in totally new applications. To illustrate this premise, let us look at two vignettes. Early in the last century, the Swiss were widely recognized as the world's preeminent watchmakers. Their spring and balance technology was considered the model for all fine watches and time-keeping. The Swiss monopolized the timekeeping field, and no one could argue that they had the best practices in their field. However, as noted by Hamel and Prahalad (1996), the perception and style of watches were changing, gradually at first and then dramatically. By the middle of the century, new applications, such as digital and battery technology, from new players on the world scene, like the Japanese, had impacted the Swiss market share. This came as a surprise to the Swiss watchmakers and, to some degree, the industry at large. But the story does not stop there; the Swiss eventually recognized the paradigm shift and adopted and ultimately advanced the new technology. They converted their processes and methods to the best practices in fine watchmaking they are known for today. A second illustration of this point is the 2008 presidential campaign. One of the most remarkable stories of this campaign, along with the numerous "firsts" that everyone acknowledges, is the fact that the most democratic (YouTube and CNN, 2007) presidential debates ever occurred through the collaboration of YouTube and CNN in the 2008 campaign. CNN reported that pointed questions posed by our nation in an Internet-based format had engaged more viewers and more voters than ever before in the history of presidential campaigns (Walton, 2007).

A second working premise, the term *improving best practices*, is not an end state but is instead a continuum, because there is always room for improvement. This is often referred to as **continuous quality improvement** (CQI). Research indicates that there is no single standardized definition for what makes up best practices in health promotion. Perhaps this is best described by a colleague of mine.

> Unlike a medication or procedure, a health promotion intervention is not intrinsically effective. It is the circumstances surrounding the intervention that determine whether or not it will be effective. Under the right circumstances or context, even a poorly designed intervention can eventually be changed to become effective. Under the wrong circumstances, a well-designed intervention will fail. Applying the methods and metrics of quality improvement to health promotion and disease prevention is a powerful way to adapt the circumstances to the intervention and the intervention to the circumstances, improving the likelihood of effectiveness (Veazie, M., personal communication, 2008).

In a similar vein, Don Berwick, one of the nation's leading authorities on health care quality and improvement has concluded that "experimentalists have pursued the single-minded thought of whether a program works at the expense of *knowing why* it works" (Berwick, 2007).

It is clear that different organizations across various sectors use different definitions and criteria for acknowledging best practices (U.S. Department of Health and Human Services, 2007). With that as a backdrop, it is appropriate to consider different models that can be applied to best practices in health promotion.

One of those models, first used widely in business and manufacturing, is now used in health care. Since the 1950s, W. Edwards Deming has had a profound effect on manufacturing and business practices. His major contribution, an approach to quality, called *total quality management* (TQM), has revolutionized quality improvement, first in Japan and then worldwide (12 Manage, 2007). TQM still resonates in the marketplace today. Deming, building upon a model first proposed by the preeminent statistician Walter Shewhart, proposed the **Deming Cycle**, PDSA cycle or PDCA cycle — terms that are often used interchangeably in the literature (12 Manage, 2007). This approach consists of a series of steps that, when taken as whole, make logical sense. The four parts of the Deming Cycle are plan (anticipate change and plan accordingly); do (implement an action in small steps); study–check (analyze what happened); and act (determine what is needed to improve the process; (12 Manage, 2007). The Institute for Healthcare Improvement (IHI) adapted the Deming Cycle to health care through an initiative known as the Collaborative Model for Achieving Breakthrough Improvement (Institute for Healthcare Improvement [IHI], 2003, see Figure 13-1).

IHI promotes the PDSA cycle, the focus area of this chapter, as a useful and practical method for analyzing a process of change where an aim or goal to improve a health care delivery process has been established. This is rele-

The Model For Improvement

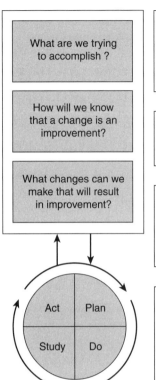

Setting Aims
Improvement requires setting aims. The aim should be time-specific and measurable; it should also define the specific population of patients that will be affected.

Establishing Measures
Teams use quantitative measures to determine if a specific change actually leads to an improvement.

Selecting Changes
All improvement requires making changes, but not all changes result in improvement. Organizations therefore must identify the changes that are most likely to result in improvement.

Testing Changes
The Plan-Do-Study-Act (PDSA) cycle is shorthand for testing a change in the real work setting—by planning it, trying it, observing the results, and acting on what is learned. This is the scientific method used for action-oriented learning.

Figure 13-1
The Model for Improvement
Source: The Model for Improvement as seen on the Institute for Healthcare Improvement website (http://www.IHI.org) was developed by Associates in Process Improvement [Langley, Nolan, Nolan, Norman, Provost. (1996). *The improvement guide.* San Francisco: Jossey-Bass Publishers].

vant to health promotion because it provides the framework for rapid improvement cycles, enabling health planners and promoters to adjust goals and strategies based on information and feedback from previous efforts (IHI, n.d.). In their adaptation of this famous model, IHI suggests that once a problem has been identified the following four steps should occur: Plan indicates a way of identifying and testing the change needed; do is implementing the change in a small observable way such as a series of pilots; study (or evaluation) is learning from the observations made; and act indicates what changes should be made to the test so that CQI occurs.

Three basic questions arise when using this model, and these constitute the guiding theme of this chapter: (1) What are we trying to accomplish and how will we know if we are successful? (2) How will we know that a change is an improvement? (3) What changes can we make that will result in improvement (IHI, n.d.)?

Now let us explore a way in which this logical model can be applied to study and advance the field of health promotion.

Planning a Health Promotion Program

**Anticipate Change
and Plan
Accordingly**

There are multiple aspects to planning a health promotion program. Green and Kreuter describe these aspects as "determining the combination of educational and ecological supports for actions and conditions of living conducive to health" (1999, p. 27). The first step is to define the health objective that the health promotion activity will address. This often requires that the needs of the target community be formally assessed. The assessment produces the project's topic or focus area. There are many methods to accomplish this initial step, and decisions made at this juncture will affect all subsequent aspects of the project; it is in many ways similar to the clinical diagnostic process. Using the phases of the PRECEDE–PROCEED Model, the process includes a social diagnosis, which defines the self-determined needs, wants, resources, and barriers affecting the target community; an epidemiological diagnosis of the target community's health problems; a behavioral and environmental diagnosis of specific behaviors that target community's environmental factors; an educational and organizational diagnosis of target community conditions that affect behavior; or an administrative and policy diagnosis of the resources needed and their availability in the targeted community.

A number of recent health promotion programs have demonstrated that in many cases a number of these diagnostic steps are needed. The Diabetes Detection Initiative was a selective screening effort to identify adults who may have undiagnosed diabetes. This national initiative was developed as a result of various "diagnostic" procedures as epidemiological, behavioral, and administrative aspects contributed to its design, implementation, and evaluation (Lanza, Albright, Zucker, & Martin, 2007). A *Purchaser's Guide to Clinical Preventive Services: Moving Science into Coverage*, a health promotion reference tool designed to improve the coverage of evidence-based screening, immunizations, and counseling, has been produced in response to a behavioral, educational, and administrative–policy diagnosis (National Business Group on Health, 2006).

Once one or more of these diagnostic procedures has been used, it is important to determine the prevention level (primary, secondary, or tertiary) of the program. Numerous sources have described these **levels of prevention** and definitions are not always consistent (Employee Benefit Research Institute, 2005). For example, based on the previously described diagnostic steps, will the program focus on a primary prevention level in which activities to control for risk factors in healthy people are directed to either all or high-risk members of the target community with the goal of stopping the occurrence of a disease *before* it starts?; Will the prevention level be secondary prevention in which activities and strategies target already diagnosed members of the community that are at *risk* of disease complications to prevent progression or serious complications?; Will the prevention level be tertiary prevention in which services are directed to diagnosed members of the target community to *reduce the extent of disability* or other negative complications of disease (Gordus, 2000)?

Importance of Goals and Objectives

There is no doubt that CQI or best practices require the setting of goals. Objectives should be specific, measurable, attainable, realistic, and time bound (Top Achievement, 2007). Goals should reflect the intended level of prevention as previously described as well as the specific population that will be affected. Any discussion of goals and objectives needs to occur cognizant of what we are trying to accomplish and how we will know if we are successful; how we will know that a change is actually an improvement; and what changes can we make that will cause an improvement. The Deming PDSA cycle facilitates the evaluation of a program's short-term goals; more rapid improvement cycles enable health planners to adjust goals based on information and feedback from previous efforts (IHI, n.d.).

Identifying the Target Community

We have already alluded to identifying the target community in the previous section. Simply stated, the target population is those members of a community that represent the conditions that have been identified in the diagnostic process. It is important to delve more deeply into this part of the planning process because it is critical. Program interventions should be designed so that they "fit" with the target population that has been identified through the assessment process. For example, if improving diabetes treatment is identified as the focus area of a health promotion program, the primary target community may be physicians who treat those who have already been diagnosed with diabetes and are at risk for complications. Similarly, the target community for the prevention of obesity in a community may be school-aged children who can be reached through the public media, as described in the CDC's VERB Youth Media Campaign (2002). There are some unique programs that target multiple levels of the community. IHI's 100k Lives Campaign is a good example of a program that has targeted clinicians, hospitals, patients, and the media with the goal of significantly reducing lethal hospital mistakes (Berwick, 2006). When discussing target community, other concepts often come into play. These concepts, borrowed from the marketing world, are related but have different forms, functions, and results. **Target segmentation** relates to the process of dividing a broader population into smaller segments. As reported by Wright and cited in McKenzie and Smeltzer (2001), these segments are more likely to have similar needs and wants and are therefore expected to react similarly to an intervention. Heitgard and Lee (2003) describe geodemographic segmentation using **PRIZM (Precise Rating Index by Zip Markets)** in an example of how health promotion programs have applied this principle. **Geodemographic segmentation** is a "multivariate statistical classification technique for discovering whether the individual or a population fall into different groups by making comparisons of multiple characteristics with the assumption that difference *within* any group should be less than differences *between* groups" (Wikipedia, 2008). Neilson Claritas, a premier market research company providing resources and solutions in consumer and business-to-business marketing, developed PRIZM to provide a standard way of sorting the U.S. population into smaller groups based on demographics, lifestyle preferences, and consumer behavior (Claritas, 2006).

A correlative concept of segmenting is *tailoring*. This pertains to an intervention activity that is designed specifically to meet the needs or wants of the segmented targeted population. The rationale for this customization is that a body of research, including research on nutrition, has demonstrated that there is a higher level of attention and awareness to information that has personal significance to the individual (Campbell, Devillis, Strecher, Develllis, & Sandler as cited in McKenzie & Smeltzer, 2001).

Importance of Relationships

Not surprisingly, relationships are essential ingredients in the best practices of health promotion. They are often a key indicator of success and are often the "circumstances surrounding an intervention," as previously described by Veazie (personal communication, 2008). This work will not chronicle the already expansive field of relationships and partnerships. We will, however, cover two critical and related areas of this topic that will ultimately lead to the success or failure of a health promotion initiative. As reported by Chapman and cited in McKenzie & Smeltzer (2001), relationships are critical in gaining the support of decision makers and community leaders who are influential in providing momentum and resources for a health promotion initiative. This support and those resources ideally need to come from both the executive as well as the "rank and file" levels of the stakeholder organizations, keeping in mind that leadership often transcends the formal designation or level of an individual in an organization. The second reason why relationships are so important to this work is the concept of interest-based negotiation and conflict resolution. As described in their work, Marcus and Dorn (2007) recognize that uni- and two-dimensional negotiation, even when executed well, are not as effective in the long term as multidimensional problem solving. This level of negotiation addresses the needs and concerns of all parties or stakeholders in the process and its outcome, ultimately resulting in a win-win approach, where the groups' interests are aligned. Gaining the support and resources of key decision makers and influencers and employing a multidimensional approach to problem solving would not be possible without the foundational step of relationship building and maintenance.

Importance of Partners

Green and Kreuter (1999) characterized health promotion as a "combination" of supports that will lead to actions. It is essential to recognize the role of partners in this area of best practices of health promotion. Because of the multiple determinants of health in any given community, health promotion often includes a wide and diverse array of stakeholders who can become partners. Green and Kreuter, as cited in McKenzie & Smeltzer (2001), have classified these partners in two basic camps: educational partners who are considered the more traditional participants in health promotion in that they determine and deliver the process of educating people about health; and ecological partners who deal with many of the more nontraditional determinants of health, such as the political, organizational, economic, environmental, and social interactions that affect health. Olson proposes a practical guide to learning about and managing these partnerships in this text's chapter on "Partnerships and Collaborations: The Keys for Reaching Our Health Goals."

Delivering a Health Promotion Program

Implementing an Action in Small Steps

To be successful, health promotion programs must be delivered. This may sound obvious; however, the planning phase of health promotion often overshadows the implementation or delivery phase. Extensive resources are allocated for planning, but resources for implementation (and even more so for evaluation) are often limited. A recent example of where a lack of implementation and planning has *not* occurred has been the CDC's VERB Campaign to increase and sustain physical activity among "tweens" (youth between the ages of 9 and 13 years). The leaders of this campaign recognized the importance of venue–community, the importance of communication, and the importance of champions–leaders in the delivery of this successful national campaign (CDC, 2002).

Importance of Small Steps

Small pilot-type steps are the foundation for the Model for Improvement (see Figure 13-1) described by IHI. This is relevant to health promotion because it provides the framework for rapid improvement cycles, enabling health planners and promoters to adjust goals and strategies based on information and feedback from previous efforts, thus treating health promotion as a more iterative rather than stagnant process.

Importance of Venue–Community

We have all seen various definitions of venue and community. Simply stated, *venue* can be defined as a "place where events are held" (Merriam-Webster, 1998, p.1311) and *community* is defined as "a group of people with similar interests who do not necessarily live in the same place" (Merriam-Webster, 1998, p. 233). VERB was a mass media campaign using airtime and advertising on such networks as Nickelodeon to promote and encourage physical activity in tweens. This campaign's delivery changed how many in the field of health promotion perceive the concepts of venue and community. One may still recall the tag line "Verb, it's what you do; what's your verb?" Therefore, the place where events were held was expanded to enable planners to consider air space and time, not simply the physical place and staging of events. The VERB campaign's program delivery reflected its view of the target community. Not confined by physical location, VERB recognized the importance of reaching a very specific subset of our nation's youth who are generally not traditional consumers of health care yet form a powerful community because of their developmental stage. Historically, marketers have not ignored this powerful group and now, through the delivery of the VERB Campaign, health promoters have not either.

Importance of Communication

Countless scholarly works have reported on and discussed the importance of communication in all human interactions. Health promotion programs that represent best practices in today's environment need to incorporate a new and more expansive vocabulary to be highly effective. For example, a health promotion program at the workplace not only needs to be structurally sound as it relates to the field of health promotion (for example, it needs to simultaneously address individual, environmental, policy, and cultural factors affecting health and productivity) but it also needs to translate and transition these processes and outcomes into terminology and concepts that are meaningful and actionable to the business community. Goetzel, et al. (2007) suggest that careful attention should be paid to terms and concepts, such as human capital, business case, return on investment, benchmarking, cost burden, and cost analysis, when determining if a work site health promotion program could be considered a best practice because this will be understood and accepted by businesses and therefore is more likely to be implemented. *A Purchaser's Guide to Clinical Preventive Services* is a good example of how the science of prevention can be translated and transitioned so the nonmedical and public health audience can understand their economic investment in health and plan accordingly. School-based and faith-based initiatives have their own set of key terms and concepts that influence how health promotion programs are delivered and how their processes and outcomes are communicated.

Importance of Champions–Leaders

Certain aspects of leadership, which can play a key role in a program's success or failure, are often overlooked in health promotion. These aspects have been described as "leading up" or "follow-ship." Useem (2001) noted that "leading up is the act of working with people above you...to help them and you get a better job done" (p. 9), and Gibson (2004) described follow-ship as simply "the art of following a leader" (p. 1). These essentially convey the same message, i.e., all empowered and engaged members of an organization can and should provide leadership to the development, implementation, and evaluation of a program that affects their community. The role of leaders or champions can be filled from many levels in an organization, but leaders are always people who impact the community, either on a formal or informal basis. Experts concur that these champions or leaders can play different roles, but the ones most often noted are the roles of gatekeepers (those who maintain focus and keep on task) and power brokers (those who exert influence to raise support; Wright, as cited in McKenzie & Smeltzer, 2001).

Two examples of community based and business leadership initiatives are as follows:

- The Steps to a Healthier U.S. program demonstrates the importance of community leadership. This program engages entities at the national, state, and local levels in coordinated efforts to address chronic disease prevention and health promotion. This integration is manifested by the decision to implement programs across numerous health conditions such as diabetes and asthma, and health risks such as being overweight or obese, tobacco use, physical inactivity, and poor nutrition. Carrying out this decision required strong leadership, champions, and commitment, as these programs are typically funded and implemented independently in a community setting. Early in the process, the leaders and champions of Steps also understood that, to be effective, the program needed to be delivered across a variety of community sectors (public health, health care, housing, education, and through the social, environmental, justice, and economic systems [CDC, 2007b].

- The Leap Frog Group is a good example of how the senior leadership of the business community decided that something meaningful, concrete, and timely needed to be done to reduce the incidence of lethal medical mistakes, as reported in the IOM's *To Err is Human: Building a Safer Health System* (Institute of Medicine [IOM], 1999). The Leap Frog Group is a voluntary initiative that uses employer health care purchasing to leverage improvements in health care, safety, quality, and customer value. This is accomplished by developing programs to reduce preventable mistakes; encouraging the public reporting of quality and outcomes; and rewarding doctors and hospitals for specific improvements (The Leap Frog Group, 2008).

Studying (or Evaluating) a Health Promotion Program

Analyze What Happened

Studying both the intended and unintended effects of a health promotion program is critical to the evaluation and is the reason why we do evaluation in the first place. In applying the Deming model to this work, the study of both the intended and unintended effects is completed in a rapid cycle. This is an important variation on the traditional approach, which often invests a considerable amount of time in the study stage. The rapid cycle process provides the opportunity for multiple midcourse corrections (the action step) because of the accelerated timing and chance to make numerous adjustments, having learned from iteration. Although this phase is conducted in an accelerated process, there are three critical elements that need to be considered: the importance of metrics, the importance of measurement methods, and the awareness of confounders and other errors.

Importance of Metrics and Measuring the Correct Things

Outcome measures can be described as the program's ability to identify their results, not their efforts or actions. This is often a very difficult task as best practice programs are able to form an understandable and feasible link between program activities and health results, taking into account the economic, social, and environmental conditions that also produce change in behavior. In other words, they are able to isolate the results that are associated with the program they have developed (Rossi, Freeman, & Lipsey, 1999).

Notwithstanding the oft quoted statement, "what gets measured, gets managed," measurements, in and of themselves, are not very enlightening. It is imperative that a set of quantitative measures be established and then studied to determine if a specific change or intervention actually causes an improvement, or if the change is a result of other factors. Similarly, simply measuring or monitoring change alone is not very helpful, as not all changes lead to improvements. It is important that an organization acknowledge the changes that are more likely to be recognized as improvements (IHI, n.d.).

Importance of Measuring Methods

Although there are significant challenges to measuring the correct things as related to program outcomes, there are a few methodological components that should be addressed. First and foremost, the outcome measures should be applied to the target audience or population. It is also essential to study the control population not exposed to the intervention to conclude that the intervention, and not some other factor, led to the change. An outcome measure, for example, the change in percentage of a community that is obese, should only be applied to those members of the target population that received the intervention. This observation relates to the second principle of measuring methods. Because randomized control trials are resource intensive and difficult to implement, most real-world health promotion programs develop outcome measures or indicators that measure pre- and postprogram results, although some experts believe this provides very weak evidence. In our obesity example, it is less critical to know the current percentage of members exposed to a program who are obese than it would be to know what percentage were obese before and after the intervention. Similarly, knowing the rate of change in obesity in a community at large and comparing that rate to the targeted community that participated in the program would be most informative. When similar changes are found in the intervention and comparison groups, one can attribute these changes to factors other than the program intervention. An additional feature to consider when determining methodology, particularly for a prevention intervention addressing a problem such as obesity, is the level of risk in the targeted audience. A percentage change in obesity levels may be a significant measure if there is a percentage of the population that was overweight and therefore at risk for becoming obese (Rossi, Freeman, & Lipsey, 1999).

Acting on, Sustaining, or Ending a Program

Determine What is Needed to Improve the Process

This is a distinct and important step from the delivery of a health promotion program in that it applies the lessons learned from delivering the program in a way that will sustain the program beyond its initial stage. Therefore, the key term in this clarification is the *improvement*, not simply the delivery, of the program.

Maintaining Support after the Thrill is Gone

There is often a great deal of attention and energy associated with the onset of a health promotion program. Media coverage is generally at its height, and key stakeholders share similar expectations and anticipation. But how is a productive level of attention and energy maintained in order to ensure that a program will meet its goals and objectives after the thrill and initial "honeymoon" period ends? One of the key features of the Deming or PDSA cycle is, when applied to a health promotion program, that program will regularly change because this model promotes rapid cycle CQI. There will be a reinvestment in the planning phase and a return to the PDSA cycle (12 Manage, n.d.). Therefore, it is essential to maintain support of the approach for continuous improvement, as it will often exhibit new features on a regular basis. This is not always an easy task but can be accomplished by recognizing the three elements of empowerment, motivation, and incentives. Understandably, the key stakeholders need to have a strong sense of "buy in" and a clear understanding of and acceptance of the approach. Strong leadership needs to maintain the motivational level of all, and initial successes can be seen as both motivators and incentives so that the support for the health promotion program can be sustained.

Understanding "Shelf Life" and Not Conveying Abandonment

Well-meaning and often very successful health promotion programs do not recognize the life span of specific programs, as this is directly dependent upon the social, epidemiological, behavioral, environmental, and educational variables that are relevant for a target community. Because of this, a program such as Racial and Ethnic Approaches to Community Health U.S., Finding Solutions to Health Disparities (formerly REACH 2010, now REACH U.S.) demonstrates the importance of empowering the community, as opposed to providing a program to the community. The REACH model is based on training and empowering dependable and long-term members of its target communities (in this case, communities and populations that have experienced significant health disparities) to encourage community members to seek better health; to bridge the gaps between the health care delivery system and the community; to change local environments and practices to overcome identified barriers to good health; to implement evidence-based public health programs to fit the local social, political, economic, and cultural circumstances; and to move beyond interventions that seek to improve individual behavior to those that influence change at the community and systems levels (CDC, 2007a). REACH U.S. also demonstrates a good example of what we can call "understanding shelf life." Although it has been operational since 1999, the program has changed significantly since then. The program is based on the current social, epidemiological, behavioral, environmental, and educational variables that are determined to be relevant to the target community. Changing the name from REACH 2010 to REACH U.S. is a basic but significant illustration of this point. Additionally, because community leaders are trained and empowered, there is far less of a sense of abandonment than there would be with a public health program that reaches the end of its funding cycle.

Looking for New Opportunities and Ventures

By definition, the Deming Cycle of Plan-Do-Study-Act is perfectly suited to provide an environment for new opportunities and improvements. It is a CQI method that uses the concepts of speed and scale to look for better ways to do something, and arguably, there are always better ways to deliver a health promotion program. The model provides a method and approach of accelerating improvement and is not meant to replace change models in which an organization may already have invested. Use of the model will require the response to three basic questions: (1) What are we trying to accomplish and how will we know that we are successful? (2) How will we know that a change is an improvement? (3) What changes can we make that will result in improvement (IHI, n.d.)? As described earlier, iterations of a health promotion program provide an opportunity for improvement, refinement, and potentially new and improved versions.

CONCLUDING REMARKS

This chapter has conveyed a logical and intuitive approach to best practices in health promotion based on the Deming Cycle and its focus on CQI. The reader will notice that we have not described how to do actual health promotion programs in the context of their status as a best practice, as this is covered in other chapters of the text, particularly Chapters 3, 4, and 6.

A best practice designation is arbitrary and subjective, as one can't argue that all practices can be improved, which is a main tenet of the Deming Cycle. Having established that it is difficult to objectively establish best practices in health promotion, we would not do this subject area justice if we did not briefly describe what evidence does exist for best practices in the areas of community-based health promotions. *The Guide to Community Preventive Services: What Works to Promote Health?* is a useful tool for all who are interested in health promotion (Zaza, Briss & Harris, 2005). Here is a sampling of this body of work in two key public health areas of diabetes control (what strategies can be employed at a population level to improve the care of those with diabetes?) and promoting physical activity (what strategies work best in helping people become more physically active?).

According to rigorous methods and reviews of the Task Force on Community Preventive Services, there is strong or sufficient evidence to provide disease and case management through the health care system to people with diabetes, and there is equally strong or sufficient evidence to provide self-management education in community gathering places and at home to people with diabetes.

Similarly, the Task Force, which consists of national leaders in the health promotion field, has supported that there is strong or sufficient evidence to support informational approaches to increase physical activity in community-wide campaigns and at point-of-decision prompts, such as a sign by the elevator encouraging use of the stairwell. In the area of behavioral and social approaches to increasing physical activity, there is strong or sufficient evidence to support individually adapted health behavior changes (e.g., coaching), school-based physical education, and nonfamily social support. Additionally, in the area of environmental and policy approaches, there is strong or sufficient evidence to support the creation of enhanced access to physical activity venues that include informational activities (Zaza, Briss & Harris, 2005). *The Community Guide* (Zaza, Briss & Harris, 2005) is the gold standard for all interventions that have evidence to support their implementation at the community level, and it is updated regularly. This information will serve as fertile ground for communities to implement what works to promote health, and the Deming PDSA Cycle can serve as a useful tool in concert with other models to accelerate and refine the improvement process.

In conclusion, we have established the following key points:

1. Best practices, or more accurately, improving best practices, need to inspire and promote change, going beyond the raising of awareness or sharing of information. We live in a world of fast information but slow inspiration.

2. There are many well-respected models to design, implement, and evaluate health promotion programs. Any of these models or approaches can be improved by applying the Deming Cycle so that refinements can be tested and developed in an accelerated time frame.

3. Although sounding like an oxymoron, improving best practices is an accurate term and concept because all health promotion practices should be viewed as a process, recognizing that there is always room for improvement.

4. Health promotion is an iterative process, and the process or journey taken by a community is at least as important as the ultimate program or destination.

DISCUSSION QUESTIONS

1. Describe the Deming Cycle and how it can be applied to health promotion.

2. What are the key elements of the cycle that changes how we currently look at health promotion programs?

3. What are the three questions that formulate the guiding theme of this chapter?

4. Do you think of best practices differently after reading this chapter?

DISCLAIMER

The findings and conclusions of this chapter are those of the author and do not necessarily represent the official positions of the Centers for Disease Control and Prevention.

REFERENCES

Berwick, D. (2006). In M. Stobbe, *Campaign against hospital mistakes says 122,000 lives saved.* Available at http://signonsandiego.printthis.clickability.com. Accessed June 15, 2006.

Berwick, D. (2007, December*). Eating soup with a fork.* Keynote speech delivered at Institute for Health Care Improvement, Orlando, FL.

Campbell, K. P., Lanza, A., Dixon, R., Chattopadhyay, S., Molinari, N., Finch, R. A., (Eds.). *A purchaser's guide to clinical preventive services: moving science into coverage.* Washington DC: National Business Group on Health; 2006

Centers for Disease Control and Prevention. (2007a). Racial and Ethnic Approaches to Community Health (REACH). Available at http://www.cdc.gov/reach/about.htm. Accessed December 28, 2007.

Centers for Disease Control and Prevention. (2007b). Steps to a Healthier U.S., CDC's Steps Program. Available at http://www.cdc.gov/steps. Accessed December 28, 2007.

Centers for Disease Control. (2002). VERB Youth Media Campaign. Available at http://www.cdc.gov/youthcampaign/. Accessed December 28, 2007.

Claritas. (2006). PRIZM. Available at http://www.claritas.com. Accessed September 15, 2008.

Employee Benefit Research Institute. (2005). *Fundamentals of employee benefit programs, part three: health benefits.* Washington DC: Employee Benefit Research Institute.

Gibson, D. (2004). *Followship.* Available at http://www.salesstar.com/mm092704.htm. Accessed December 28, 2007.

Goetzel, R. Z., Scechter, D., Ozminkowski, R. J., Marmet, P., Tabrizi, M., & Roemer, E. C. (2007). Promising practices in employer health and productivity management efforts: Findings from a benchmarking study. *Journal of Occupational and Environmental Medicine, 49* (2), 111–130.

Gordus, L. (2000). *Epidemiology* (2nd ed.). Philadelphia, PA: WB Saunders Company.

Green, L. W., & Kreuter, M. W. (1999). *Health promotion planning: An educational and ecological approach* (3rd ed.). Mountain View, CA: Mayfield Press.

Hamel, G., & Prahalad, C. K. (1996). *Competing for the future.* Boston, MA: Harvard Business School Press.

Heitgard, J. L., & Lee, C. V. (2003). A new look at neighborhoods near national priorities list sites. *Social Science & Medicine, 57,* 1117–1126.

Institute of Medicine. (2004). *To err is human: building a safer health system.* Washington DC: National Academy of Sciences Press.

Institute for Healthcare Improvement. (n.d.). How to improve. Available at http://www.ihi.org/IHI/Topics/Improvement/ImprovementMethods/HowToImprove. Accessed September 12, 2007.

Institute for Healthcare Improvement. (2003). *Innovation Series 2003. The breakthrough series: IHI's collaborative model for achieving break through improvement.* Cambridge, MA: Institute for Healthcare Improvement.

Knowledge @ Wharton. (2001). Leading up: The art of managing your boss. Available at http://knowledge.wharton.upenn.edu/article.cfm?articleid=350. Accessed December 28, 2007.

Lanza, A., Albright, A., Zucker, H., & Martin, M. (2007). The Diabetes Detection Initiative: A pilot program of selective screening. *American Journal of Health Behavior, 31*(6), 632–642.

12Manage. (n.d.). Deming Cycle (PDSA). Available at http://www.12manage. com/methods_demingcycle.html. Accessed August 28, 2007.

Marcus, L. J., & Dorn, B. C. (2007). *The walk in the woods: A step by step approach to multi-dimensional problem solving.* Unpublished manuscript.

McKenzie, J. F., & Smeltzer, J. L. (2001). *Planning, implementing and evaluating health promotion programs, a primer* (3rd ed.). Needham Heights, MA: Allyn & Bacon.

Merriam-Webster. (1998). *Merriam-Webster's Collegiate Dictionary* (10th ed.). Springfield, MA: Merriam-Webster, Incorporated.

Rossi, P., Freeman, H., & Lipsey, M. (1999). *Evaluation: A systematic approach* (6th ed.). Thousand Oaks, CA: Sage Publications.

Task Force on Community Preventive Services. (1996). U.S. Department of Health and Human Services.

The Leap Frog Group. (2008). Available at http://www.leapfroggroup.org. Accessed October 21, 2008.

Top Achievement. (2007). Creating S.M.A.R.T. goals. Available at http://www. topachievement.com/smart.html. Accessed December 28, 2007.

U.S. Department of Health and Human Services. (2007). Identifying and promoting promising practices overview. Available at http://www.acf.hhs.gov/programs/ ccf/resources/gbk_bp/bp_gbk_ov.html. Accessed October 26, 2007.

Useem, M. (2001). In *Knowledge @ Wharton: Leading up: The art of managing your boss.* Available at http://knowledge.wharton.upenn.edu/article.cfm? articleid=350. Accessed December 28, 2007.

Walton, J. (2007). *The CNN YouTube debates.* Available at http://www.cnn.com/ 2007/POLITICS/0704/youtube.debates/index.html. Accessed December 27, 2007.

Wikipedia website. (2008). *Geodemographic segmentation.* Updated March 24, 2009. Available at http://en.wikipedia.org/wiki/Geodemographic_segmentation. Wikipedia, the free encyclopedia. Accessed Jan 30, 2008.

Winslow, C. E. (1920). The untilled field of public health. *Modern Medicine,* 2183–2191.

Zaza, S., Briss, P., & Harris, K. (Eds.). (2005) *The guide to community preventive services: What works to promote health?* New York, NY: Oxford University Press.

Evidence-Based Health Promotion Programs

Bernard J. Healey, PhD

OBJECTIVES   After reading this chapter, you should

- Understand the need to be able to prove the value of health promotion efforts
- Be able to define and explain the components of the development of an evidence-based health promotion effort
- Be aware of the need for evidence-based health interventions
- Understand the problems associated with the implementation of a complete smoking cessation program

KEY TERMS   Clinical preventive services   Healthy lifestyle
Cost-benefit analysis   Positive locus of control
Evidence-based health promotion   Type 2 diabetes

Introduction

The cost of health care services is expected to continue its upward trend over the next 10 years. A recent press release issued by *Health Affairs* revealed that health spending in the United States will reach $4.1 trillion in 2014, doubling today's rate of spending on this service. The average growth rate of health spending is expected to average almost 7% each year for the next 10 years. The out-of-pocket cost for health services for consumers will also increase to $440.8 billion by the year 2016. The rising cost of health care services has increased the demand for accountability in the use of scarce resources to pay for these services.

President Obama has begun discussion with Congress about the need for some type of reorganization of our health care system to offer access to everyone in need of health care services. Several states are attempting to follow the lead of Massachusetts in offering their residents health insurance coverage no matter what their income or employment status.

Americans are not asking for access to medical care, but they are asking for access to good health. Access alone will not guarantee anyone good health, especially if they are practicing high-risk health behaviors. People are also not asking for entrance to a hospital or a visit to a physician. Rather, they are asking for good health and protection from the enormous costs associated with entering the health care system if they become ill. They certainly do not want to encounter poor health, but they would rather remain healthy until they die from old age. They really want information on how to stay well.

I have flood insurance on my home and personal belongings because I live in a flood prone area. I certainly do not pay my yearly premium for this insurance in hopes that my development will become the victim of a disastrous flood. I do want the government to expand the flood protection in my area and have in place an early warning system in the event that a flood becomes eminent. Ideally, I should stop practicing my high-risk behavior of living in a flood plain and move to higher ground.

Health promotion experts are convinced that prevention programs are the answer to all of the problems found in our current health care delivery system. The question becomes, What prevention programs work and at what cost in terms of the use of scarce resources? Whether it is called **evidence-based health promotion** or best practices in health promotion, it stands to reason that those working in the field of health promotion need to work with programs that have achieved past success.

There needs to be a comprehensive assessment of the health of the community and the use of the best health promotion practices to share information about the prevention of health problems to the members of the community. Fielding and Briss (2006) believe that there needs to be urgency in sharing scientific discoveries concerning the causes of poor health within the community. There is no excuse for public health to not prioritize health promotion efforts to all community members utilizing the emerging methods of communication. Those working in health promotion know what needs to be done, and they have the evidence to support their decisions; now the resources need to be made available to implement evidence-based health promotion programs.

Evidence-Based Medicine

McKenzie, Pinger, and Kotecki (2005) describe evidence-based practice as utilizing scientific evidence that demonstrates a service will actually work before utilizing that service. Fielding and Briss (2006) argue that the improvement of the health of the population can be accomplished through the introduction of evidence-based policies that have an impact on the process of acquiring disease. This is especially relevant when dealing with chronic diseases and prevention programs that are used to educate the population about these diseases. They also define evidence-based public health as the utilization of science-based decisions to improve the health of populations. Evidence-based medicine can help the health promotion specialist in the prioritization of the choice of disease and high-risk health behaviors on which to concentrate the limited program resources.

Maciosek et al. (2006) completed a study that identified the most important preventive services that can be offered in a medical practice. Many of these services require the consumer to have information to be able to ask questions of his or her health care professional. The consumer also needs to know what works when attempting to practice a **healthy lifestyle**. Coffield et al. (2001) argue that recommended **clinical preventive services** are not being utilized by physicians and are not being requested by consumers. There is a tremendous need for information concerning the value of certain prevention procedures that are capable of reducing disease and disease complications in our population.

According to Satcher (2006) "in the United States, more money is spent on treating diseases and their complications than on preventing them in the first place" (p. 1009). Those individuals given the responsibility to promote good health for populations need to be given the best evidence on what works and what costs are associated with the preventive program in order to make good choices in the use of scarce resources.

Those individuals developing health promotion efforts need to be aware of what interventions have the best chance of success so they can prioritize their actions. If they have the scientific evidence that a prevention program will work, it becomes that much easier to attract the resources and talent needed to ensure successful intervention.

Clancy and Cronin (2005) argue that there is increased interest in the development of the best science for utilization in making decisions about care that is provided by our health care system. This need for cost effective medical decisions is of great importance when confronting the challenges of treating chronic diseases.

According to CDC (2005) preventive services have been evaluated and ranked according to benefit and cost. This Community Guide to Preventive Services revealed that the three most valuable preventive health services that can be offered in medical practice today are discussing daily aspirin use with at-risk adults to prevent cardiovascular disease, immunizing children, and helping tobacco users to quit the habit. These recommended procedures have the greatest impact on health for the lowest cost. It is this type of prevention effort that can be the catalyst to best practice health promotion programs.

Clancy and Cronin (2005) argue that there has been an explosion in the amount of information available to assist clinicians in making evidence-based decisions that have the best chance of helping their patients maintain good health. This information is meant to be an adjunct to the expert opinion of the clinician. This same information and technology needs to be made available and further developed for use in the development, implementation, and evaluation of health promotion programs. This evidence-based health information also needs to be made available to consumers so they are more knowledgeable when dealing with their physicians.

There has been a movement throughout the health services sector of our economy to compare the costs of alternative courses of action with the outcomes associated with these choices. McKenzie, Neiger, and Thackeray (2009) argue that this movement is forcing funders to apply the same measurement techniques to health promotion programs.

Chronic Diseases

Morewitz (2006) argues that chronic diseases represent the leading cause of mortality each year, and over 25 million Americans currently have at least one chronic disease. The increased life expectancy of most Americans coupled with the increased prevalence of chronic diseases are forcing the health care delivery system to consider the use of best practices to prevent the complications associated with these chronic diseases. Health promotion programs that have demonstrated success in preventing these complications are growing in demand in order to stabilize the costs of health delivery in this country.

Morewitz (2006) points out that three of the most prevalent chronic diseases—cardiovascular disease, cancer, and diabetes—cost this country over $700 billion every year. The costs of these diseases are so high because of the complications resulting from living with these diseases. These complications can be reduced or even prevented with better education for those afflicted with the diseases.

Those utilizing the results of evidence-based findings in the development of health promotion programs need to realize that there are limitations in this procedure. Glanz and Saraiya (2005) point out that the major limitation is found in the fact that lack of sufficient evidence about a certain intervention does not mean the intervention is not worthy of consideration. There needs to be more evaluation and the gathering of more data concerning the intervention. Evidence-based health promotion must be considered a work in progress.

The use of evidence-based health promotion programs offers those in public health the opportunity to better the outcomes of the proposed programs while also to reduce the costs of these interventions. An example of two chronic diseases and the largest contributor to chronic diseases is capable of demonstrating this evidence-based process to readers. The chronic diseases are **Type 2 diabetes** and skin cancer. The largest contributor to chronic diseases, tobacco use, will also be evaluated using evidence-based methods. Kongstvedt (2007) argues that most of the mortality and, therefore the health care costs, could have been prevented. The modifiable risk factors that helped to produce these chronic diseases include tobacco use, physical inactivity, and poor dietary habits.

Kongstvedt (2007) argues that there needs to be an organized and strategic focus on prevention efforts if this nation is ever going to be able to deal with the enormous costs associated with chronic diseases and their complications. These prevention programs include well-developed health promotion programs that have provided evidence that they work at a reasonable cost. These preventive services have been shown through **cost-benefit analysis** to be cost effective.

The major goals of prevention programs are to encourage the practice of healthy lifestyles, to identify individuals who could benefit from intervention for a condition for which they are unaware, and to prevent complications among individuals who already have an established disease. There is tremendous value in the promotion of preventive services. These services must really be considered an investment of current resources with payment found in the reduction of the costs associated with future disease and the health complications associated with that disease.

For example, the promotion of never starting tobacco use or quitting the habit can result in individuals avoiding tobacco-related diseases altogether. Preventive services can also discover disease at a very early stage when it is curable. Several chronic diseases lend themselves to evidence-based support.

Diabetes

The Issue Diabetes mellitus is a prevalent, expensive chronic disease that is increasing in the United States every year. Diabetes is the seventh leading cause of death and approximately one-third of those with this disease are unaware that they have the condition. Over 90% of those with diabetes have type 2 diabetes, which is caused by lifestyle behaviors. These high-risk behaviors include poor diet, obesity, and physical inactivity.

Individuals with diabetes are at higher risk of heart disease, stroke, kidney disease, blindness, amputations, and several other medical complications. Morewitz (2006) points out that people with type 2 diabetes have a 2- to 4-fold increase in coronary heart disease and a 4-fold increase in mortality from coronary heart disease. The American Diabetes Association reports that in 2002 the cost of health care for a person with diabetes was $13, 243, as opposed to $2,500 for a person without diabetes. Type 2 diabetes can be prevented, and the complications from this type of diabetes can be eliminated or postponed if healthy behaviors are practiced.

The Evidence Intervention programs can delay the onset and slow the progression of complications, which in turn reduces the costs associated with this disease. There needs to be a complete plan involving increased physical activity and improved nutrition established in individuals' daily activities before they are diagnosed with diabetes, and it needs to be continued even if it is discovered that they already have diabetes. The goal needs to include glycemic control, decreased complications and mortality, and improved individual quality of life. These programs are rather expensive to develop and implement. They also take years to show definitive results. But, given time and resources, they can most certainly prove their worth.

Although type 2 diabetes represents a potentially enormous cost to employers in terms of increased health insurance costs and reduced productivity by the affected employees, it also offers a very real opportunity for employers and employees to work together to ensure that proper management of this chronic disease reduces the human and economic impact on employees and the business.

Akinci, Healey, and Coyne (2003) argue that diabetes does not have to cause long-term complications if the disease is managed properly. Control of the progression of diabetes has been demonstrated in several studies to delay the onset and to slow the progression of complications, which in turn reduces the costs associated with the disease. The American Diabetes Association (2002) argues that less than 50% of individuals with diabetes receives the 3 recommended screenings every year to prevent the complications from this very dangerous chronic disease. These screenings include blood sugar test, foot examination, and eye examination.

Morewitz (2006) argues that a **positive locus of control** may be the key to coping strategies that help the person with diabetes avoid the complications from this disease. The evidence suggests that a very important component in helping the person with diabetes practice self-care behaviors is social support. This social support involves the offering of information and motivational support in dealing with the disease. Therefore, the attendance at diabetes education programs and exercise and weight loss programs with others who have diabetes have been proven to do very well in preventing the complications from diabetes.

The health promotion program for people with diabetes needs to include a multifaceted approach to the disease. This effort needs to include counseling, group education sessions, self-care training, stress management, nutritional counseling, and weight management.

Cancer

The Issue   Cancer is now the leading cause of death in the United States. This disease, also called *malignant neoplasms*, occurs when cells in the body lose control over their growth and division. Many of the various forms of cancer are available for prevention or cure if detected in an early stage. Skin cancer is the most common form of cancer found in this country.

There are three major types of skin cancer: basal cell, squamous cell, and malignant melanoma. Basal cell and squamous cell cancers are highly curable, while malignant melanoma diagnosed at a late stage is most likely to spread to other sites in the body.

Glanz and Saraiya (2005) found that in 2004, more than 1 million individuals were diagnosed with squamous cell or basal cell carcinoma, resulting in more than 2,200 deaths. Approximately 65% to 90% of melanoma is caused by ultraviolet radiation (UVR). Morewitz (2006) points out that there are a number of genetic factors that predispose an individual to being more susceptible to developing skin cancer including fair complexion, family or personal history of skin cancer, history of sunburns early in life, and a large number of moles, atypical moles, and freckles.

Skin cancer, although it is the most common form of cancer, is largely preventable. The key to preventing this form of cancer lies in protection from the sun and awareness of the risk factors for this disease. Having said that, what is the most effective way to share this information with individuals at risk at the lowest cost?

The Evidence   Skin cancer is a very preventable form of cancer requiring knowledge about individual risk factors and knowledge about the disease. The evidence suggests that exposure to UVR of the sun appears to be the most important factor in the development of this form of cancer.

Reviews of evidence of the effectiveness of intervention for reducing UVR exposure to prevent skin cancer were conducted by the task force on Community Preventive Services in 2004. This task force evaluated several settings where intervention in preventing skin cancer could take place by health promotion programs. These settings include day care centers, recreation centers, primary schools, work sites, community-wide programs, and media campaigns. According to Glanz and Saraiya (2005), only two of these settings provided evidence that was strong enough to support intervention. They were primary schools and recreation–tourism areas.

Glanz and Saraiya (2005) argue that absence of data to prove efficacy of an intervention effort could mean that more data needs to be gathered. Because the available data does support concentration of resources in primary schools and outdoor recreation programs, these areas should be the focus of health promotion efforts until more data is available.

Tobacco

The Issue   According to the CDC (2005), cigarette smoking is the leading preventable cause of death, causing 438,000 deaths per year and 38,000 of these deaths are the result of secondhand smoke. This high-risk health behavior costs $167 billion each year, which includes $92 billion in lost productivity and $75.5 billion in health care costs. This product is responsible for 30% of cancer deaths and also contributes to deaths from heart disease, stroke, and chronic obstructive pulmonary disease. The CDC (2005) also reports that 21% of adults and 22% of American high school students continue this deadly habit every year.

The rates of smoking tobacco have been on the decline for the last several years, but more needs to be done to virtually eliminate this dangerous habit over the next several years. This is clearly a high-risk behavior that lends itself to well-developed health promotion programs. There are resources available for health promotion programs to reduce the use of tobacco, but these resources need to be utilized on programs that offer the greatest chance of success at the lowest cost. The IOM (2000) argues that tobacco control programs are an excellent example of the successful use of multifaceted health promotion programs.

The Evidence   The best practices for comprehensive tobacco control programs put forth by the National Institutes of Health (2006) emphasizes:

- preventing the initiation of tobacco use among young people,
- promoting cessation among young people and adults,
- eliminating nonsmokers' exposure to secondhand smoke, and
- identifying and eliminating the disparities related to tobacco use and its effects among different population groups.

The National Institutes of Health (2006) also recommends that states establish tobacco control programs that contain the following elements:

- Community programs to reduce tobacco use
- Chronic disease programs to reduce the burden of tobacco-related diseases
- School programs
- Statewide programs
- Countermarketing efforts
- Tobacco cessation programs
- Surveillance and evaluation
- Administration and management

The National Institutes of Health (NIH; 2006) evaluated the best practices available to prevent tobacco use in adolescents and young adults. This conference pointed out that the research strongly suggests that tobacco use usually begins during adolescence. School-based intervention programs emphasizing tobacco prevention are effective in the short run. In the long run, there needs to be a change in community norms through community-driven systems that create environments where it is uncommon to see, use, or be negatively impacted by tobacco products and tobacco smoke pollution.

Kongstvedt (2007) argues that group intensive counseling has been found to be the most effective cessation program but is only practiced by 5% of participants. There is also interest in Internet-based cessation programs. They have resulted in one-third of the participants quitting or reducing the number of cigarettes smoked per day. Almost 80% responded that the program had strengthened their desire to quit the habit.

The NIH (2006) found that despite strong evidence that a variety of pharmacologic and behavioral interventions work, only a small proportion of tobacco users ever try them. Most adult smokers want to quit, and effective interventions exist; however, only a small proportion of smokers ever use the treatment. Well-developed health promotion programs regarding the health effects from tobacco use needs to be expanded.

CONCLUDING REMARKS

The escalating costs associated with the delivery of health care services are providing opportunities for the development of cost-effective health promotion programs. There is ample evidence that disease can be prevented, and if disease does occur, the complications from the disease can be reduced significantly if healthy behaviors become the norm. The problem has always been that our health care delivery system has always been fixated on curing diseases rather than preventing their occurrence in the first place. In fact, the majority of the finances available to health care in our country have always been allocated to the part of the system that attempts to cure health problems, leaving precious little for the prevention part of health care budgets.

The benefits of healthy practices must be communicated to Americans who need to understand the difference between living longer lives and living longer healthy lives. Those working in health promotion programs need to continuously evaluate what they do and how they do it in order to improve the process of educating individuals about how to prevent disease and the complications associated with disease.

It is time to take evidence-based medicine results to evidence-based health promotion efforts. The results of this effort should produce better health and allocation of scarce resources for successful health promotion initiatives. In order to continue or expand health promotion programs, there must be solid evidence that these programs are effective and efficient.

DISCUSSION QUESTIONS

1. Please offer a complete explanation of evidence-based medicine.
2. Offer an explanation of the costs and benefits of many of the major health prevention efforts currently being used in the United States.
3. What are the most important preventive services that can be offered by a physician's office? Explain.
4. Why is so little attention paid to prevention programs by our current medical care delivery system?

REFERENCES

Akinci, F., Healey, B., & Cotne, J. (2003). Improving the health status of UD working adults with type 2 diabetes mellitus. *Disease Management Health Outcomes, 11*(8), 489–498.

American Diabetes Association. Economic consequences of diabetes mellitus in the United States in 1997. Diabetes Care 1998:21:269-209.

American Diabetes Association. Standards of medical care for patients with diabetes mellitus. Diabetes Care 2002: 25 (1): 213-29.

Centers for Disease Control and Prevention. (1995). Assessing the effectiveness of disease and injury prevention programs: costs and consequences. *Morbidity and Mortality Weekly Report, 44*(RR-10), 1–11.

Centers for Disease Control and Prevention. (1986). Premature mortality in the United States: Public health issues in the use of years of potential life lost. *Morbidity and Mortality Weekly Report, 35*, 1–11.

Centers for Disease Control and Prevention. (2005). CDC Evaluation Working Group. Available at http://www.cdc.gov/eval/index.htm. Accessed August 28, 2006.

Clancy, C. M., & Cronin, K. (2005). Evidence-based decision making: Global evidence, local decisions. *Journal of Health Affairs, 24*(1), 151–162.

Coffield, A. B., Maciosek, M. V., McGinnis, M., Harris, J. R., Caldwell, M. B., Teutsch, S. M., et al. (2001). Priorities among recommended clinical preventive services. *American Journal of Preventive Medicine, 21*(1), 1–9.

Fielding, J. E., & Briss, P. A. (2006). Promoting evidence-based health policy: Can we have better evidence and more action. *Health Affairs, 25*(4), 969–978.

Glanz, K., & Saraiya, M. (2005). Using evidence-based community and behavioral interventions to prevent skin cancer: Opportunities and challenges for public health practice. *Preventing Chronic Disease Public Health Research, Practice, and Policy, 2*(2), 1–5.

National Institutes of Health. (2006). *National Institutes of Health State-of-the-Science conference statement: tobacco use: Prevention, cessation, and control*. Paper presented at the *Ann Intern Med*. June 12–14, 2006, 145.

Health Affairs. (2007). Health care spending projected to pass $4 trillion mark by 2016. Available at http://content.healthaffairs/org/cgi/content/abstract/hthaff.26.2.w242

Institute of Medicine. (2000). *Promoting health intervention strategies from social and behavioral research*. Washington DC: National Academy Press.

Kongstvedt. P. (2007). *Essentials of managed health care* (5th ed.). Sudbury, MA: Jones and Bartlett Publishers.

Maciosek, M. V., Coffield, A. B., Edwards, N. M., Flottemesch, T. J., Goodman, M. J., & Solberg, L. I. (2006). Priorities among effective clinical preventive services results of a systematic review and analysis. *American Journal of Preventive Medicine, 31*(1), 52–62.

McKenzie, J.F., Neiger, B. L., & Thackeray, R. (2009). Planning, implementing and evaluating health promotion programs: A primer (5th ed.). San Francisco, CA: Pearson/Benjamin Cummings.

McKenzie, J. F., Pinger, R. R., & Kotecki, J. E. (2005). *An introduction to community health* (5th ed.). Sudbury, MA: Jones and Bartlett Publishers.

Morewitz, S. J. (2006). *Chronic diseases and health care*. New York, NY: Springer Publisher.

Satcher, D. (2006). The prevention challenge and opportunity. *Health Affairs, 25*, 1009–1011.

Partnerships and Collaboration: Critical Components to Promoting Health

Sarah J. Olson, MS, CHES

OBJECTIVES

After reading this chapter, you should

- Be able to describe why partnership and collaboration are an important strategy to achieving the nation's health goals
- Be able to identify the important characteristics of successful partnerships
- Be able to identify and describe five steps and key activities of planning and implementing a successful partnership
- Be able to describe the unique characteristics and strategies for partnering with business, education, health care, and faith-based organizations

KEY TERMS

Business partnerships	Partners
Education partnerships	Partnership
Faith-based organizations partnerships	Partnership evaluation

Introduction: Rationale for Partnerships and Collaboration

Despite enormous strides in public health that have resulted in a greatly extended life span, the quality of these extra years of life is jeopardized by increasingly complex threats to the public's health and safety. A one-time immunization is not available for most of today's threats—cancer, heart disease, HIV–AIDS, injuries, obesity, and risky behavior. These threats can only be reduced by the sophisticated use of a large number of prevention measures that rigorous scientific evaluations have shown to be effective. Effective prevention measures typically work by changing individuals' behaviors and by helping people and organizations make better choices that affect health. Rarely can prevention measures be forced or mandated; most public health agencies—state, local, and even the Centers for Disease Control and Prevention (CDC)—have little (if any) regulatory authority. Moreover, those agencies and organizations often have far fewer resources than are needed to implement optimal prevention programs. Because public health agencies have limited resources and little regulatory authority, they must work closely with private citizens and with public- and private-sector organizations in order to improve health outcomes. Why should public and private organizations and agencies work together on common prevention activities, especially because they have different organizational goals and objectives that may not even have health as a central component?

> "... partnerships successfully bring people together, expand resources, and focus on a problem of community concern better than any single group or agency could do alone. ..."
>
> —Frances Butterfoss,
> *Coalitions and Partnerships in*
> *Community Health,* 2007

The answer is that the problems affect all of us, and it will take our working together to solve them.

As stated by Tennyson in *The Partnering Toolbook* (2003), "The hypothesis underpinning a **partnership** approach is that only with comprehensive and widespread cross-sector collaboration can we ensure that sustainable development initiatives are imaginative, coherent and integrated enough to tackle the most intractable problems"(p. 3).

Many organizations in different market segments (e.g., business, education, faith-based, and community organizations) have different missions, goals, and objectives and may not have health as a primary part of their mission at all. Despite these differences, there is a space in which public and private entities share a common interest. For example, reducing absenteeism and health care costs can be motivators for improving the health of employees. This "common interest" or overlapping space with public health is the environment in which public–private partnerships may evolve. The goal is to make the common interest space as large as possible (see Figure 15-1).

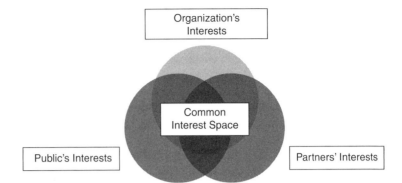

Figure 15-1
Common Interest Space

Potential Benefits of Partnering and Collaborating

Before entering into a new partnership (or continuing an existing one), all **partners** should assess the benefits and risks that may arise from being involved in a partnership of any type if they are going to commit to their partners and support the principle of mutual benefit. Partnerships are not always the right strategy. Potential benefits must outweigh the potential risks.

Tennyson (2003) lists the following potential benefits:

- Unable to optimize the public's health without partners
- Leveraging—maximizing resources—increase cost-effectiveness by pooling talents and resources; few organizations or agencies possess resources to address all health issues
- Improving reach to the community
- Minimizing duplication of efforts
- Generating broad-based support
- Increasing credibility beyond that of individual organizations
- Being more appealing to funders because they represent diverse agencies and organizations

Cohen, L., Aboelata, M., Gantz, T. L., and Van Wert, J. (2003a) list the following potential risks:

- Implementation challenges—new challenges and commitments will emerge once the partnership is formed and project implementation begins
- Conflicts of interest
- Drain on resources
- Possible negative reputation impact
- Loss of autonomy
- Reduced independence

Lastly, by engaging and addressing the competing interests, it is possible to develop a better product–program–intervention because it more realistically addresses the world as it really is. By ignoring competing interests and real-world complexity, the product will not be as good and will likely fail. The need to touch base is really to be able to develop a product–program that has a chance to succeed in an increasingly complex, sophisticated, and skeptical environment.

Definitions

Terms related to partners are often used in different ways in the literature. Before going into the details about creating partnerships, let us define the terms as they will be used in this chapter and as they will relate to health-related partnerships and collaborations.

Partners are individuals, organizations, or groups who work collaboratively to achieve a shared goal to protect and promote the safety and health of the public. (Note: Organizations often have different missions, but they can still have a common goal; they collaborate by being willing to commit time, money, skills, staffing, knowledge, or intellectual capital, or other resources toward achieving this common goal.)

Partnerships are collaborations in which two or more organizations or individuals agree to work together through trust, shared vision, investment, risk, responsibility, evaluation, management, and governance to achieve shared or complementary goals.

What Makes Partnerships Successful: General Guidelines

Effective partnerships do not just happen. There are design principles and strategic steps that create them. The following general principles for creating effective partnerships have been identified by numerous researchers, including Cohen (2003a), Foley (2002), Gardner (2005), Tennyson (2003), and the University of Kansas' *Community Toolbox* (2005):

- Build trust. No partnership can be successful without trust. Trust is one of the most often listed components in published literature of effective collaboration. Openness and honesty in working relationships are preconditions of trust. Honoring commitments and being honest about plans, available resources, and resource requirements can expand and deepen trust. Partners need to be honest and frank about what their interests are and what they need to get from the collaboration. From the beginning, they should build into the action plan what each partner needs. When a partnership is first being considered, the partners should explicitly identify actions of each partner that could damage the partnership, and they should build a mechanism to reduce the likelihood of such damage. For example, organizations often share proprietary information and resources with a partner, trusting that those resources will not be misused. Methods to protect those treasured organizational resources must be defined at the outset, and rules that govern their use must be agreed upon, usually in writing in a memorandum of understanding or similar document. When such resources are shared, partnerships often need to build a mechanism to monitor compliance with partnership agreements. Even when the partnership structure is designed with trust in mind, trust takes time to build. Partners must keep their commitments and promises.

- Have champions. The partnership should be sponsored and promoted by committed leaders with the power to legitimize its role or value. Although there is no single, perfect governance structure, the most effective partnerships are typically led by influential and trustworthy leaders—elected officers, grassroots organizers, or key leaders through status or knowledge.

- Begin with the ends in mind. It is critical to have a clear agreement about shared missions and goals at the beginning of the relationship. It is wise to start with clearly defined, achievable results and work backward to develop an action plan to get there, including the rules and responsibilities of partners. It is usually necessary to collect baseline data to assess progress and outcomes. Participants should resist the urge to start activities until the goals, objectives, action plan, and responsibilities have been developed and agreed upon. It is especially risky to launch a partnership hoping that, by working together, it will be easier to resolve those disagreements. In such settings, the disagreements often harden.

- Make good use of data. Successful partnerships typically use data to set reasonable goals and mobilize support. Reliable shared data can be used to plan, evaluate, and understand trends. Data can make the case for continued involvement, organizational support, and continued or expanded financial support. Partnerships also need to have firm agreements about data security, ownership, and access.

- Distribute accountability among partners. Under a guiding principle of shared (not necessarily equal) accountability, stakeholders can jointly assess effectiveness and identify who has responsibility for doing what, how it will be measured, and what needs to be improved. Each common goal should be framed broadly enough so that all the players can support it and/or have a clear role to play in meeting it.

- Ensure mutual benefit. If all partners are expected to contribute to the partnership, they should also benefit from the partnership. A healthy partnership will work toward achieving specific benefits for each partner over and above the common benefits to all partners.

- Plan for organizational competence. In addition to the goals of the partnership, the governance structures and principles of the partnership itself should be clearly articulated so that basic tasks can be performed effectively and efficiently. An effective partnership must establish strong leadership and determine how decisions will be made, who will provide staff services, and what the communication processes will be to keep the members informed. Actions to be addressed include (1) administrative responsibility, (2) meeting logistics and follow-up, (3) membership recruitment and support, (4) research and data collection, (5) public relations and public information, (6) coordination of activities and events (including media, if appropriate), and (7) fundraising. Lack of structure can lead to difficulties in retaining members, thus undermining mutual accountability and limiting meaningful cooperation.

- Ensure that meetings are productive. Meetings should have key outcomes and action steps, with responsibilities and dates for completion clearly delineated. Paying attention to efficient meetings goes a long way. Examples include the following: agree how decisions will be made; establish ground rules for meeting procedures, behaviors, and frequency; solicit members' input on the agenda; ensure all attendees are actively engaged in the process; clarify decisions and resulting tasks, timetables, responsibilities, and follow-up; begin and end on time; and allow opportunities for social interaction and networking. It is wise to pay attention to the meeting location(s), time of day, and comfort of the site. Make sure the partnership is moving forward—do not have a meeting just to meet, or attendance and participation will decline.

- Address the issues of equity and inclusion and how money relates to membership. Equity implies an equal right to be at the table and a validation of those contributions that are not measurable simply in terms of cash value or public profile. Equity means fair distribution but does not necessarily mean equal roles, responsibilities, or authority. Strive for broad representation of individuals and organizations that look at problems and solutions differently and yet permit the partnership to move forward. This will help forge joint solutions and comprehensive approaches to the problems or issues being addressed and reduce the likelihood that other groups will openly oppose activities. Start by identifying organizations that already work on the issue, and then look for other organizations or individuals that have an interest in the issue and can help be part of the solution.

- Be realistic about progress and celebrate "quick wins." Effective partnerships acknowledge the incremental progress they make and celebrate the quick wins. Leaders should emphasize the hope and accomplishments of the group, as well as the progress (Foley 2002).

- Take steps to address and diffuse "turf" issues. When forming partnerships, often there are expectations of self-sacrifice from individuals and organizations as they move toward solutions. It is a good idea to be explicit about the areas and issues of sacrifice and investment. These may include competition from the same pool of resources, issues relating to recognition and publicity, and which will be the specific approaches to the problem being addressed by the partnership. Instead of instructing members to "leave turf at the door," a more realistic approach is to acknowledge that turf issues will challenge the group and blend the pursuit of individual interests with the greater good, identifying and addressing the issues explicitly. There is no one-shot formula to avoid turf struggle. Working collectively takes hard work and requires a combination of strong relationships, planning for sustainability, and focusing on the big picture. Effective turf management tips from Cohen and Gould (2003b) include the following: (1) acknowledge potential turf issues, (2) talk details, (3) shape the collective partnership identity and share the limelight, (4) make fair decisions, (5) seek funding for coordination of the partnership, (6) reward members and celebrate successes, (7) build bridges, (8) remind participants of the big picture, (9) make struggles overt (acknowledge conflicts and discuss solutions), (10) encourage flexibility and compromise, and (11) foster joint problem solving.

One final general recommendation includes the following:

- Use theories to guide planning and implementation of the partnership. Theories are useful in providing context and understanding of the potential contribution of a partnership. As stated in Glanze and Rimer's *Theory at a Glance* (2005), theories and models "provide a road map for studying problems, developing appropriate interventions, and evaluating their successes"(p. 5). They provide context and theoretical guidance on how partnerships can approach public health problems as well as the forces which affect the partnership's functioning and ultimate success. Theories help integrate planning, implementation, and evaluation. They guide strategies that will reach the target audiences and have an impact. They help set priorities for efficiently allocating resources. They help identify which indicators should be monitored and used for evaluation. There are many books and publications that focus solely on models and theories related to public health and can provide insight and guidance and would be worth considering for guiding the partnership, especially *Community Coalition Action Theory, Social Network Theory, Community Empowerment and Community Engagement Models*, and *Social Marketing*, to name a few. The reader is encouraged to seek out information on theories and models and use them to help plan his or her partnership activities.

Summary of Success: Factors of a Successful Collaboration

Mattessich, Murray-Close, and Monsey (2001) conducted a meta-analysis of 133 studies to identify factors related to successful collaboration. They identified 20 success factors, grouped into 6 categories: environment, membership characteristics, process and structure, communication, purpose, and resources. These factors serve as an effective summary of the general guidelines for success and are as follows:

- History of community collaboration and cooperation in the community
- Seen as a legitimate community leader in the community
- Favorable political and social climate
- Mutual respect, understanding, and trust
- Appropriate cross-section of members representing community segments
- Collaboration seen by members as being in their self-interest
- Ability to compromise

- Members share stake in both process and outcome
- Multiple layers of participation from organizations
- Flexibility
- Clear roles, rights, and policy guidelines
- Adaptability
- Appropriate pace of development
- Open and frequent communication
- Established informal relationships and communication links
- Concrete, attainable goals and objectives
- Shared vision
- Unique purpose
- Sufficient funds, staff, materials, and time
- Skilled leadership

Steps in Building a Partnership

Building a successful partnership is not an overwhelming task if it is done strategically and systematically. The following information is a distillation of information from a number of sources developed by thoughtful researchers who have studied successful and unsuccessful partnerships and who have identified the critical elements and processes that have made them so. This section breaks down the partnering process into five steps that will help to maximize your efforts, resources, and outcomes. It is important to realize, although the steps below are depicted in a linear fashion, in actuality, the activities may occur simultaneously, in a different order, or may even be repeated as the effort goes forward.

An overview of the five steps and significant activities for each is depicted in Figure 15-2. This section of the chapter will then discuss each step and activity in more detail. Each activity is numbered to indicate the step and the activity under that step (e.g., the first activity under Step 1 is 1.1, the second activity is 1.2).

Step 1:
Prepare–
Groundwork

1.1   Determine public health problem, goals, and affected populations. Assemble data that makes the case for and inform the need of a collaborative effort to address a public health problem.

1.2   Conduct a preliminary analysis of the problem. Identify assets and gaps—needs related to the problem and what needs to be done to address it.

1.3   Assess the need for a partnership. A partnership may not be the best way to address a potential public health problem. Determine if a partnership is appropriate and the best strategy for your organization.

1.4   Assess if proposed partnership meets organizational policies and guidelines. Ensure that collaborating with any of the potential partners is not against the guidelines or policies for your agency or organization.

Building a successful partnership is not overwhelming if it is done strategically and thoughtfully. This will help maximize effective use of resources and outcomes.

1. Prepare	2. Plan	3. Implement	4. Evaluate	5. Sustain
1.1 Determine public health problem, goals, and affected populations	2.1 Convene an initial meeting of the partnership	3.1 Implement the action plan and monitor progress	4.1 Develop evaluation plan	5.1 Focus on team building, decision making, and consensus development
1.2 Conduct a preliminary analysis of the problem	2.2 Systematically assess the problem	3.2 Develop and maintain tracking system to record progress of partnership	4.2 Evaluate progress of goals and objectives	5.2 Adhere to established ground rules
1.3 Assess the need for a partnership	2.3 Identify leverage points and shared investments	3.3 Adjust goals, objectives, and steps as necessary	4.3 Record and track data according to established timeline	5.3 Monitor progress of activities
1.4 Assess if proposed partnership meets organizational polices and guidelines	2.4 Define a shared vision, mission, and goals that are supported by all members	3.4 Provide oversight to partner commitments and ensure adherence to action plan	4.4 Share results with the partners	5.4 Be able to document or demonstrate outcomes of the partnership
1.5 Identify potential partners/stakeholders	2.5 Develop an action plan	3.5 Reward and recognize contributions of partners	4.5 Compare results to project goals to determine level of achievement	5.5 Secure resources from internal an/or external sources
1.6 Assess potential partners' appropriateness	2.6 Identify quick wins	3.6 Maintain consistent communication	4.6 Use evaluation findings to inform the partnership, programs, and projects, and to direct improvements in the programs and activities	5.6 Review the range of partners
1.7 Convene a core group of potential partners	2.7 Ensure the partnership has characteristics for success not failure	3.7 Ensure regular opportunities for informal contact	4.7 Write evaluation report	5.7 Create processes for recognizing and celebrating collective achievements
1.8 Develop a draft mission statement and goals	2.8 Ensure partner needs are met	3.8 Publicize successes	4.8 Promote the partnership by sharing achievements with partners, the public, funders, the press, and stakeholders	5.8 Communicate clearly and frequently with members
1.9 Identify other potential members	2.9 Delineate roles responsibilities, and commitments	3.9 Share new materials and information that are relevant to their organization and partnership		5.9 Communicate with the public and the press, when appropriate
1.10 Determine type of partnership and follow organizational policies and guidelines for approval	2.10 Delineate financial needs and resources			5.10 Record case study for documentation and use by others
1.11 Ensure variety and diversity among potential partners to enable a comprehensive understanding of issues being addressed	2.11 Prepare appropriate legal documents and obtain necessary approval/clearance			
	2.12 Establish clear ground rules or by-laws			
	2.13 Establish procedures that will minimize the barriers to successful partnerships			

Figure 15-2 Steps in Building a Partnership

1.5   Identify potential partners–stakeholders.

Many organizations critically involved in advancing the goals may not be a traditional public health partner.

Determine key organizations already working on the identified issue and then look more broadly. Consider organizations and individuals who are experts or leaders. These core leaders can meet to discuss whether it is worthwhile to pursue forming a partnership. Categories of potential partnership members may include business, health, education, faith-based organizations, community and nonprofit organizations, government (local, state, federal), or foundations.

1.6   Assess potential partners' appropriateness. Evaluate potential partners' history, direction, capabilities, resources, and fit. For example, do they have a good track record, reasonable standing–respect in the sector or community, access to the priority population, access to relevant information–resources–experience, record of financial stability, and reliability?

1.7   Convene a core group of potential partners. Share the preliminary data and concerns and explore their level of interest in collaborating. Articulate benefits to the partner(s).

1.8   Develop a draft vision and mission statement and goals:
- A vision statement is a future-looking ideal of what an organization desires to become, achieve, or create. A vision proposes a state beyond current position or capabilities; it is a picture of the desired future.
- A mission statement expresses clear and compelling goals. It states the purpose, what the partnership will do, and why. It is more directly actionable than a vision. It should be concise.

1.9   Identify other potential members. List organizations–individuals–agencies–stakeholders who will be invited to be members of the partnership effort (see Steps 1.5 and 1.6). This preliminary discussion among foundational partners can identify which stakeholders or opinion leaders in the community are missing. The larger group will then convene in Step 2 to more fully plan for the partnership.

1.10   Determine type of partnership. Partnerships vary in their complexity, intensity, and formality. The broader the scope of the problem and the longer the projected lifetime of the partnership, the more complex, tightly linked, and formal a partnership should be. More limited and short-term partnerships may require a less formal, less complicated approach. Himmelman (2001) describes partnerships as being on a continuum from simple networking to formal collaboration, as shown in Figure 15-3.
- Networking: provides a forum for the exchange of ideas and information for mutual benefit, often through newsletters, conferences, meetings, and electronic information sharing. It is one of the least formal forms of partnership and requires little time or trust among partners.

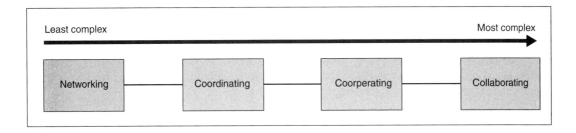

Figure 15-3 Variations in Partnership Types

- Coordinating: involves exchanging information and altering activities for a common purpose.
- Cooperating: involves exchanging information, altering activities, and sharing resources. It requires a significant amount of time, high level of trust, and sharing of turf.
- Collaborating: includes enhancing the capacity of the other partner for mutual benefit and a common purpose, in addition to the above activities.

1.11 Ensure variety and diversity among potential partners to enable a comprehensive understanding of issues being addressed. Diversity includes stakeholders and organizations who represent, advocate, or have access to those at greatest risk, e.g., low socioeconomic status (SES), age, ethnicity, gender.

Are you ready to move on to Step 2, Action Plan–Organize the Partnership? **Please see the Step 1 Checklist in Appendix C.**

Step 2: Create Action Plan–Organize Partnership

This step involves two simultaneous activities: (1) creating an action plan and (2) organizing the partnership. Both are critical to success.

It is wise to resist the temptation to just get started without thoroughly and systematically creating a plan to guide the activities of the partnership, based on data and guided by theory. Otherwise, key components of the problem and strategies to address them may not be identified and addressed, and the partnership will have less of a chance of success before it even gets started.

Step 2A: Create an Action Plan

2.1 Convene an initial meeting of the partnership

2.2 Systematically assess the problem. Analyze data; conduct an asset and gap analysis; identify partner interests, capabilities, and resources; and identify modifiable components.

2.3 Identify leverage points and shared investments. Highlight skills and resources that partner members bring to the solution.

2.4   Define a shared vision and mission and goals that are supported by all members and meet member organizations needs. Goals should be
   - realistic and attainable within the time frame of the project,
   - supported as feasible by the largest segment of the community, and
   - based on data research that attainment will improve the health of the population or community.

2.5   Develop a SMART action plan. Outline specific objectives and steps to achieve each goal and set a time frame for each objective. Objectives should
   - be specific, measurable, appropriate, realistic, and time framed (see Step 4, Evaluation, for more details);
   - use multiple strategies; and
   - specify what will happen, the target, a time frame, and who is responsible for each step.

2.6   Identify quick wins. Decide which goals will be addressed first. Achieving a quick win will get some positive momentum going for the partnership and help get the group working together. A quick win will help cement dedication to the goals and create a desire to continue to stay involved.

Step 2B: Organize the Partnership—Build Trust and Ownership

The second part of Step 2 is to specifically address how the partnership will be organized and managed. Often the functioning of the partnership is not specifically addressed or well articulated when it is being formed, and this can lead to a less than successful endeavor.

2.7   Ensure the partnership has characteristics for success, not failure.

   Kreuter and Lezin (1998) and others list characteristics for success and failure in partnerships (see Figure 15-4):

2.8   Ensure that partners' needs are met. Identify areas of common interest and complementary mission and goals of individual partners and those of the partnership.

2.9   Delineate roles, responsibilities, and commitments.

2.10 Delineate financial needs and resources. Outline monetary and non-monetary resources required. Determine channels through which to obtain necessary resources.

2.11 Prepare appropriate legal documents and obtain approval and clearance, if appropriate.

2.12 Establish clear ground rules or by-laws and processes to promote effectiveness. For example, governance structure; stable and committed leadership; roles, responsibilities, and expectations of partners; decision-making processes; frequency, location, and duration of meetings; partners' involvement in planning and priority setting; how work

Characteristics of Failed Partnerships	Characteristics of Effective Partnerships
• Unclear, unrealistic, vague goals	• Mutual respect and trust
• Unclear, unrealistic, vague roles	• Well-defined, specific issue
• Responsibility without authority	• Shared vision and goal(s)
• Top-down, external mandates	• Group seen as legitimate leader
• Unrealistic timeframes for success	• Clear roles, rights, and policy guidelines
• Low trust	• Appropriate cross-section of members
• Poor communication	• Open and frequent communication
• Costs to members exceed benefits	• Flexible and adaptable

Figure 15-4
Characteristics
of Partnerships

will be done (e.g., work groups, committees); how progress will be communicated; how basic tasks will be accomplished (e.g., clerical, meeting logistics, membership recruitment, research and data collection, public relations and public information, fundraising); crediting of members' contributions; and clear lines of communication.

2.13   Establish procedures that will minimize the barriers to a successful partnership. Kreuter and Lezin (1998) offer the following recommendations and procedures:
  • Formal and informal processes for resolving disputes
  • Strategies to ensure expression of alternative views
  • Strategies to address differences in organizational priorities and those of the partnership
  • Core leadership that is stable and committed to the partnership
  • Meetings that are not bogged down in procedures or poor group dynamics
  • Partnership that does not focus on too many long-term goals without short-term objectives to identify early wins
  • Adequate planning and resources, or the activities will be ineffective and unsuccessful

Are you ready to move on to Step 3, Implement?

Please see the Step 2 Checklist in Appendix C.

**Step 3:
Implement**

3.1   Implement the action plan and monitor progress.

3.2   Develop and maintain tracking system to record progress of partnership. Update tool to keep a running view of key activities, messages, time frame of communication, and feedback.

3.3 Adjust goals, objectives, and steps as necessary.

3.4 Provide oversight to partner commitments and ensure adherence to action plan through already defined monitoring and evaluation process.

3.5 Reward and recognize contributions of partners (e.g., during partnership meetings, press releases, and media events).

3.6 Maintain consistent communication. Keep partners informed through regular meetings, newsletters, conference calls, and letters; provide regular status updates.

3.7 Ensure regular opportunities for informal contact. Maintain communication between leadership, staff, and partners.

3.8 Publicize successes.
  - Give partners credit in news releases and other publicity
  - Send partners copy of any publicity

3.9 Share new materials and information that are relevant to the partnership member organizations.

Are you ready to move on to Step 4, Evaluate?

Please see the Step 3 Checklist in Appendix C.

Step 4: Evaluate   **Partnership evaluation** should be planned from the beginning when the action plan is being developed, not left until the end. It should be an ongoing process throughout the life of the partnership. Increasingly, there is a public and organizational clamor for greater efficiency, effectiveness, and economy; alignment of interventions with goals and performance measures and accountability. The key to meeting this expectation is monitoring and evaluation. Some types of partnerships will have a relatively simple evaluation process, whereas other more complex partnerships may have a more elaborate, or formal evaluation process. If the objective is a big one, the effectiveness of the partnership can sometimes be determined by the degree to which the goal is met. The most challenging evaluations are those where there are many variables or difficult-to-measure contributions or outcomes. The complexity of the evaluation is determined by which outcomes to assess. Select the degree of formality and complexity–elaborateness appropriate for your partnership.

Why evaluate? Evaluation

- aids in the development of reasonable–measurable goals, objectives, and steps;
- produces data to document whether objectives are achieved;
- determines partnership's progress–success at reaching its goals;
- tracks effectiveness of the process—what has worked and what has not;
- helps hold people and groups accountable for the progress;
- meets demands for public and fiscal accountability, especially to funders or the partnership's constituency;

- provides supportive evidence for, and improves the credibility of the partnership;
- builds a case for continued support, especially to move on to next steps;
- creates a process to acknowledge the importance of the skills and contributions of the members;
- provides positive publicity of important successes; and
- assists with future planning.

Steps

4.1 Plan and implement an evaluation plan before the activities begin. Determine what will be measured, when, how, and by whom.
   - What: the target health problem or health service–activity to be addressed
   - How much: the quantity of change in a health problem or the amount of activity to be performed or utilized
   - Who: the target population that will benefit from the change in health status or health service
   - Where: the geographical area in which the target population is located
   - When: the time (month, fiscal year, calendar year) by or during which the objective should be achieved
   - Who: the person(s) or organization(s) responsible for the objective activity.

   The evaluation plan should include details of the following:
   - Develop work plan (goals, objectives, methods, activity schedule, budget and resources, evaluation plan)
   - Identify questions for each objective and activity
   - Identify data or indicators for each question and determine data sources and measurement methods
   - Identify criteria for measuring progress toward each indicator
   - Identify time frames for benchmarks
   - Complete a final assessment of usefulness, feasibility, propriety, and accuracy of methods
   - Determine the types of reports to be generated and in what form the results will be disseminated
   - Determine the function of the evaluation report—decision making about current and future activities, public relations, different audiences (different reports may be required for different recipients)
   - Determine the time frame for data collection, analysis, reporting, and action
   - Determine roles and responsibilities for conducting the evaluation (e.g., data collection, analysis, reporting); determine if a consultant is needed to complete the analysis
   - Analyze and interpret findings
   - Provide results to funders–members–constituents

- Use results to improve program–partnership
- Clarify who has control of data and will write reports

Resources needed for evaluation:
- Possible budgetary allocation
- Staff time to conduct evaluation–and provide data
- Expertise for technical aspects

4.2   Evaluate progress of goals and objectives (process, impact, and outcome).
- Process evaluation looks at the implementation process (as it was designed or amended for better effectiveness) and who participated, not whether the goals were reached. It is conducted during the program or partnership, rather than afterward. This is "quality control" and provides feedback to the program as it progresses, e.g., appropriateness of the program site location and times, level of community support, number of people reached, resources, interactions between staff and participants, and amount of staff time and resources required. Process data include number of participants, number of programs–activities, letters of recommendations, participant comments, purchase orders, and attendance sheets. Process looks at the following: How well is the partnership adhering to its plans? How well is the action plan being implemented (e.g., were meetings held as planned, did partners complete their responsibilities on time, is participation consistent or is it declining)?
- Impact evaluation measures the early effects or influence of the program–partnership on the target audience and reaching stated goals. This type of evaluation determines if the program–partnership's objectives have been achieved and which interventions are effective. Impact measures four categories of information: knowledge, skills, attitudes, and behaviors. Data includes pre- and posttests, questionnaires, observations and simulation of skills, self-report inventories and diaries, surveys, and observations and interviews related to behaviors. Data is analyzed to gain information on personal opinions and percent change. It includes follow-up data after the intervention, e.g., at 6 months or 1 year later. Impact looks at the following: Did the methods and activities result in the desired immediate change or initial effect (e.g., did more people get immunized or get a mammogram)?
- Outcome evaluation gauges the long-term effects of the program–partnership—did it produce improvements in health status or quality of life? This type of evaluation is more difficult and expensive and takes a longer period of time. It is measured by data such as morbidity and mortality.

4.3   Record and track data according to established timeline.
- Quantitative data provide information that is quantifiable, measurable, and objective, such as the number of individuals reached; number of programs; number of people by age, gender, and race;

and numerical assessment of pre- and posttest scores before and after an intervention. Quantitative data can be obtained through questionnaires, structured interviews, observations, physiological measurements, project records, surveys, and objective tests such as pre- and posttests.

- Qualitative data relates to the target population's attitudes, beliefs, insights, and views, and usually does not have a numerical value. This information is useful in facilitating decision making about program strategies and the target population. This is sometimes called "soft" data. Qualitative data can be obtained by focus groups, interviews, case studies, and observations.

4.4 Share results with the partners. Publicize the important successes of the partnership.

4.5 Compare results to project goals to determine level of achievement.

4.6 Use evaluation findings to inform the partnership, programs, and projects and to direct improvements in the programs and activities.

4.7 Write evaluation report.

4.8 Promote the partnership by sharing achievements with partners, the public, funders, the press, and stakeholders.

Are you ready to move on to Step 5, Sustain?

Please see the Step 4 Checklist in Appendix C.

Step 5: Sustain Many of the factors important in the planning and implementation continue to play a role in maintenance of a partnership, e.g., leadership, degree of formalization, membership, management conflict, difference in member contributions and involvement. Sustainability may relate to the partnership until or unless it meets the goals, or it may expand further to sustaining the partnership to address other key issues, once the original goals of the partnership are reached and an effective working relationship is achieved. Once a project or program is underway, partners are often ready to move on to new things, especially if the partnership is deemed a failure, and may not want to continue the relationship. Other times, partners become more engaged in the project,and the partnership (as trust is built), and the partners may want to continue involvement in the partnership, whether the goals remain the same or not.

Common organizational problems that arise once the partnership commences operation include the following:

- Actual costs are greater than the benefits
- Lack of administrative support for partnership activities
- Threats to the autonomy of the members
- Lack of consensus about membership criteria or partnership structure
- Disagreements about responsibilities for service provision
- Inadequate attention to members' other priorities

Steps:

5.1 Focus on team building, decision making, and consensus development.

5.2 Adhere to established ground rules. Maintain lines of authority that were established when the partnership was formed.

5.3 Monitor progress of activities. Track evaluation measures to make sure that activities stay on track, and keep members informed through newsletters, special mailings, distribution of minutes, and/or conference calls.

5.4 Be able to document or demonstrate outcomes of the partnership.

5.5 Secure resources from internal and/or external sources. Besides getting resources from the organizations making up the partnership, other sources of support may include grants, cooperative agreements, foundations, local–state–federal governments, and community funding sources (e.g., United Way). Often new funding sources will become available to continue a partnership if you can document success of reaching the original partnership's goals.

5.6 Review the range of partners. Monitor contributions and fulfillment of roles and responsibilities. As new or amended goals are developed, review partners and stakeholders and identify key organizations that are not currently participating and explore inviting them to join the partnership.

5.7 Create processes for recognizing and celebrating collective achievements.

5.8 Communicate clearly and frequently with members in a variety of ways, both formal and informal.

5.9 Communicate with the public and the press, when appropriate.

5.10 Record case study for documentation and use by others. Documenting the history, processes, benchmarks, and outcomes can be useful to obtaining continued funding, support, and participation by current and future partners. The documentation should be collected throughout the life of the partnership and might include basic information (e.g., name–partners–stakeholders, key dates, key issues that led to the partnership); history (e.g., original issues and goals, who started it, first steps); activities (e.g., activities, outcomes); roles (e.g., key individuals and organizations and responsibilities); accountability (e.g., how was accountability defined–assigned–tracked–measured to assess impact and outcome, decision-making processes); challenges (e.g., main challenges and how they were addressed); resources (e.g., cash–in-kind, staffing, funding—what was renewable and what was one time); future plans (e.g., immediate and long-term future plans, issues); and achievements (e.g., key successes, outcomes, and impact) and how it was communicated and how credit was given.

Please see the Step 5 Checklist in Appendix C.

Summary: Steps in Building a Partnership

The information presented in this section of the chapter is a distillation of the results of researchers and practitioners who have studied partnerships and collaborations that have been successful, as well as those that have not reached their goals. Much can be learned from both.

Health promotion is both an art and a science. Although the steps just discussed are listed in a sequential manner in this publication and are based on science, the art of utilizing them may include using one's judgment in employing the steps and activities (sometimes simultaneously) or even looping back to redo some of them. Further, the recommendations and checklists are not like a recipe, where a dish being prepared may fail if all the ingredients are not included. Rather, the steps and activities are options to consider for usefulness, much like the components of a toolbox, where tools are a resource for the partnership to choose to use or not, as deemed appropriate.

How to Partner with Specific Market Segments

Previous information in this chapter consisted of general guidelines and steps applicable to all partnerships. However, different groups (or market segments) have unique characteristics, needs, behaviors, or cultures that may require additional considerations for the partnership to be successful. This differentiation of groups, or market segmentation, is one of the key principles of social marketing. Market segmentation will help to develop strategies and interventions that will resonate with each group's values, desires, and needs and will increase chances of success. You will be better able to communicate in the ways preferred by the market segment, are sensitive to their unique culture, and relate to their goals and priorities, motivations, and stage of problem recognition.

There are two major types or market segments of partnerships for public health:

- Traditional public health partners (e.g., health departments, health care, and health-related organizations) for whom health is a major goal or part of their mission.
- Nontraditional public health partners. Examples of nontraditional partners include business, education, faith-based groups, nongovernment community and professional organizations, and sports–entertainment, where health is not a major part of their mission or goals. However, they do have areas of common or overlapping interest that include health. For example, looking at businesses, their fundamental goals may include profitability, shareholder value, and product development. They may also be concerned with absenteeism or workforce productivity and lower health care costs for which the business may be partially responsible through paid health insurance. Public health goals include improved health of the public, effective health monitoring, enhanced prevention, sound public health policies,

and health impact. At first glance, these may look completely different; however, business's workforce productivity (including absenteeism due to illness), health care costs, improved health of the public (including employees and their families), and health impact are areas of common interest and overlap. This is the common interest space and the basis for collaborating on a common problem or issue. Working together creates a win-win situation, with everyone getting key goals and issues addressed.

The next section of this chapter contains specific tips from the field on working with unique market segments. This information was gathered from interviews with multiple practitioners who have significant experience collaborating with each of the market segments: business, education, health care, and faith-based groups. These tips are presented in a chart format and contain specific recommendations related to the culture, processes, and communication for that segment. Some additional resources and guidance from published materials are included, as well.

Keys to Success with Business

As stated in a report by the Washington Business Group on Health for the W. K. Kellogg Foundation (2000), "The health of a community impacts the economic health of its businesses and corporations are able to play a unique role in the development of a community's health and continued vitality." Increasingly, businesses are searching for new approaches that will improve the overall health, functioning, and productivity of their employees, dependents, and retirees. In the same report, they found the interdependence of a company with its community can be expressed in two ways: (1) the health of a community impacts the economic health of its businesses and (2) corporations are able to play a unique role in the development of a community's health and continued vitality. Additionally, corporate social responsibility emerged as a strong and central value that is reflected in their mission statements. They believe it is good for business (see Figure 15-5).

Key Observations   The National Business Coalition on Health conducted a needs assessment and published a report, written by Mercure, in 2000. Some key points include the following:

- Businesses need business case development tools and health information that are flexible to use and adaptable to a variety of workforce and industry scenarios.
- Businesses are concerned about value, which they describe as the combination of quality and cost with the expectation that quality improvements will lead to cost avoidance and/or reduction.
- Businesses need a trusted source for evidence to assist in their purchasing decisions (e.g., health insurance) and for their employees and family members for consumer health decisions. The "Purchaser's Guide to Clinical

Business Culture

- Businesses' chief goal/mission may not exclusively be health-related, but they are concerned about rising health care costs and the health of workers (relates to absenteeism, "presenteeism," and productivity). Address "What's In It For Me? (WIIFM)
- This partner may perceive that they have other, higher priorities.
- Businesses need practical information that tells them the implications and actions of the partnership.
- Businesses may not always feel comfortable sharing information—be aware of proprietary interests.
- Sometimes, formalizing the relationship through MOUs, contracts, etc., can mitigate some of these difficulties.

Process

- Learn the business sector culture, including differences in public health versus private sector language, acronyms and norms. Speak their language, don't expect them to learn yours.
- Tell your partners up front the anticipated length of time for the partnership.
- Make the business case; routinely evaluate and report partnership benefit and value compared to cost (ROI-Return on Investment).
- Be aware of the partners' business cycles and impact on implementing change and times when funding is allocated.
- Be clear on your goals and on what you can bring to the table to accomplish those goals.
- Establish measurements of progress and success.
- Timeliness is essential, especially in the business world.
- Promptly respond to phone calls and e-mails even if requested information is not yet available.
- Develop definite timelines and make sure you can meet them.
- Identify key leadership.

Communication

- Communications should be succinct and to the point; one-page summaries that include bullets are best.
- State the problem, potential solutions/past successes, and how the partnership is going to implement the plan and measure the outcome.
- Provide practical, understandable, and actionable advice.
- Information should be easy to read, without jargon and technical terms.
- Be collaborative, listen, adapt.
- Assist partners by sharing your insights/knowledge, but also learn from them. Think of the exchange of ideas and approaches that can be mutually beneficial.
- Relate to the concept of "corporate social responsibility," contributing to economic development while improving the quality of life of the workforce, their families, and the local community.

Figure 15-5
Business

Preventive Services," produced by the National Business Group on Health (2006), in collaboration with the Centers for Disease Control and Prevention and other partners provides the science and cut-and-paste information for businesses to use in health insurance design and contracting.

- Businesses want a broad approach to assess disease burden that allows them to select conditions for their population for programs delivered through their health plans and/or the work site.
- Businesses and coalitions have differing needs and approaches to dealing with health care cost and quality, suggesting that flexibility is needed in services, information, and tools.

Seven Opportunities for Business-Community Collaboration

The Washington Business Group on Health document for the W. K. Kellogg Foundation (2000) lists the following eight challenges to business-community collaboration:

1. Lack of communication opportunities (lack of avenues and opportunities for communication between business and public health; no natural intersections)
2. Lack of a common working language and assumptions
3. Lack of clarity about whom to contact in business, especially large corporations
4. Lack of clarity about whom to contact about a community's health, especially if multiple communities and states are covered
5. Unclear information on available community health programs; available programs are not "packaged to go"
6. Absence of information on a program's impact on the business productivity (e.g., gains in employee productivity and bottom line gains)
7. Limited ability to attract and initiate grant-based projects by businesses, therefore usually have to fund internally
8. Lack of clarity in determining when to activate business participation, identifying when is the most appropriate developmental stage in which to engage the employer.

The same report lists the following eight potential opportunities for engaging business in community health development:

1. Build consensus around health priorities for the community. Participate in local, regional meetings of business leaders, health providers, and public health officials to prioritize specific issues in the community, especially schools. Businesses have an interest in improving the curriculum for its diet and physical activity programs that affect the health of the families they insure (and the children who are their potential future workforce).
2. Develop consumer-responsive programs. It is all about the health care consumer. Know your market, your population's health needs.
3. Develop web-based direct-to-consumer health information. Web information is "hot." Employers want their employees to use it, and people

tend to trust nonprofit community groups as a source of information that is likely to be evidence based.

4. Approach local business groups and coalitions for assistance. Community health initiatives staff should engage local business groups, business coalitions, and chambers of commerce.

5. Use business to help promote and disseminate health messages to the public. Large and medium-size employers can be a primary information source on health care for their employees. Business can be a critical channel for reaching a community, including employees, dependents, and retirees.

6. Develop web-based portals for employers to get data on local and regional health issues. Make the data available that describes the local or regional health needs and concerns for employers so that they will become engaged in local community health initiatives. The data needs to include local demographics and epidemiology.

7. Develop research with emphasis on productivity, disability, and lost time from jobs. Develop or add to the research that other groups have done.

8. Fund and develop programs via local nonprofits to extend grant monies into the workplace. Government grants are usually not available to employers. The public agencies that receive these grants may be able to partner with business and can implement the project through the workplace.

Keys to Success with Education

Good health is necessary for effective learning. Education is the factor consistently linked to longer, healthier lives in every country where it has been studied. According to Wong, et.al. (2002), graduation from high school is associated with an increase in average life span of 6 to 9 years. A large portion of the U.S. population can be reached through schools—including students, staff, and parents. People with higher levels of education are associated with better health across all ages and incomes and are far less likely to participate in government-funded social programs like Medicaid, school lunch programs, and food stamps.

Before partnering, define the answers to these three questions:

- What do I want from schools?
- What can I offer schools?
- How is my agenda related to what's important to education leaders?

The education sector factors to keep in mind can be found in Figure 15-6.

School-Business Partnerships: Seven Strategies for Success

School-**business partnerships** have been flourishing for more than 30 years. Since the 1970s, partnership programs have evolved from one-sided "adopt-a-school" efforts to mutually beneficial partnerships that provide advantages to both schools and businesses. According to the Daniels Fund (2005), schools and students benefit from additional human and financial resources from business partnerships. Partnerships offer business leaders and their employees an opportunity to contribute to increasing the skills and knowledge of the community's future work force, influencing understanding and advocacy for public education, and boosting employee morale through meaningful volunteerism. There is truly a confluence of interests among public health, schools, and business; the very things that businesses want from the schools—

Education (K-12) Culture
- Recognize that education's chief goal/primary mission is not health-related.
- Focus on the educational impact and frame your arguments for partnerships in educational outcomes. For example, impacting student health reduces absenteeism and increases academic achievement.
- Education and implementing quality school health programs are primarily state and local school district responsibilities.
- School leaders tend to be wary of controversy.

Process
- Learn the nomenclature and current terminology used by policy-makers (e.g. "No Child Left Behind," annual yearly progress).
- Respect the hierarchy. For example, to work with teachers, you must have the permission of the principal.
- Work with educational and professional associations as they will reach more people and provide you with broader exposure, which will in turn improve your program's credibility.
- State level: governors, legislators, state boards of education, chief state school officer.
- School level: school boards, superintendents, and central office staffs.
- Engage students in public-hearing agendas, research, etc.

Communication
- Link communications about desired programming to the state and national education standards and current terminology.
- Communications should be short, succinct and to the point and address the educational mission.
- Provide practical advice identifying research-based successes/ best practices.
- Provide specific conclusions and policy options.
- Information should be easy to read, without jargon and technical terms.
- Be collaborative, listen, adapt.
- Already prepared curricula and lesson plans, with links to required standards, will be more likely to be used—teachers do not have time to develop new materials.

Figure 15-6
Education

smart, healthy future employees—are the same priorities for public health—smart, healthy children. The Daniels Fund researched why some school partnerships are more effective than others. Its report highlights seven strategies for successful partnerships based on the findings:

1. Ensure student learning and achievement are the focus of every partnership.
2. Develop a well-defined and well-managed program that supports school-based partnerships.
3. Make strategic matches between schools and businesses that advance a school's improvement goals.
4. Set clear expectations for schools and businesses.
5. Provide training for school staff and business employees.
6. Create a meaningful process for communicating about the program and recognizing the contributions of business partners.
7. Regularly monitor and evaluate each partnership and the overall program.

An excellent resource for partnering with education is available from the National Association of State Boards of Education, titled *How Schools Work and How to Work with Schools*, originally developed in 1991 and revised in 2003. It includes detailed information about how education works at the school, district, state, and national levels. It also provides practical tips for working with educators, administrators, and policy makers.

Keys to Success with Health Care

The health care delivery system is complex and consists of many distinct types of organizations, including hospitals and health systems; health care professionals (e.g., physicians, nurses, pharmacists, occupational and physical therapists); accrediting organizations; quality improvement organizations (e.g., NCQA); insurance companies—HMOs; payers; and regulators.

Factors to keep in mind for partnering with health care can be found in Figure 15-7.

Community and nongovernment professional organizations (e.g., American Cancer Society, American Heart Association, American Diabetes Association, Senior Centers, Boys and Girls Clubs of America) have a number of programs that provide direct support, education, and guidance for individuals that address common conditions and issues. They have the potential to play an important and complementary role to the health care provider and to assist people to optimize the health and their health care. An excellent resource is *Partnering Physicians with Community Organizations, A Toolkit for Physician Champions*, developed by the National Council on Aging in 2005.

Health Care Culture
- Recognize that the sector is very diverse and has varying interests, bottom-lines, and motivators.
- Do your research early. Determine what is happening in the organization and make sure that your partnership project aligns with their priorities and projects. Connect with the organization(s) early in the process.
- Adjust your discussion to the interests of your partner/potential partner.
- Research the sector and determine which group is best to target and how.
- Conduct an in-depth environmental scan, including political culture, to gain a better perspective on the sector's priorities. Make sure that you are partnering rather than imposing.

Process
- Working through the larger organizations and professional associations will give you greater reach. Even within these groups, however, there can be multiple priorities and mindsets. You need to have multiple approaches.
- Understand their priorities before you push your own agenda. A failure to do so will make your message irrelevant in their minds.
- Listen to what they want; take into account what their daily life is like.
- Multiple priorities and mindsets require a variety of approaches and strategies.
- Start with the leadership. If there is a champion for the partnership issue in the organization, work with that person to gain organizational support.

Communication
- Keep all written communication under two pages in length.
- Work on building relationships; this is the most effective approach to building true partnerships. Find out what they want from you and how they want to receive further communication.

Figure 15-7
Health Care

Keys to Success with Faith-Based Organizations

Over 180 million people in the United States are allied with Christian, Jewish, Muslim, Hindu, or other congregations (Pew forum (2008). Faith-based organizations can be important partners in improving the nation's health, in part because they play an important role in ensuring equitable access to health systems and have direct access to individuals for information and support. Many faith-based organizations participate in initiatives to improve health in international settings, as well as in communities in the United States. They are also a key component in preparing for and responding to natural disasters and emergencies. They play an essential role in shaping the public's knowledge, attitudes, beliefs, and behaviors. Partnerships with this group must be based on sound science, well-defined health issues, and the public good. The goal in partnering should be getting health information and evidence-based interventions to people in the communities that need them, especially those at greatest risk.

Factors to keep in mind when partnering with this sector can be found in Figure 15-8.

Faith-Based Organizations Culture
- Recognize that this sector is very diverse and widespread in our society. For example:
  - There are differences between faiths, within the same faith, and even within the same denomination or congregation. Be careful about making assumptions and generalizations within and across groups.
  - People of faith are members of, and interact within, multiple sectors. For example, they may be members of a congregation, but may also be leaders in business, education, government and/or other sectors.
  - Organizations can also vary broadly in organizational structure, race and ethnicity, education, and other areas.
- Show respect to what they value (e.g., religious duty/obligation, trust, integrity, honesty, equity, and fairness).
- Consider the broader sociopolitical context. Social and political issues occurring locally, domestically, and globally may personally impact individuals' lives. Be aware of and sensitive to these issues.
- Keep a humble, respectful, demeanor and maintain neutrality. Be honest if you are not familiar with a particular culture or faith.
- Be careful about making assumptions and generalizations within and across groups. Express your interest in learning and ask questions in a respectful manner.
- Lack of impartiality can damage a team's internal dynamics. It is important to foster a connection without creating the impression that you (especially if you work for the government) are sponsoring, endorsing, or inhibiting religion generally, or favoring or disfavoring a particular religion.

Process
- Begin the relationship by understanding and recognizing the strengths of faith-based organizations and their potential to contribute to community health and wellness. For example, these organizations may have the following:
  - leadership and infrastructure to work with local and state public health agencies
  - communications networks that are credible and trusted to address rumors and misinformation
  - ability to reach persons with special needs (e.g. elderly, disabled, indigent or limited English speakers), etc.
- Learn and respect a potential partner's mission, hierarchy, organizational structure, communication practices and level of community interaction. For example, while the Salvation Army is known for its social programs and community outreach, it is actually a church. This shapes the organization and influences its community work.

(continues)

Figure 15-8
Faith-Based
Organizations

- Identify common areas of interest, such as healthy minds, bodies, environments, and communities as a foundation for a mutually beneficial partnership.
- Consider the potential partnership objectively. Consider various possibilities: formal partnership (e.g. cooperative agreement, MOU), informal partnership (e.g. networking), or no partnership.
- Consider starting with collaboration around a small, well-defined project where values and mission are most clearly aligned. Monitor for potential risks and benefits.
- Remember that trust is built over time.
  - Involve the partner from the beginning of the planning and implementation process to the end of the project.
  - Be explicit and transparent about what resources and strengths each partner can contribute.
  - Be willing to contribute to the relationship without expectations of immediate benefit.
  - Maintain and nurture a healthy relationship once projects are complete.
- If federal funding is provided for a project, keep in mind that the recipient is not allowed to use federal funds for any inherently religious activities such as worship, religious instruction or proselytization, and cannot discriminate against a program beneficiary based on their religion or religious belief. Where a religious organization receives direct government assistance, any inherently religious activities that the organization offers must be offered separately, in time and/or location, from the activities supported by direct government funding.

Communication

- Be explicit and transparent.
- With faith-based organizations, acknowledge and respect the organization's spiritual or religious focus while maintaining your own neutral, public health focus.
- Understand and clearly communicate the rules, guidelines and legal boundaries with potential partners early in the process. Clearly distinguish between public health issues and religious issues.
- Communicate what you can and cannot provide (scientific information, technical assistance, referral and networking with other groups, potential for or lack of resources/funding).
- Avoid the use of technical jargon.
- Avoid language that implies one-sided partnerships.
- Communicate that both sides are searching for mutually beneficial relationships.
- Make sure that partnership expectations are clarified and understood by all parties.
- It is particularly important to be clear about the potential (or lack of potential) resources or funding, as an expectation of funding can be problematic.
- Keep partners informed through regular meetings, newsletters, and/or conference calls. Provide regular status updates. Face-to-face meetings interspersed with conference calls and emails are useful for communicating ideas and progress.

Figure 15-8
(Continued)

CONCLUDING REMARKS

Why is it worth the extra time and energy to organize and implement collaborations and partnerships to achieve health goals? The answer is that the goals cannot be reached by a single act or a single group. The health issues facing the United States and the world are complex, without a single magic bullet to cure them—heart disease, diabetes, HIV–AIDS, cancer, injuries, to name a few. No one organization or agency "owns" the problems, nor does any one have the resources to single handedly address them. The solution is to create synergy by working across agencies, across market segments, and across borders—to collaborate and partner with other stakeholders at all levels to make health the "default choice" for all people and all communities.

Our current system is not designed to encourage alignment of individuals or organizations. Although the United States invests more than any other country on health care, the nation is not as healthy as most developed nations. Our health system is not delivering the value it could. Many experts feel that fundamental transformation of our health system is necessary. We need to invest more in protecting health—through health promotion, prevention of disease and injuries, and preparation for new threats. This can only be achieved by working together to create a comprehensive and widespread cross-sector collaboration, with health as the goal for all people and all communities.

DISCUSSION QUESTIONS

1. Describe why collaboration and partnerships are an important strategy to achieving public health goals.
2. Identify five characteristics of effective partnerships.
3. Identify and describe the five steps and at least five activities in the partnership planning and implementation process.
4. Describe five characteristics and tips for partnering with the following market segments: business, education, health care, and faith-based organizations.

REFERENCES

Bogden, J. (2003). *How schools work and how to work with schools.* Alexandria, VA: National Association of State Boards of Education.

Butterfoss, F. D. (2007). *Coalitions and partnerships in community health.* San Francisco, CA: Jossey-Bass.

Cohen, L., Aboelata, M., Gantz, T. L., & Van Wert, J. (2003a). *Collaboration math: Enhancing the effectiveness of multidisciplinary collaboration.* Oakland, CA: Prevention Institute. Available at http://www.preventioninstitute.org

Cohen, L., & Gould, J. (2003b). *The tension of turf: Making it work for the coalition*. Oakland, CA: Prevention Institute. Available at http://www.prevention institute.org.

Daniels Fund. (2005). *School-business partnerships: Seven strategies for success*. Denver, CO: Available at http://www.danielsfund.org. Accessed November, 2008.

Foley, E. (2002). *Developing effective partnerships to support local education*. Providence, RI: School Communities that Work Task Force. Annenburg Institute for School Reform at Brown University

Gardner, D. (2005). Ten lessons in collaboration. *Online Journal of Issues in Nursing, 10*(1). Available at http://www.nursingworld.org/ojin/topic26/tpc26_1.htm. Accessed June, 2005.

Glanz, K., & Rimer, B. (2005). *Theory at a glance: A guide for health promotion practice* (Pub No 05-3896). National Cancer Institute, National Institutes of Health, DHHS.

Himmelman, A. T. (2001). On coalitions and the transformation of power relations: Collaborative betterment and collaborative empowerment. *American Journal of Community Psychology, 29(2)*, 277–284.

Kreuter, M., & Lezin, N. (1998). Are consortia/collaboratives effective in changing health status and health systems? Atlanta, GA: Health 2000, Inc.

Mattessich, P. W., Murray-Close, M., & Monsey, B. (2001). *Collaboration: What makes it work?* (2nd ed.). Saint Paul, MN: Fieldstone Alliance.

Mercure, S. (2000). *Needs assessment results report*. Washington, DC: National Business Coalition on Health.

National Business Group on Health. (2006). *A purchaser's guide to clinical preventive services: Moving science into coverage*. Washington, D.C. Available at http://www.businessgrouphealth.org/prevention/purchasers or http://www.cdc.gov/business.

National Council on Aging. (2005). *Partnering physicians with community organizations: A toolkit for physician champions*. Washington, DC: National Council on Aging.

Tennyson, R. (2003). *The partnering toolbook*. London, UK: The International Business Leaders Forum, The Partnering Initiative.

University of Kansas. (2005). Community toolbox. Available at http://www.ctb.ku.edu. Accessed June, 2005.

U.S. Department of Health and Human Services. (2006). National institutes of health state-of-the-science conference statement on tobacco use: Prevention, cessation, and control. *Ann Intern med, 145,* 839–844.

Washington Business Group on Health. (2000). *The business interest in a community's health*. Washington, DC: Author: Michael Britt and Claire Sharda.

Wong, M., Shapiro, M., Boscardin, W. & Ettner, S. (2002) Contribution of major diseases to disparities in mortality. *New England Journal of Medicine, 347,* 1585–1592.

Economic Evaluation of Health Promotion Programs

Bernard J. Healey, PhD

After reading this chapter, you should

- Understand the need to evaluate health promotion programs
- Be able to define the various methods of performing an economic evaluation of health promotion programs
- Be aware of the BASICC approach to evaluation
- Understand the need for evidence-based decisions in the funding of health promotion programs

BASICC approach
Cost-benefit analysis
Evidence-based decisions

Gross domestic product
Prescription for the American People
Years of potential life lost

Introduction

In order to better evaluate the seriousness of public health problems, there is a need to quantify the importance of at least a few of the major causes of premature death in this country. The CDC offers its own measurement of the cost of premature mortality. The CDC (1986) defines **years of potential life lost** (YPLL) as a measure of premature mortality, which is usually presented for persons under age 75 years because that is the present average age of life expectancy in this country. When this calculation is compared over dynamic populations, it is helpful to calculate the rate per 1,000 people in each age group. Over the last several years, YPLL has been increasingly utilized by public health officials in intense evaluation of prevention programs.

Although there are disputes about how valuable the measure really is, it does show that some health problems like injuries and early complications from chronic diseases manifest themselves in the working age population with disastrous results. According to the CDC (1986), this simple index of premature mortality is easy to comprehend, and it effectively emphasizes deaths of younger persons, in contrast to usual mortality statistics, which tend to focus on the elderly.

Employer Health Insurance Costs

Health insurance coverage is one of the most important benefits currently provided to the majority of employees in this country. It is one of the benefits that attracts and retains employees for a business. Unfortunately, the benefit has become costly to maintain and remain competitive. Many businesses are passing a larger percentage of these insurance costs on to their employees. The health insurance coverage issue has become a nightmare for most employers and employees in this country.

Employer-paid health insurance plans were an outgrowth of government wage and price controls of the 1950s. These relatively new benefits were used to attract and retain good workers and were also seen as a tax advantage for employers and employees alike. In lieu of wage increases, businesses showered their employees with nontaxable benefit packages that were popular with everyone concerned.

The cost of providing health insurance to employees is one of the largest costs of doing business in the United States. It is currently consuming 16% of **gross domestic product** in this country. An analysis completed on data from the U.S. Bureau of Labor Statistics (BLS) in 2004 found that health insurance benefits accounted for 23% of nonwage employee compensation in 2004. These costs are projected to continue increasing every year well into the future. This report also discovered that employers spent an estimated $330.9 billion to fund employee health insurance benefits in 2003, representing an increase of 12.1% over 2002 and a 51.4% increase since 1998.

According to a survey conducted by Price Waterhouse Cooper (2008) the increasing costs of health insurance is a major problem for employers and workers in the United States. Over the last 20 years, two major trends were developing in the delivery of health insurance to employees. One of the trends involved a significant decrease in the number of workers receiving health insurance from their employers, and the other was a sharp increase in the insurance premiums paid by workers.

The Kaiser Family Foundation (2005) reports that the number of firms offering health benefits is unchanged from last year even though it has declined over the last few years. This decline in health insurance coverage over the last several years is most profound in the small employer segment of American business, but all companies are feeling the pressure. Overall, the percentage of small firms offering health benefits has dropped by 9 percentage points in the last 6 years, according to a new survey completed by the Kaiser Family Foundation in 2005. The firms not offering employees health insurance cite high premiums as the most important reason for not doing so. If the costs of health insurance could be controlled or reduced, businesses seem interested in continuing the insurance coverage.

Shi and Singh (2005) argue that preventive and health promotional efforts need to be adopted to significantly improve the health of Americans. According to Dr. David Satcher (2006), former surgeon general, "this country spends more money treating disease and their complications than on preventing them in the first place" (p. 1009). He offers the *Surgeon General's* **Prescription for the American People** involving the following four recommendations:

- Moderate physical activity
- Consume at least five servings of fruits and vegetables per day
- Avoid toxins like tobacco, alcohol, and illicit drugs
- Practice responsible sexual behavior

This prescription needs to be dispensed before the Medicare years and the earlier in life the better. If the goal can be accomplished in the workplace, the costs of providing health insurance coverage to employees should decrease to a more manageable level.

The question that needs to be asked over and over by employers is, "What are the major triggers that lead to illness, injury, and disability for my employees?" This leads to the more important question, "Which preventive programs give me the greatest return for my investment?" This is where economic analysis needs to enter the employer decision-making process when it comes to keeping employees' health costs at a reasonable rate.

The Purpose of Economic Evaluation

The CDC (1995) argues that decision makers in public health are faced with the need to consider the costs and effectiveness of these choices when it comes to offering preventive services to Americans. The decision makers need to consider not only what preventive programs work but also the additional costs associated with the use of these interventions. Businesses are also charged with finding affordable ways of keeping their workforce healthy and productive. The expense of providing health insurance to their workers is a good investment only if the workers remain healthy and productive.

Fielding and Briss (2006) argue that improvements in the health of the population can be achieved through better use of **evidence-based decisions** concerning the use of finite resources in order to do the right thing at the right time. What is needed is faster and better use of scientific information that increases the return on the investment by having the desired effect on the health of the public.

The Burden of Workplace Injury and Illness

Injuries represent one of the most serious public health problems facing our country and especially our workplace. Finkelstein, Corso, and Miller (2006) argue that injuries impact our society through premature death, disability, medical costs, and lost productivity like no other health problem facing our nation today. Making matters worse, workers with chronic diseases also represent a significant cost to employees.

Businesses in the United States spend billions of dollars each year for employee health insurance that is apparently doing very little to keep these employees healthy. When these employees become ill, their productivity usually drops because of absenteeism from the job, and the employer's costs of insuring their health continues to rise. Insurance companies historically have not paid enough attention to the development of preventive health programs to keep the employees free of injuries and illness in their working years.

Prevention programs should (1) improve the quality of life, (2) reduce the incidence or severity of a disease or injury, and (3) reduce premature death through early detection or interventions to reduce risks or exposures associated with incidence.

In the workplace, more attention must also be paid to the true costs associated with poor health. A prevention program should have a specific objective: to avert or reduce the occurrence of a specific health outcome. Prevention effectiveness analyses are generally incidence based; therefore, the analysis should include all adverse health outcomes that are caused or prevented during the lifetime of the participant as a result of the prevention program. Fielding and Briss (2006) explain the fact that many improvements in health result from evidence-informed programs that affect the likelihood of acquiring a disease, the severity of the disease, and the receipt of appropriate and timely medical care.

The CDC (1995) offered a basic assessment scheme for the evaluation of costs and consequences of preventive health programs. The requirements offered in Table 16-1 offer a very rational approach to developing a prevention strategy for workplace wellness programs. Although other evaluation methods will be discussed in this chapter, they all revert back to many of the components found in the **BASICC approach** developed by the CDC in 1995.

Requirements of a Prevention Program

A successful prevention effort requires a well-developed plan of action. This plan must be developed by stakeholders of the program and include someone with public health expertise. Table 16-1 includes the various requirements for a prevention program. If these requirements are met, the program has a very good chance of achieving a successful outcome.

Table 16-1 Requirements	• A complete description of the program, the units in which the service(s) are provided, and the time frame of the program • Health outcome(s) averted by the prevention program and the estimated time between its implementation and when the health outcome is averted • The rates and societal burden of the health outcome • The preventable fraction for the health outcome, with the program in place and used in a realistic manner (i.e., the proportion of the health outcome averted through the program) • Intervention costs per unit of intervention, including the cost of any intervention side effects • Direct medical treatment cost of the health outcome prevented

Source: Centers for Disease Control and Prevention. (1995). Assessing the effectiveness of disease and injury prevention programs: Costs and consequences. *Morbidity and Mortality Weekly Report,* 44(RR-10), 1–11.

The success of prevention activities can be defined by whether they delay or avert morbidity and mortality from illness or injury.

Types of Economic Analysis

Efficacy has been defined by the CDC, in 1995, as the scientific basis for "what works" in reducing adverse health outcomes. These evaluations attempt to discover the value or efficacy of certain interventions in an attempt to keep individuals healthy at a reasonable cost. Evaluating efficacy allows us to see evidence of improvement in health as a result of resources being allocated to a prevention strategy or intervention. There are several economic tools available to measure these improvements and to rank them in some logical order of success. The major methods used in economic evaluations are cost analysis, cost-effectiveness analysis, cost-utility analysis, and **cost-benefit analysis**.

Cost Analysis (CA) This type of analysis includes the cost of total illness estimates, including direct and indirect costs of the problem. It represents an economic evaluation technique that involves the systematic collection, categorization, and analysis of program costs. The results are actually a measure of the burden of disease for some period of time.

Cost-Effectiveness Analysis (CEA) This type of analysis compares the costs of intervention with the resulting improvement in health. It is an analysis used to compare the costs of alternative interventions that produce a common health effect. Table 16-2 shows the value of various health interventions to offer to the population that are cost effective. The study was completed by the Partnership for Prevention and was published in the July 2006 issue of the *American Journal of Preventive Medicine*. According to the study, the most cost effective preventive health services that can be offered in medical practice are smoking cessation, aspirin therapy, and pneumococcal immunization. This study is a good example of using economics to assist in making decisions about the utilization of scarce health resources.

Nas (1996) argues that because of the difficulty in identifying and quantifying outcomes, health care services research usually uses CEA or cost-utility analysis (CUA) when determining value in the use of health resources. CEA provides a good measurement tool for determining the efficiency of a particular procedure or program in meeting its goal. The outcome in CEA is usually represented by a single health outcome, such as years of life saved or improvement in health status.

Cost-Utility Analysis (CUA)

This is a special type of cost-effectiveness analysis that uses years of life saved combined with quality of life during those years as a health outcome measure. These measures allow direct comparison.

Table 16-2
Cost-Effective Preventive Health Services

1. Aspirin therapy
2. Childhood immunizations
3. Tobacco use screening, intervention
4. Colorectal cancer screening
5. Measuring blood pressure in adults
6. Influenza immunizations
7. Pneumococcal immunization
8. Alcohol screening and counseling
9. Vision screenings for adults
10. Cervical cancer screening
11. Cholesterol screening
12. Breast cancer screening
13. Chlamydia screening
14. Calcium supplement counseling
15. Vision screening in children
16. Folic acid
17. Obesity screening
18. Depression screening
19. Hearing screening
20. Injury prevention counseling
21. Osteoporosis screening
22. Cholesterol screening for high-risk patients
23. Diabetes screening
24. Diet counseling
25. Tetanus-diphtheria boosters

Source: Johnson T. (2006). Preventive services a good investment for health. *The Nation's Health.*

**Cost-Benefit
Analysis (CBA)**

This is a type of economic analysis that compares both costs and benefits in dollar terms. They are adjusted to their present value through a process called *discounting*. If a program demonstrates a net benefit after computations, the program is considered to provide a good economic value and should be continued or, perhaps, expanded.

Consumers continually use economic evaluation techniques every day. Whenever they shop for a product or service, they usually compare price with value before making a purchase decision. The free market economy usually allocates resources based on information that becomes available through the price system. This market efficiency operates under conditions first described by an Italian economist named Vilfredo Pareto. Nas (1996) defines Pareto optimality as an efficiency norm where no one can be made better off without first making someone worse off.

Nas (1996) argues that the impact of CBA grew significantly in the 1960s because the federal Office of Management and Budget made cost benefit a principal tool of evaluation of government programs. Using economic theory to evaluate performance in the Flood Control Act of 1936, the government developed a standard guide for water resources. In the 1960s, the Planning Programming and Budgeting System (PPBS) adopted a system of analysis in the Department of Defense using economic evaluative methods.

The CDC has been using CBA for years to justify the costs and potential benefits of prevention programs. These justifications can be easily applied to illness and injury programs in the workplace. The CDC (1995) pointed out that prevention effectiveness analysis methods, a form of CBA, could be used to measure the effects of public health programs. In order to compare different prevention strategies, there is a need for reliable and consistent cost and effectiveness data. This information is necessary to document which programs and activities provide the greatest benefit for the funds expended. Table 16-3 shows how each of these analysis methods can be applied to document economic effectiveness of programs.

Target Areas for Economic Evaluation

The resources to be used in wellness initiatives are finite and, therefore, must be used in an efficient manner. It is helpful to target a few areas of intervention where programs have been put in place in many businesses and to evaluate their success in some way to see if they are having a positive impact. This is difficult because there is a long time gap between the implementation of a wellness program and the ability to demonstrate positive results from that program.

Some of the interventions lend themselves to pure economic evaluation using CBA or CEA criteria. Other programs are currently using qualitative analysis until true costs and benefits can be determined. Much more research is necessary because we are dealing with issues like quality-of-life

Table 16-3
Overview of Economic
Evaluation Methods

Economic Evaluation Method	Comparison	Measurements of Health Effects	Economic Summary Measure
Cost Analysis	Used to compare net costs of different programs for planning and assessment	Dollars	Net cost Cost of illness
Cost-effectiveness analysis	Used to compare interventions that produce a common health effect	Health effect, measured in natural units	Cost-effectiveness ratio Cost per case averted Cost per life-year saved
Cost-utility analysis	Used to compare interventions that have morbidity and mortality outcomes	Health effects, measured as year of life, adjusted for quality of life	Cost per quality-adjusted life year (QALY)
Cost-benefit analysis	Used to compare different programs with different units of outcomes (health and nonhealth)	Dollars	Net benefit or cost Benefit-to-cost ratio

Source: Centers for Disease Control and Prevention. (1995). Assessing the effectiveness of disease and injury prevention programs: Costs and consequences. *Morbidity and Mortality Weekly Report, 44*(RR-10), 1–11.

measurements, which are very subjective and difficult to place a monetary value on. Program areas in which this has already been demonstrated include smoking cessation, diabetes prevention, and injury prevention.

Smoking Cessation Programs

Tobacco use is clearly one of the most important triggers to illness, disability, and death in this country. It is also linked with a tremendous loss of productivity in the workforce. There is no doubt that this dangerous product is responsible for a dramatic reduction in the profits of many companies in America, and unfortunately, many companies are not even aware of the loss.

Tobacco use by workers results in poor health, lost wages, and lost productivity. The CDC (2005) reports that smoking costs the nation about $92 billion in the form of lost productivity in the years 1997 to 2001, up from $10 billion from the annual mortality related productivity losses for the years 1995 to 1999. The new lost productivity estimate combined with smoking-related health care costs, which was reported at $75.5 billion in 1998, exceeds $167 billion per year in the United States. This represents an enormous loss in profits for American businesses.

There are only two ways to reduce consumption of this deadly and costly product in the workplace. They are regulation of the use in the workplace or smoking cessation programs that include education and therapy.

Simon and Fielding (2006) point out that since 1965 the smoking rate has been reduced from 42% of the population to 21% in the United States through regulation, taxes, and social marketing programs to discourage tobacco use. During that same time period, a more aggressive program in California reduced tobacco use to just 15% of the population. These lower smoking rates were achieved in California through higher taxes, creative anti-smoking ads, and a more aggressive regulation of a smoke-free workplace.

There are a variety of tools available to help smokers quit the deadly habit. The experience in California certainly demonstrated that a variety of public policies encourage individuals to never begin the habit in the first place. Based on the California experience, it seems that working with a regulatory approach in the workplace seems to produce the greatest success.

On the other hand, programs that assist young and adult smokers to quit can produce a more rapid quit rate than any other component of a tobacco control program. The CDC (2005) reports that smokers who quit before age 50 years cut in half their risk of dying in the next 15 years. Smoking cessation programs are more cost effective than many other clinical prevention services.

Identification of smokers during a clinical visit costs $1 per person. Provision of motivational counseling programs to the smokers would cost $2. A full range of cessation services would cost $275 per smoker served per year. The problem with this intervention is that only 10% of all smokers aged 18 years and older would most likely use this service.

Ong and Glantz (2005) compared the cost effectiveness of a free nicotine replacement therapy (NRT) with a mandatory statewide smoke-free workplace policy in Minnesota. This study used the numbers that quit smoking and the quality adjusted life years as the measures of benefit.

The final results of this study revealed that a smoke-free workplace policy was 9 times more effective than a NRT program. The raw data reported the cost for quitters was $12,500 with NRT at a cost of $7,020 per quitter and $10,400 for quitters with a smoke-free workplace at a cost of $799 per quitter. Although both programs were cost effective, it is clear that the smoke-free workplace should be the public health priority program.

Epidemic of Type 2 Diabetes   The CDC (2005) reports that from 1980 through 2004 the number of individuals with diabetes in this country doubled, rising from 5.9 million to 14.7 million Americans with diabetes. Diabetes is the seventh leading cause of death affecting 6% of the total population, and over one-third of those with this disease are unaware that they have diabetes and what the future complications might entail.

Majority of Diabetes Cases Linked to Poor Lifestyle Choices

The vast majority of these people with diabetes have type 2 diabetes, which is usually related to lifestyle and not hereditary factors. Death rates are twice as high for middle-aged persons with diabetes as for those in the same age group without diabetes. The other potential complications from diabetes, like amputations, blindness, stroke, kidney disease, high blood pressure, and nervous system disease, also affect the middle-aged individual at a more rapid rate. Making matters worse, the lifestyle behaviors that predispose one to diabetes—physical inactivity and diet—are very difficult to change as one grows older.

The American Diabetes Association (2002) reports that the national cost of diabetes was $132 billion—$92 billion in direct medical costs and $40 billion in indirect costs. The indirect costs were related to lost days from work, restricted activity, premature mortality, and permanent disability. These indirect costs are borne primarily by employers in terms of higher health insurance costs and reduced worker productivity.

Table 16-4 demonstrates that many interventions, especially self-management of diabetes, can be developed and utilized in the community. There is mounting evidence of the cost-effective results obtained from diabetes prevention efforts. The question becomes what type of intervention will yield the greatest impact at the lowest cost?

Intervention programs can delay the onset and slow the progression of complications, which in turn reduce the costs associated with this disease. There needs to be a complete plan involving increased physical activity and improved nutrition established in daily activities before individuals are diagnosed with diabetes, and the plan needs to be continued even if it is discovered that they already have diabetes. The plan needs to control glycemia,

Table 16.4
Diabetes Evaluation

Source: Centers for Disease Control and Prevention. (2001). Strategies for reducing morbidity and mortality from diabetes through healthcare interventions and diabetes self-management education in community settings. *Morbidity and Mortality Weekly Report,* 50 (RR-16), 1–15.

Health Care System Interventions	
Disease Management	Recommended (strong evidence)
Case Management	Recommended (strong evidence)

Self-Management Education	
Community gathering places	Recommended (sufficient evidence)
Home-type 1 diabetes	Recommended (sufficient evidence)
Home-type 2 diabetes	Insufficient evidence to determine effectiveness
Recreational camps	Insufficient evidence to determine effectiveness
Work site	Insufficient evidence to determine effectiveness
Education of school personnel	Insufficient evidence to determine effectiveness

decrease complications and mortality, and improve the individual's quality of life. These programs are rather expensive to develop and implement. They also take years to show definitive results. But, given time and resources, they can most certainly prove their worth.

Akinci, Healey, and Coyne (2003) argue that diabetes does not have to cause long-term complications if the disease is managed properly. Diabetes education programs can go a long way in teaching the individual the many benefits of self-management of his or her diabetes.

Injury Prevention Programs

The CDC (1999) reports that over the last 60 years, work-related unintentional injury death in the United States has decreased nearly 90% from 37 injuries per 100,000 workers in 1933 to 4 injuries per 100,000 workers in 1997. Despite these facts, injuries still remain a tremendous source of morbidity, mortality, and economic cost to American businesses. Finkelstein, Corso, and Miller (2006) point out that injuries are still one of the most serious public health problems facing this country. They are still the leading cause of death in individuals between the ages of 1 and 44 years.

Simon and Fielding (2006) argue that worker productivity has improved because of the reduction in injuries. This reduces the cost to business due in large part to public health interventions that are low cost compared with the medical care that would have been utilized if the injury had not been prevented.

Although the decline in injuries since 1970 seems to have resulted from a variety of factors, some sources point to the Occupational Safety and Health Act of 1970, which created the National Institute for Occupational Safety and Health (NIOSH) and the Occupational Safety and Health Administration (OSHA) as the reason for success in this area. Since 1971, NIOSH has investigated hazardous work conditions, conducted research to prevent injury, trained health professionals, and developed educational materials and recommendations for worker protection. OSHA's regulatory authority for work site inspection and development of safety standards has brought about safety regulations, mandatory workplace safety controls, and worker training. During 1980 through 1996, research findings indicated that training creates safer workplaces through increased worker knowledge of job hazards and safe work practices in a wide array of work sites.

Work-related health problems, such as coal workers' pneumoconiosis (black lung) and silicosis—common at the beginning of the century—have come under better control. Severe injuries and deaths related to mining, manufacturing, construction, and transportation also have decreased; since 1980, safer workplaces have resulted in a reduction of approximately 40% in the rate of fatal occupational injuries

Smith et al. (2006) found that injuries on the job comprise about 30% of all medically treated injuries to adults aged 18 to 64 years. This fact alone makes it most important that workplace conditions are examined in an effort to reduce the impact of injuries on society. Christoffel and Gallagher (2006) believe that evaluation of the effectiveness of injury prevention programs should be done on a routine basis. Unfortunately, one does not always have the luxury of engaging in carefully designed and controlled studies, and it is not always easy to offer quantitative data to prove the worth of injury control programs.

Workplace Wellness Programs

It is not very difficult to make the case that healthy employees are less likely to use expensive health services and that healthy employees are usually more productive. The employer not only wants but needs healthy employees in order to remain competitive. Wilson, Holman, and Hammock (1996) found most of the research evidence supports the effectiveness of work site wellness programs in keeping employees healthy. They caution that the quality of work site research and evaluation needs to be significantly improved before it can show cause and effect. On the other hand, Jeffrey et al. (1993) found that over 70% of the work sites eligible to participate in wellness programs declined for one reason or another. The fact that the incidence of workplace injuries has dropped to such a great extent over the last several years is indicative that current injury control programs are working, and the fact that injuries still pose a substantial problem shows that more can still be done.

Educating the worker about his or her health is a mammoth task because the current system of health care has no incentives for the individual to be knowledgeable about his or her health. Good health is generally taken for granted in that we are usually healthy when we are born and remain that way as we grow older. Our mentality regarding illness developed around the occurrence of communicable diseases in which we see a doctor, take some medication, and rest until we get better. We have also been conditioned to having health insurance to pay for the health problem. It is interesting to note that even if one has complete health insurance coverage, it does not guarantee good health. The health insurance alone does not guarantee that he or she has the knowledge to make the right choices about his or her personal health at the right time.

The workplace offers a place where everyone has incentives to remain healthy. The employer desires a well-trained, healthy workforce that is capable of producing profits.

The employee desires a fair wage and a benefit package that includes health insurance paid predominantly by the employer. Most employees desire to remain healthy as they grow older, allowing them to enjoy life to its fullest. These dual incentives offer a very unique opportunity for employer and employee to join forces in the focus on good health for everyone in the place of employment.

There is a need for strong leadership in health promotion programs in the workplace in order to achieve and maintain wellness. Someone in top management needs to become convinced that workplace wellness programs are worth the investment of time and money necessary to develop fertile ground in the company to seize this opportunity to keep workers well. Workplace leaders of the future will be involved in building cultures that guide others to achieve good health.

Jeffrey et al. (1993) point to the many positive aspects of employer-based wellness initiatives. They include convenient access to populations in need, the presence of social support systems, and the potential to recover costs through reduced absenteeism and health care expenditures. Wilson et al. (1996) argue that the number of organizations offering health promotion programs has grown exponentially since 1980 with over 80% of work sites offering some type of health promotion program. Evaluation of the success or failure of workplace wellness programs is extremely difficult for many reasons. Many work sites may offer wellness programs, but their sophistication is so low that it is difficult if not impossible to measure achievement.

Over the years, there has been an evolution of four generations of wellness programs with very few programs reaching the fourth generation of sophistication. The fourth generation would encompass a comprehensive approach to all health aspects of employees, family, and the wider community. Another problem is that although work sites want to offer quality programs, they usually do not have the resources to support theoretical research to document the program's outcomes. These facts make it very difficult to evaluate the success or failure of workplace wellness programs. Their mere existence is a testament to a belief that if given time and resources, employers could become a catalyst in helping to keep their employees healthy and in reducing the rising costs associated with providing health insurance for their employees.

Discussion of Grant Writing

Health promotion programs are heavily dependent on private and public grants for start-up and expansion. A health promotion program requires resources to accomplish the goals set forth by the health promotion specialist. These resources can be obtained from the government, foundations, and businesses. In order to obtain these funds, the potential program must be able to develop and submit a successful grant application.

According to Ward (2006), a successful grant application usually includes the following:

- Need statement
- Objectives
- Activities
- Personnel
- Evaluation method
- Budget

Grant approval is usually denied because they are poorly developed and not supported by demonstrated need and the document simply does not make sense to those evaluating the proposal. The most important piece of the grant proposal is the needs assessment. This document explains how the proposed program can meet the priorities of the funding agency. The needs statement also explains how the proposed program will offer a solution to the problem under consideration. The grant application has to be written in a way that makes funders comfortable that the new program has the capability of solving the problem.

An equally important part of the proposal is the development of objectives and how the program will evaluate success or failure of the proposed program. An objective is nothing more than the intent of the program. In other words, the objective must be a very clear representation of what the program is going to attempt to accomplish. Therefore, the objective has to be concise, measurable, and time bounded. The health promotion specialist is attempting to show potential funders how the new program will produce the desired results.

A great deal of attention must be paid very early in program development on how the program will be evaluated. Ward (2006) points out that for the last 20 years the evaluation part of the proposal has become one of the most important parts of the grant proposal. Potential funders want proof that the dollars given to health promotion programs have been used effectively.

CONCLUDING REMARKS

Economic evaluation of illness and injury reduction programs makes good sense in order to prove their worth and attract new interest and resources for their expansion. The costs of supplying health insurance to workers in this country is increasing at such a rapid rate that many businesses are passing more and more of the costs of health insurance on to the employee. At the same time, the workers' productivity is decreasing because of poor health due to the effects of chronic diseases developed and manifested during the working years.

Employers are looking for help in order to confront these workplace issues, to retain their employees, and to keep their workers healthy and productive. Health promotion programs have the requisite tools to help employers develop workplace wellness initiatives, implement these initiatives, and prove their worth through qualitative and quantitative evaluation techniques.

The purpose of economic evaluation is to make value judgments about intervention strategies. In other words, if the company is attempting to improve the health of the workers, they need to know the value of the intervention and the costs associated with the intervention in order to determine if it is a good investment for the company.

This approach has been called evidence-based health care, population-based medicine, and cost-effectiveness analysis. Whatever it is called, both OSHA and NIOSH can take a leadership role in its use in the work-place initiatives to reduce injury and illness in the workplace.

DISCUSSION QUESTIONS

1. Please offer an explanation of how to conduct an economic evaluation of health promotion programs.
2. Explain the difference between cost-benefit analysis and cost-effectiveness analysis.
3. What is the value of using the BASICC approach developed by CDC when evaluating health promotion programs?
4. Explain the *Prescription for the American People* developed by the former Surgeon General, Dr. David Satcher (2006).

REFERENCES

Akinci, F., Healey, B, & Cotne, J. (2003). Improving the health status of UD working adults with type 2 diabetes mellitus. *Disease Management Health Outcomes, 11*(8), 489–498.

American Diabetes Association. (2002). Standards of medical care for patients with diabetes mellitus. *Diabetes Care, 25*(1), 213–229.

Centers for Disease Control and Prevention. (2005). Annual smoking-attributable mortality, years of potential life lost, and productivity losses–United States, 1997–2001. *Morbidity and Mortality Weekly Report, 54*(25), 1–2.

Centers for Disease Control and Prevention. (1995). Assessing the effectiveness of disease and injury prevention programs: Costs and consequences. *Morbidity and Mortality Weekly Report, 44*(RR-10), 1–11.

Centers for Disease Control and Prevention. (1986). Premature mortality in the United States: Public health issues in the use of years of potential life lost. *Morbidity and Mortality Weekly Report, 35*, 1–11.

Centers for Disease Control and Prevention. (1999). Ten great public health achievements—United States, 1900–1999. *Morbidity and Mortality Weekly Report, 48*(12), 241–243.

Christoffel, T., & Gallagher, S. (2006). *Injury prevention and public health: Practical knowledge, skills and strategies.* Sudbury, MA: Jones and Bartlett Publishers.

Community Partnerships. (n.d.) A guide to community preventive services. Available at http://www.thecommunityguide.org. Accessed August 5, 2006.

Fielding, J., & Briss, P. (2006). Promoting evidence-based public health policy: Can we have better evidence and more action? *Health Affairs, 25*, 969–978.

Finkelstein, E., Corso, P., & Miller, T. (2006) *The incidence and economic burden of injuries in the United States.* New York, NY: Oxford University Press.

Heath Affairs. (2006). Medicare beneficiaries treated for five or more chronic conditions account for virtually all program spending growth. Available at http://content.healthaffairs.org/index.dt1. Accessed August 5, 2006.

Jeffery. R. W., Forster. J. L., French S. A., Kelder. S. H. and Lando. H. A. (1993). The Healthy Worker Project: A worksite intervention for weight control and smoking cessation. *American Journal of Public Health, 83*, 395–401.

Kaiser Family Foundation. (2005). *Employer health benefits 2005 annual survey.* Menlo Park, CA: Henry J. Kaiser Family Foundation. Available at http://www. kff.org/insurance/7315/upload/7315.pdf. Accessed January 2, 2009.

Nas, T. (1996). *Cost benefit analysis theory and application.* Thousand Oaks, CA: Sage Publications Inc.

Ong, M. & Glantz, S. (2005). Free nicotine replacement therapy program vs implementing smoke-free workplaces: A cost-effectiveness comparison. *American Journal of Public Health, 95,* 969–975.

Price Waterhouse Coopers. (2008). *The price of excess identifying waste on health care spending.* Available at www.pwc.com/healthindustries. Accessed February 3, 2009.

Satcher, D. (2006). The prevention challenge and opportunity. *Health Affairs, 25,* 1009–1011.

Shi, L., & Singh, D. (2005). *Essentials of the U.S. health care system.* Sudbury, MA: Jones and Bartlett Publishers.

Simon, P., & Fielding, J. (2006). Public health and business: A partnership that makes cents. *Health Affairs, 25*(4), 1029–1039.

Smith, G., Wellman H., Sorock. G., Warner. M., Courtney. T., Pransky. G. Fingerhut M. L. (2005). Injuries at work in the U.S. adult population: Contributions to the total injury burden. *American Journal of Public Health, 95*(7), 1213–1219.

U.S. Bureau of the Census. U.S. Census Figures 2006. Available at http://www. census.gov/. Accessed August 29, 2006.

U.S. Bureau of Labor. (2004). Health Insurance Coverage 2004. Available at http:// www.bls.gov/pub/cwc/cm2007 u28arolpl.htm. Accessed August 20, 2006.

Ward. D. (2006). Writing grant proposals that work. Sudbury, MA: Jones and Bartlett Publishers.

Wilson, M., Holman, P., & Hammock, A. (1996). A comprehensive review of the effects of worksite health promotion on health-related outcomes. *Science of Health Promotion, 10,* 429–435.

MAPP: A Strategic Approach to Community Health Improvement

Julia Joh Elligers, MPH

After reading this chapter, you should

- Be able to explain why MAPP is a process for community health planning and improvement
- Understand the seven principles that underlie the MAPP process
- Be able to describe the six phases of the MAPP process
- Be able to explain how MAPP provides a strategic framework for achieving health promotion goals

Assessment	National Association of County and
Dialogue	City Health Officials (NACCHO)
Local public health system	Partnerships
MAPP	Strategic planning

Introduction

The **National Association of County and City Health Officials (NACCHO),** the Public Health Practice Program Office at the CDC, and a work group comprised of local health officials, CDC representatives, community representatives, and academicians developed Mobilizing for Action through Planning and Partnerships (**MAPP**) between 1997 and 2000.

MAPP is a strategic approach to community health improvement. This [process] helps communities improve health and quality of life through community-wide strategic planning. Using MAPP, communities seek to achieve optimal health by identifying and using their resources wisely, taking into account their unique circumstances and needs, and forming effective **partnerships** for strategic action (NACCHO, 2004, p. 3).

This chapter will describe how MAPP can help communities achieve their health promotion goals and can provide a framework for thinking about health promotion in the context of local public health systems and community health planning and improvement.

MAPP is not a health promotion tool per se; however, it can provide a framework for reaching health promotion goals. Through dialogue, collaboration, partnership building, **assessments**, and strategic thinking, the MAPP process assists communities in developing, implementing, and evaluating community health plans. By going through the MAPP process, health promotion activities resulting from a community's health plan are well informed by the community, address the actual needs of the community, and capitalize on the assets already available for health promotion.

The philosophy underpinning the MAPP process aligns well with the theoretical foundations of health promotion. As described in earlier chapters, health promotion works to improve the population's health by identifying the determinants of health; by using data to identify needs; by involving community participation; and by incorporating root-cause analysis and evidence-based practices into strategies to ultimately change behavior and improve health. MAPP incorporates these aspects of health promotion throughout the six phases of the process. In particular, community involvement and collaboration drives each phase of the MAPP process. The data collected and analyzed using mixed method approaches help identify health issues and the strategies for addressing them. MAPP also incorporates both root-cause analysis into identifying critical community health issues and plans for intervention and evidence-based practices in formulating, implementing, and evaluating health improvement efforts. Moreover, the framework for planning and action outlined in the MAPP process focuses on populations as opposed to individuals in promoting health.

Principles Underlying the MAPP Process

The MAPP process is based on a broad definition of health. As defined by the World Health Organization (1998), "Health is a dynamic state of complete physical, mental, spiritual and social well-being and not merely the absence of disease or infirmity," and according to the Institute of Medicine (IOM, 2001, p. 28), public health is "what we as a society do collectively to assure the conditions in which people can be healthy." Public health is not limited to the provision of health services, health insurance, health education, and disease surveillance. It also includes broader issues, such as mitigating environmental health threats, improving land use and community design, and addressing conditions attributed to poverty, race, and class. At the same time, public health does not only serve the disadvantaged and poor. Public health services such as restaurant inspections, water quality maintenance, school immunizations, bioterrorism planning, and community mobilization protect everyone regardless of social class.

Improving health is a shared responsibility. As noted by the IOM (1997), in addition to health care providers and public health officials, a variety of other actors in the community contribute to the health of populations. Protecting the public's health requires the expertise of a variety of actors in the community who contribute to the well-being of individuals and populations. For instance, police, fire, and emergency response prevent and respond to emergencies that threaten personal safety. Teachers, school nurses, and parents protect the heath and safety of children. City planners, transportation authorities, neighborhood associations, and businesses work to ensure access to services that promote and support healthy lifestyles, such as safe parks and recreational facilities, bus routes to health care providers, and vendors that sell nutritious foods. The judicial and penal systems also contribute to the public's health not only in terms of the health of the individuals who use their services but also in identifying potential risk factors and health trends such as increases in drug abuse, domestic abuse, and personal injury. Moreover, community groups like churches, home owners associations, and civic organizations provide insight into the quality of health and services in a community. In sum, all the entities that contribute to the public's health in some capacity comprise the **local public health system** (LPHS). Figure 17-1 depicts how different private, public, and voluntary entities responsible for ensuring the public's health interact within the LPHS.

Local Public Health System

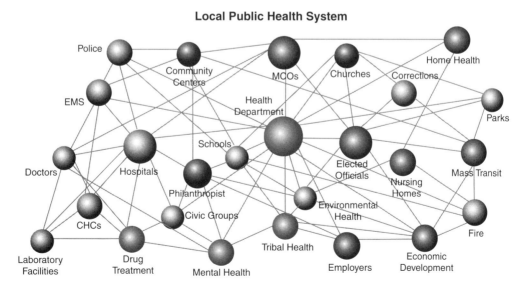

Figure 17-1 Local Public Health System
Source: CDC.

MAPP is not a **strategic planning** tool only for the health department; rather, MAPP is a health improvement process for the entire community, which involves coordinated planning among all LPHS entities. As noted in the MAPP web-based tool, MAPP focuses on the system instead of a public health agency and "promotes an appreciation for the dynamic interrelationship of all components of the local public health system required to develop a vision for a healthy community." This system approach also recognizes that health promotion "requires consideration and a better understanding of the various components that determine good or poor health," as noted in Chapter 1.

In addition to being a process organized by the LPHS, MAPP is a community-driven process. In order to implement MAPP, the facilitating body mobilizes and engages the community so that the process and its outcomes have credibility within the community. Without this engagement, the community may not fully embrace identified priority issues and related health promotion activities. Community members are involved in every phase of the process. They participate on committees that plan and evaluate the process. They help design the assessment methods used to collect data, such as focus groups, surveys, interviews, town hall meetings, and task forces. Then, through these methods, they share their perceptions and insights into why public health issues exist in their communities and what assets the community has to address public health issues. In addition to their involvement in the assessment phase, community members also help analyze and synthesize all the assessment data to develop and implement a strategic plan. Community engagement and mobilization is important because the wisdom found within communities is as important as the technical expertise found among health professionals. As noted in *Achieving Healthier Communities through MAPP: A User's Handbook*, "Technical knowledge does not address the essential questions of what values and vision to pursue and what issues are important for community health" (NACCHO, 2004, p. 110). In effect, MAPP elicits collective thinking that results in effective, innovative, and sustainable solutions to complex problems that are important to the community.

It is important to note that even though LPHS entities are members of the community and community groups are entities within the LPHS, the terms LPHS and community are not exactly synonymous. LPHS entities provide services and help ensure the public's health; whereas, the community refers to those who reside or work in a community and use public health services. Community members may contribute to the public's health, but collectively, they do not represent the LPHS; however, references to the community also include LPHS partners. Therefore, referring to MAPP as a community-driven tool indicates that the community, which includes the LPHS, drives the process.

Community-driven processes like MAPP can be challenging to facilitate because they require the cooperation and collaboration of competing interests and different stakeholders; however, a community-driven approach should result in greater benefits than agency-focused or agency-dominated health improvement efforts. As noted in the MAPP guidance,

> Creating healthy communities and strong local public health systems requires a high level of mutual understanding and collaboration. To accomplish this, communities must find ways of working together that create stronger connections throughout the community and provide access to the collective wisdom necessary to address community concerns (NACCHO, 2004, p. 110).

In order to both foster and sustain mutual understanding and collaboration among community members and LPHS entities, successful MAPP communities have used dialogue skills. **Dialogue** is the development of shared understanding by simply holding differences together in a way that is open, empathetic, and equal. Dialogue is a methodology that (1) encourages the broadest possible participation by the various parties; (2) validates the legitimacy and equality of divergent perspectives; and (3) allows new ideas, solutions, and even wisdom to emerge that may well have been previously unseen or never before articulated. Thus, dialogue assists in ensuring respect for diverse voices and perspectives during a collaborative process and uncovers the collective wisdom of a community. Dialogue is also instrumental in surfacing long-held cultural assumptions that, for example, may have considered quantitative data as somehow more important, more equal, than the qualitative data that is revealed when a community begins to voice its own wisdom.

A community's collective wisdom is combined with other types of information, which are used to ensure that a community's health plan is strategic and well informed. One of the hallmarks of the MAPP process is the use of four different types of assessments. The four assessments, which will be described in more detail in the next section, provide a comprehensive picture of the health of a community; the assets and resources available to address public health issues; the capacity of the LPHS to provide public health services; and future trends that may influence health and public health capacity in a community. The collection of a comprehensive set of data helps communities create strategic community health plans that address the most important community health problems effectively.

Strategic thinking is a critical component of the MAPP process. As defined by Liedtka (1998), "Strategic thinking is built on the foundation of a systems perspective. A strategic thinker has a mental model of the complete end-to-end system of value creation, his or her role within it, and an understanding of the interdependencies it contains" (p. 31). In understanding a community's public health issues and the overall system, thinking strategically means looking at multiple sources of information, such as local perceptions about health and the community, public health data and trends, information about how the public health system is operating and gaps in services, and forces of change such as new legislation or changes in state funding for public health. Strategic thinking accommodates divergent interests and values that arise within the system, which helps facilitate communication and participation and foster orderly decision making and successful implementation. Strategic thinking involves an exploration of alternatives to public health problems with an emphasis on the future implications of present decisions. By looking at multiple sources of information, thinking about future implications of decisions, and using broad input, communities develop stronger health improvement plans that have a greater likelihood for success and sustainability.

Overall, MAPP is a strategic process that reflects a paradigm shift in public health practice. First, public health has historically focused on the public health agency and has not regularly looked to the community or the entire LPHS for guidance and knowledge. The philosophy behind MAPP incorporates a community's knowledge and wisdom, which entails a shift from an "agency knows all" perspective to the belief that "everyone knows something." Second, MAPP reflects a change from day-to-day operational planning to more broad, information and vision driven strategic planning. Third, the process is a shift away from a biomedical model of health that emphasizes individual health behaviors and health outcomes—like poor nutrition and infectious diseases—to a model that encompasses a broad definition of health that recognizes the multiple determinants of health in the prevention of disease. Finally, in order to understand the state of health in a community and to identify possible solutions, MAPP does not only focus on assessing needs but also emphasizes assessments of existing assets and resources. By gathering all of the assets and resources within the community, the community is able to determine how best to use all of the wisdom to create a healthier community. Collectively, these characteristics of MAPP reflect a paradigm shift in the business and practice of public health.

Even though MAPP can be thought of as a paradigm shift in public health practice, the principles and the components of the MAPP process are not novel. Surveying and engaging community members, conducting assessments, creating visions of healthy communities, and applying a broad definition of public health are common in public health practice. However, what makes MAPP unique and effective is the integration of these practices under a solid philosophical framework that is grounded in best practices and professional expertise. As noted by Patrick Lenihan (2005):

> The success of MAPP as a planning tool is based on both building on the history of planning in public health and on introducing new approaches that connect public health agencies to the challenges of today and to the partners they will need to meet those challenges (p. 385).

In sum, MAPP brings together successful public health practices into a model for community health improvement.

Overview of the MAPP Phases

Two graphics illustrate the six phases of the MAPP process. In the MAPP model (see Figure 17-2), the phases of the MAPP process are shown in the center of the model, while the four MAPP assessments—the key content areas that drive the process—are shown in the four outer arrows. In the illustrated

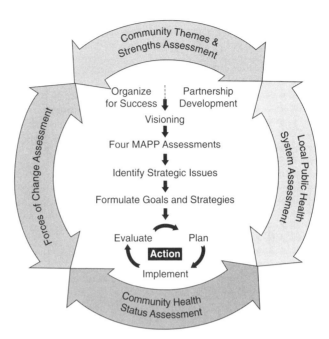

Figure 17-2
MAPP Model

Source: National Association of County and City Health Officials.

"community roadmap," (see Figure 17-3) the process is shown moving along a road that leads to a healthier community.

To initiate the MAPP process, lead organizations in the community begin by organizing themselves and preparing to implement MAPP through the first phase, Organize for Success–Partnership Development. Community-wide strategic planning requires a high level of commitment from partners, stakeholders, and community residents who are recruited to participate. The second phase of the MAPP process is visioning. A shared vision and common values provide a framework for pursuing long-range community goals. During this phase, the community answers questions such as, What would we like our community to look like in 10 years?

Next, the four MAPP assessments are conducted, providing critical insights into challenges and opportunities throughout the community:

- The Community Themes and Strengths Assessment provides a deep understanding of the issues residents feel are important by answering the following questions: What is important to our community? How is quality of life perceived in our community? What assets do we have that can be used to improve community health?
- The Local Public Health System Assessment (LPHSA) is a comprehensive assessment of all of the organizations and entities that contribute to the public's health. The LPHSA answers the following questions: What are the activities, competencies, and capacities of our local public health system? How are the essential services being provided to our community?

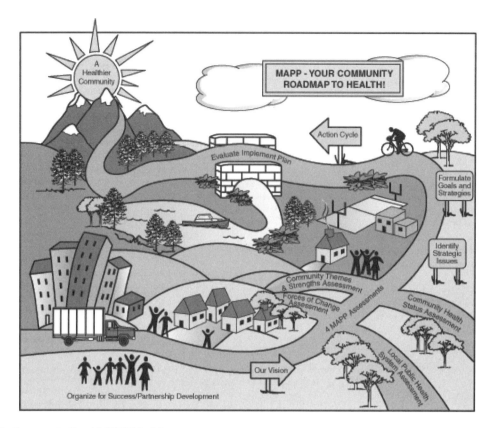

Figure 17-3 Community Road MAPP Model
Source: National Association of County and City Health Officials.

- The Community Health Status Assessment identifies priority issues related to community health and quality of life. Questions answered during the phase include the following: How healthy are our residents? What does the health status of our community look like?
- The Forces of Change Assessment focuses on the identification of forces such as legislation, technology, and other issues that affect the context in which the community and its public health system operates. This answers the following questions: What is occurring or might occur that affects the health of our community or the local public health system? What specific threats or opportunities are generated by these occurrences?

Once a list of challenges and opportunities has been generated from each of the four assessments, the next step is to identify strategic issues. During this phase, participants identify linkages between the MAPP assessments to determine the most critical issues that must be addressed for the community to achieve its vision. After issues have been identified, participants formulate goals and strategies for addressing each issue. The final phase of MAPP is the Action Cycle. During this phase, participants plan, implement, and evaluate their efforts to achieve their goals.

Implementing the MAPP Process

Phase 1: Organize for Success– Partnership Development

A successful community-wide strategic planning process requires careful preparation. The purpose of this phase is to lay out a planning process that builds commitment, engages participants, uses participants' time well, and results in a plan that can be implemented successfully. These activities are crucial to putting a community on the path toward a successful community health improvement process.

Two interrelated activities occur during this phase:

- Organize for success: A decision is made to undertake MAPP, and the planning process is outlined.

- Partnership development: Participants, including the MAPP Committee, are identified and recruited.

Step 1: Determine the necessity of undertaking the MAPP process

The first step in organizing the MAPP process is gaining a clear understanding of why such a process is needed. This understanding helps focus planning efforts and assists in the recruitment and sustained involvement of participants. In addition to identifying reasons for initiating MAPP, participants should also consider the benefits they hope to gain from the process and the obstacles that may be encountered along the way.

Step 2: Identify and organize participants

During this step, careful consideration should be given to identifying and recruiting participants. Conveners should seek broad representation from LPHS partners, other community organizations, and community residents. Participants' expectations, time commitments, and logistics should determine how the group will be organized. While the MAPP Committee will provide oversight throughout the process, subcommittees should be identified to carry out specific activities.

Step 3: Design the planning process

Designing a process involves answering several related questions: What will the process entail? How long will it take? What results are we seeking, and how will we know when we are finished? Who will do the work? All of the MAPP phases should be carefully reviewed and used to develop a timeline and work plan that meets the community's needs.

Step 4: Assess resource needs and secure commitment

While the principal resources for the planning effort will be time and energy contributed by the participants, other resources will be needed as well. Some of these include meeting space, refreshments, report production and printing, and costs associated with information gathering and data collection. Participants should identify resource needs and determine sources for meeting those needs. Some resources may be available through in-kind donations from participating organizations.

Step 5: Conduct a readiness assessment

The information collected in the previous four steps should provide a clear picture of the community's preparedness to begin the MAPP process. As a final review, the readiness assessment should ensure that all of the critical elements are in place.

Step 6: Manage the process

The final step in organizing the MAPP process is to consider how the process will be managed as it moves forward. This involves paying attention to the many details that may affect the success of a community planning process. Tools such as a project proposal, master calendars, and meeting agendas should be developed. A process for clarifying assignments and managing the work should also be outlined. Careful preparation puts the community on the path to a successful MAPP process.

Phase 2: Visioning   The second phase of MAPP, visioning, guides the community through a collaborative and creative process that leads to a shared community vision and common values. Vision and values statements provide focus, purpose, and direction to the MAPP process so that participants collectively achieve a shared vision of the future. A shared community vision provides an overarching goal for the community—a statement of what the ideal future looks like. Values are the fundamental principles and beliefs that guide a community-driven planning process. Because visioning is done at the beginning of the MAPP process, it offers a useful mechanism for convening the community and building enthusiasm for the process, setting the stage for planning, and providing a common framework throughout subsequent phases.

Step 1: Identify other visioning efforts and make connections as needed

The MAPP Committee should revisit the inventory of other community initiatives to see whether or not visioning efforts have taken place. It is a good idea to rescan community efforts to ensure that no similar efforts have emerged since the Organize for Success phase occurred. If a similar visioning process is in progress or has been completed, try to link it with the MAPP process.

Step 2: Design the visioning process and select a facilitator

Visioning can be conducted through either of the following approaches:

- Community visioning: a broad-based process with 40 to 100 participants. Community visioning is useful for engaging and mobilizing the broader community but can be more challenging to manage and may require more resources to implement.

- Advisory committee–key leadership visioning: participants include members of the MAPP Committee, as well as other key leaders in the community. This type of visioning process may be easier to manage and requires fewer resources but will not include the ideal level of broad involvement. Once an approach is selected, a small group is charged with preparing the visioning sessions, identifying and working with the facilitator, recording the results of the sessions, and drafting the resulting vision and values statements.

Step 3: Conduct the visioning process

Visioning sessions are conducted using the method described on the MAPP website or another approach. As the process is implemented, it is important to ensure that broad ranges of participants are included in the effort. Both a shared vision and common values should be identified through brainstorming and open discussions.

Sample questions for brainstorming a shared vision:

1. What does a healthy Anywhere County mean to you?
2. What are important characteristics of a healthy community for all who live, work, and play here?
3. How do you envision the LPHS in the next 5 or 10 years?

Sample questions for brainstorming common values:

1. Taking into consideration the vision that has been developed, what key behaviors will be required from the LPHS partners, the community, and others in the next 5 to 10 years to achieve the vision?
2. What type of working environment or climate will be necessary to support these behaviors and to achieve the vision?

Step 4: Formulate vision and values statements

A small group formulates the vision and values statements based on the outcomes of the visioning session(s). The vision statement should be strong and powerful and represent the ideal future outlined during the visioning process. The values statement should emphasize a positive climate and supportive behaviors that contribute to the achievement of the vision.

Step 5: Keep the vision and values alive throughout the MAPP process

As the community moves through the MAPP process, it is important to ensure that the vision statement continues to drive the MAPP effort. Ways to keep the vision and values alive include reading the statements at meetings or including them on informational materials. Both may be refined as the community progresses through the planning process.

Phase 3 (MAPP Assessments): Community Themes and Strengths Assessment

The Community Themes and Strengths Assessment answers the following questions: What is important to our community? How is quality of life perceived in our community? What assets do we have that can be used to improve community health? The Community Themes and Strengths Assessment is a vital part of a community health improvement process. During this phase, community thoughts, opinions, and concerns are gathered, providing insight into the issues of importance to the community. Feedback about quality of life in the community and community assets is also gathered. This information leads to a portrait of the community as seen through the eyes of its residents.

By including Community Themes and Strengths in the MAPP process, several benefits are gained.

- Community members become more vested in the process when they have a sense of ownership in and responsibility for the outcomes. This occurs when their concerns are genuinely considered and visibly affect the process.
- The impressions and thoughts of community residents help to pinpoint important issues and highlight possible solutions.
- The themes and issues identified here offer additional insight into the findings uncovered in the other assessments.

Listening to and communicating with the community are essential to any community-wide initiative. Mobilizing and engaging the community may be a daunting task; however, when successful, it ensures greater sustainability and enthusiasm for the process.

Step 1: Prepare for the Community Themes and Strengths Assessment

Establish a subcommittee to oversee the Community Themes and Strengths Assessment. This subcommittee should determine the most effective approaches for gathering community perspectives. Possible approaches include the following:

- community meetings
- community dialogue sessions
- focus groups
- walking or windshield surveys
- individual discussions–interviews
- surveys

The subcommittee should carefully select a variety of approaches that will best reach broad segments of the population, then identify the skills and resources needed to conduct the activities.

Step 2: Implement information-gathering activities

When implementing selected activities, the broadest participation possible should be included. The subcommittee should identify groups or individuals whose voices are not being heard. Also, the subcommittee should ensure that the logistics—how, when, and where the meetings are held—promote good participation.

Three levels of information-gathering occur during the Community Themes and Strengths Assessment:

- Open discussion to elicit community concerns, opinions, and comments in an unstructured way: Asking open-ended questions ensures that issues of concern and interest to the community are raised. If concerns are properly addressed, this activity can raise the credibility of the process and underscore its community-driven nature.
- Perceptions regarding community quality of life: Questions about quality of life in the community help pinpoint specific concerns. This may highlight aspects of neighborhoods and/or communities that either enhance or diminish residents' quality of life.
- A map of community assets: Asset mapping is an important tool for mobilizing community resources. Through this process, the capacities of individuals, civic associations, and local institutions are inventoried.

Step 3: Compile the results of the Community Themes and Strengths Assessment

The subcommittee should keep a running list of ideas, comments, quotes, and themes while the activities are being implemented. Subcommittee members should also note possible solutions to identified problems or innovative ideas for providing public health services. The results of this phase are compiled into one central list.

Step 4: Ensure that community involvement and empowerment is sustained

Although the specific activities conducted (i.e., focus groups, windshield surveys) occur on a finite timeline, the dialogue that has opened up within the community should be never-ending. Participants involved in the community themes and strengths activities should continue to be involved throughout the remaining phases of the MAPP process.

Phase 3 (MAPP Assessments): The Local Public Health System Assessment

The LPHSA answers the questions, What are the components, activities, competencies, and capacities of our LPHS? and How are the essential services being provided to our community? The LPHSA focuses on the LPHS—all organizations and entities within the community that contribute to the public's health. The LPHSA uses the essential public health services as the fundamental framework for assessing the LPHS. The essential services list the 10 public health activities that should be undertaken in all communities.

Step 1: Prepare for the LPHSA

A subcommittee should be established to oversee the LPHSA process. Subcommittee members should represent diverse segments of the LPHS. Once the subcommittee is convened, members review LPHSA steps and tools and plan how each step will be implemented.

Step 2: Discuss the essential services and identify where each organization–entity is *active*

The first LPHSA meeting should focus on orienting participants to the essential services (see Table 17–1). After a brief overview of the essential services framework, each participant shares information about where his or her organization is active. Posting the information on flip charts can be a fun and easy way to do this. The last part of the meeting should be devoted to a dialogue about the essential services and how each organization contributes to them. This discussion will help identify opportunities for collaboration, gaps in service provision, and overlapping activities.

Table 17-1
Essential Public Health Services

1. Monitor health status to identify community health problems.
2. Diagnose and investigate health problems and health hazards in the community.
3. Inform, educate, and empower people about health issues.
4. Mobilize community partnerships to identify and solve health problems.
5. Develop policies and plans that support individual and community health efforts.
6. Enforce laws and regulations that protect health and ensure safety.
7. Link people to needed personal health services and assure the provision of health care when otherwise unavailable.
8. Assure a competent public health and personal health care workforce.
9. Evaluate effectiveness, accessibility, and quality of personal and population-based health services.
10. Research for new insights and innovative solutions to health problems.

Source: Harrell, J. A., & Baker, E. L. (1994). The essential services of public health. *Leadership Public Health, 3,* 27–30.

Step 3: Discuss and complete the performance measurement instrument

During the next step, the MAPP Committee discusses and completes the performance measures instrument. The instrument provides two to four indicators (or activities) under each essential service. By responding to the questions related to each indicator, participants get a good idea of the activities, capacities, and performance of the LPHS. To respond to the instrument, the MAPP Committee should discuss the information in the tool until a consensus emerges. This discussion should include perspectives from the organizations conducting public health activities as well as community resident input.

Step 4: Review the results and determine challenges and opportunities

During this step, participants discuss the results and identify challenges and opportunities. The results of the previous steps should highlight activity levels and coordination among partners. Through discussion, participants should be able to categorize the indicators (from the performance measures instrument) into a list of challenges and opportunities. The list should be comprehensive enough to include the issues identified in the assessment but short enough (i.e., 10 to 15 items) for the LPHS to address many of them.

Phase 3 (MAPP Assessments): The Community Health Status Assessment (CHSA)

The Community Health Status Assessment (CHSA) answers the questions, How healthy are our residents? and What does the health status of our community look like? The results of the CHSA provide the MAPP Committee with an understanding of the community's health status and ensure that the community's priorities consider specific health status issues, such as high lung cancer rates or low immunization rates.

The CHSA provides a list of core indicators (data elements) for 11 broad-based categories (see Table 17-2). Communities may also select additional indicators. By gathering data for each of the categories and assessing changes over time or differences among population subgroups or with peer, state, or national data, health issues are identified.

Step 1: Prepare for the Community Health Status Assessment

A subcommittee should be designated to oversee the CHSA. Members should include individuals that can assist with access to data as well as data collection, analysis, and interpretation. Community representatives also provide an important perspective. Once the subcommittee is assembled, members should review the CHSA steps and identify the skills and resources needed to conduct the activities.

Step 2: Collect data for the core indicators on the CHSA indicator list

During this step, data related to the MAPP core indicators should be collected, including trend and comparison data. Trend data will help to identify changes in data over time, while comparison data will measure a community's health status against other jurisdictions. Data collection may require considerable time and effort; therefore, it is important to begin this activity early in the MAPP process.

Step 3: Identify locally appropriate indicators and collect the data

The selection of locally appropriate indicators helps the MAPP Committee better describe the community's health status and quality of life in terms that are of particular interest to the community. Additional indicators might be selected related to community interest in a specific topic, demographics in the area (e.g., an aging population), or information found in the core indicators (e.g., the need to look closer at cancer rates). To keep data collection efforts reasonable in terms of time and resources, select indicators of high priority and relevance only.

Step 4: Organize and analyze the data, develop a compilation of the findings, and disseminate the information

Individuals with statistical expertise should analyze data. Disparities among age, gender, racial, and other population subgroups are especially important. Once the data is analyzed, a compilation of the findings or a "community health profile" should be developed. The community health profile should include visual aids, such as charts and graphs that display the data in an understandable and meaningful way. The community health profile should be disseminated and shared with the community.

Table 17-2
Categories of Data
Collected in the CHSA

Who are we and what do we bring to the table?
1. Demographic characteristics
2. Socioeconomic characteristics
3. Health resource availability

What are the strengths and risks in our community that contribute to health?
4. Quality of life
5. Behavioral risk factors
6. Environmental health indicators

What is our health status?
7. Social and mental health
8. Maternal and child health
9. Death, illness, and injury
10. Infectious disease

Source: National Association of County and City Health Officials. (2004). *Achieving healthier communities through MAPP: A user's handbook.* Washington, DC: Author.

Step 5: Establish a system to monitor the indicators over time

During this step, the subcommittee establishes a system for monitoring selected indicators. This helps to ensure that continuous health status monitoring occurs and establishes baseline data upon which future trends can be identified. This system will also be instrumental in evaluating the success of MAPP activities.

Step 6: Identify challenges and opportunities related to health status

The CHSA should result in a list of challenges and opportunities related to the community's health status. Data findings should be reviewed to identify challenges, such as major health problems or high-risk behaviors, and opportunities, such as improving health trends. Ideally, the final list will include 10 to 15 community health status issues that will be more closely examined in the Identify Strategic Issues phase of MAPP.

Phase 3 (MAPP Assessments): Forces of Change Assessment

During the Forces of Change Assessment, participants answer the following questions: What is occurring or might occur that affects the health of our community or the LPHS? What specific threats or opportunities are generated by these occurrences? The Forces of Change Assessment should result in a comprehensive, but focused, list that identifies key forces and describes their impacts.

Although it may not seem obvious at first, the broader environment is constantly affecting communities and LPHSs. State and federal legislation, rapid technological advances, changes in the organization of health care services, shifts in economic forces, and changing family structures and gender roles are all examples of forces of change. These forces are important because they affect—either directly or indirectly—the health and quality of life in the community and the effectiveness of the LPHS.

During this phase, participants engage in brainstorming sessions aimed at identifying forces. Forces are a broad, all-encompassing category that includes trends, events, and factors.

- *Trends* are patterns over time, such as migration in and out of a community or a growing disillusionment with government.
- *Factors* are discrete elements, such as a community's large ethnic population, an urban setting, or the jurisdiction's proximity to a major waterway.
- *Events* are one-time occurrences, such as a hospital closure, a natural disaster, or the passage of new legislation.

Step 1: Prepare for the Forces of Change Assessment

During this step, a small group responsible for overseeing the Forces of Change Assessment should prepare for the brainstorming sessions. This group determines who will facilitate the process and how the sessions will be run. Additionally, each member of the MAPP Committee should begin thinking about the major forces that affect public health or the community. This helps to ensure that everyone comes to the meeting prepared.

Step 2: Convene a brainstorming session to identify forces of change

The MAPP Committee should hold a brainstorming session to identify forces of change. Through facilitated and structured brainstorming discussions, committee members share ideas, identify new forces, and develop a comprehensive list.

Once a comprehensive list of forces has been developed, the MAPP Committee (or a small group of designated individuals) reviews and fully discusses each item on the list. An organized list is developed by combining forces that are similar or linked. Other items on the list may need to be deleted, added, or further refined.

Step 3: Identify potential threats and opportunities for each force of change

Committee members evaluate each force, and for each, identify associated threats and opportunities for the community and the LPHS. In some cases, a force might only be identified with a threat, while in other instances, it may be perceived as both a threat and an opportunity.

The final list is tabled until it is time to conduct the Identify Strategic Issues phase of the MAPP process. Participants then review each of the issues identified in the other MAPP assessments in light of the forces of change and discuss the associated threats and opportunities. This activity ensures that strategic issues are relevant to the changing environment.

Phase 4: Identify Strategic Issues

During this phase of the MAPP process, participants develop an ordered list of the most important issues facing the community. When addressing strategic issues, a community is being proactive in positioning itself for the future, rather than simply reacting to problems. Strategic issues are those fundamental policy choices or critical challenges that must be addressed for a community to achieve its vision. Strategic issues should reflect the results of all of the previous MAPP phases. Up to this point, the process has largely focused on developing a shared vision and identifying challenges and opportunities for improving community health. Strategic issues reveal what is truly important from the vast amount of information that was gathered in the four MAPP Assessments. Identifying strategic issues can be compared to pouring the assessment findings into a funnel—what emerges is a distilled mix of issues that demand attention.

Step 1: Brainstorm potential strategic issues

Participants should begin by reviewing the shared vision, common values, and results of the four MAPP assessments. They should ask, What factors identified in the assessments must be addressed in order to achieve the vision? As participants discuss this question, they should try to identify where results converge. Each potential strategic issue should be phrased as a question.

Step 2: Develop an understanding about why an issue is strategic

After strategic issues are identified, participants should discuss each issue until they understand why it is strategic. The definition and criteria for strategic issues—provided on the MAPP website—is a useful resource. This discussion will help to separate strategic issues from other problems. Participants must understand the issues to be able to make wise decisions about how to address them.

Step 3: Determine the consequences of not addressing an issue

Participants should consider each strategic issue and ask, What are the consequences of not addressing this? This will help participants determine whether or not action is required. Strategic issues may have significant consequences for the community or the LPHS, and failure to address them could lead to serious repercussions.

Step 4: Consolidate overlapping or related issues

At this point, a large number of strategic issues may have been identified. Participants should examine all of these issues and consolidate them into a limited number of nonoverlapping issues. Ideally, a community should have no more than 12 strategic issues; the fewer, the better.

Step 5: Arrange issues into an ordered list

Finally, the strategic issues should be ordered into a list. When developing this list, participants determine if certain issues should be addressed first, if there are issues with immediate consequences, or if there are timelines or upcoming events that may help or hinder addressing an issue. In some cases, communities may decide to address simpler issues first in an effort to build the necessary momentum and teamwork for addressing more complex, controversial issues.

Phase 5: Formulating Goals and Strategies During this phase, participants formulate goals and specific strategies for each of the strategic issues identified in the previous phase. Goals and strategies provide a connection between the current reality (what the LPHS and the community look like now) and the vision (what the LPHS and community will look like in the future). Together, the goals and strategies provide a comprehensive picture of how LPHS partners will achieve a healthy community. In developing goals and strategies, communities answer the following questions:

- Goals: What do we want to achieve by addressing this strategic issue?
- Strategies: How do we want to achieve it? What action is needed?

Step 1: Develop goals related to the vision and strategic issues

Participants begin by revisiting both the vision and the strategic issues. By identifying how the strategic issues link to the vision, participants develop goals that will be achieved when those issues are resolved. Whereas the vision presents what the community wants to ultimately achieve in an idealistic manner (e.g., healthy children), goals capture these results in more concrete terms (e.g., age-appropriate vaccinations for all children). This activity may be best accomplished by a small group that later presents its results to the MAPP Committee for discussion.

Step 2: Generate strategy alternatives

During this step, participants identify potential strategies for achieving goals and attaining the community vision. Several strategies should be identified for each strategic issue. These strategy alternatives reflect the range of choices from which the community may select to reach its vision. Strategy alternatives should build upon strengths and opportunities while also countering the threats reflected in the strategic issues. This step may be undertaken through small group brainstorming discussions.

Step 3: Consider barriers to implementation

The small groups continue brainstorming discussions in an effort to identify barriers to implementation. Barriers may take the form of insufficient resources, lack of community support, legal or policy impediments to authority, or technological difficulties. Barriers will not necessarily eliminate strategy alternatives; however, they should alert the community to obstacles that may be encountered if that alternative is pursued.

Step 4: Consider implementation details

The small groups flesh out details related to implementing each strategy alternative. Participants should explore issues, such as needed activities, timelines, participation, and resources. Thinking about implementation details at this stage helps to identify and refine the best strategies. It also lays the groundwork for the next phase, the Action Cycle.

Step 5: Select and adopt strategies

After the previous steps have been completed, the best strategy alternatives should become clearer. At this point, participants should examine the alternatives together to understand their relationships to one another. Understanding the interrelationship between strategies offers a comprehensive picture of the larger strategy that the community will implement to achieve the vision. Next, participants test the strategy alternatives against agreed-upon selection criteria. Once the strategies are selected, they should be adopted.

Step 6: Draft the planning report

The final step is to develop a draft planning report. A written planning report serves as a reference; tests consensus about agreements; and communicates the vision, goals, and strategies to partners and the broader community. Once the document is complete, it should be adopted by the MAPP Committee. This step marks the completion of the planning process and a time to celebrate the hard work. The plan should also be disseminated and shared throughout the community.

Phase 6: The Action Cycle

The Action Cycle links three key activities: planning, implementation, and evaluation. Each of these activities builds upon the others in a continuous and interactive manner. The Action Cycle may be the most satisfying and challenging phase of the MAPP process. During this phase, the efforts of the previous phases begin to produce results, as the LPHS develops and implements an action plan for addressing the strategic issues. Yet, this is where it becomes increasingly important to sustain the process and to continue implementation over time.

The Action Cycle can be summarized as follows:

- Planning: determining what will be done, who will do it, and how it will be done
- Implementation: carrying out the activities identified in the planning stage
- Evaluation: determining what has been accomplished

Step 1 (Planning for Action): Organize for action

The first step in this phase is organizing for action. A subcommittee should be designated to oversee the implementation and evaluation activities. This subcommittee prepares for the subsequent steps and plans and how they will be implemented. If key participants—those who will play a role in implementing and evaluating strategies—are not currently involved in the MAPP process, they should be recruited to participate.

Step 2 (Planning for Action): Develop objectives and establish accountability

For successful implementation, it is important to know where you are headed, who is responsible for getting you there, and how you are going to get there. To accomplish this, MAPP participants develop measurable outcome objectives for the identified strategies. Participants then agree on accountability or responsibility for each objective.

Step 3 (Planning for Action): Develop action plans

The outcome objectives must now be translated into specific action plans to be carried out by accountable participants. Action planning will help to identify specific activities, time frames, and needed resources. Action plans may be organization specific or may call for collective action from a number of organizations.

Step 4 (Implementation): Review action plans for opportunities for coordination

After individual and collective action plans have been developed, the MAPP Committee reviews them to identify common or duplicative activities and seeks ways to combine or coordinate the use of limited community resources. A quick review of the four MAPP assessments may be useful for exploring assets, strengths, and opportunities.

Step 5 (Implementation): Implement and monitor action plans

Each MAPP participant should be involved in implementing a minimum of one strategy. In addition, MAPP participants should regularly consider whether other organizations or individuals should be brought on board to more effectively implement strategies. Community awareness and participation ensures that action plans are appropriately and effectively implemented.

Step 6 (Evaluation): Prepare for evaluation activities

When preparing for evaluation, participants should first consider what they are evaluating. An evaluation of the entire MAPP process and each strategy should be conducted. Next, participants should think about the stakeholders that should be involved. These may include individuals whose professional work relates to the activity being implemented or people who will be affected by its implementation.

Step 7 (Evaluation): Focus the evaluation design

The next step is to design the evaluation. At this stage, the evaluation team should select the questions that the evaluation will answer, the process for answering these questions, the methodology to be used in collecting answers, a plan for carrying out the evaluation activities, and a strategy for reporting the results of the evaluation.

Step 8 (Evaluation): Gather credible evidence and justify conclusions

During this step, MAPP participants collect data to answer the evaluation questions. Once credible data is gathered, the evaluation team decides what the data indicates: Did the activity do what it set out to do? How effective was it? The evaluation team should also justify its conclusions.

Step 9 (Evaluation): Share lessons learned and celebrate successes

Finally, results of the evaluation are used and shared with others. Evaluation results can improve existing processes and help create new strategies and activities.

Evaluation results may also pinpoint successes and positive results. Participants should celebrate these successes. Continuous celebration and recognition of the hard work will go a long way toward sustaining momentum and keeping the process alive.

MAPP and Health Promotion

Instituting a strategic planning and community health improvement process like MAPP provides a framework for achieving health promotion goals. As defined earlier, health promotion is therefore a mechanism to empower large numbers of people in the school, workplace, and community to remain healthy and avoid illness and disease. This goal is accomplished through the sharing of accurate information about the long-term effects of high-risk health behaviors (see Chapter 1). MAPP addresses these key aspects of health promotion in four ways. First, MAPP provides a structure for leveraging the power that already exists within communities. In implementing MAPP, the community does more than "buy into" the process; rather, the community owns the process and is able to use its power to effect change. The community creates the vision, identifies health problems, formulates solutions, and takes action. Second, MAPP involves the sharing of accurate information through the completion of four assessments. Not only does the MAPP process help communities collect data on high-risk health behaviors but completion of the four assessments also provides information about why high-risk behaviors may be prominent in a community. The data collected through the process uncovers ways to address public health issues and help assess the LPHS's existing capacity for health promotion. Third, as a strategic planning process, MAPP acknowledges the long-term effects of high-risk behaviors. MAPP does not focus on day-to-day public health issues; rather, it is a long-term process that works toward a broad, long-term vision of community health improvement. Finally, like health promotion activities, MAPP ultimately works to improve health and help communities prevent root causes of illness and disease.

The MAPP process in Nashville, Tennessee, provides an example of how MAPP can help achieve health promotion goals (Dias, Judy, personal communication, July 2007). Like many local communities, Nashville wanted to reduce obesity, increase physical activity, and improve healthy eating; however, unlike traditional health promotion efforts, Nashville identified these health issues and the strategies for addressing them through its MAPP process. The four MAPP assessments revealed that Nashville had high rates of obesity and other conditions related to physical inactivity and unhealthy eating. The community validated health status data indicating it wanted to improve health education to ensure healthy lifestyles. The assessment data also indicated that certain populations were disproportionately affected by obesity. In addition, the community identified barriers to physical activity, such as inadequate walkways and bike routes, and a need to improve joint community collaborations and the quality of health education.

Not only did MAPP provide a comprehensive picture of the health issues in Nashville; the process also helped devise solutions based on the assets already available in the city. The community was actively involved in developing the Healthy Nashville Steps program, which worked with an existing effort called Tennessee on the Move to help residents track their physical activity and eating behavior. The leadership council responsible for the community effort worked with the department of public works and planning commission to improve the walk-ability of the community. The business community provided financial incentives to increase physical activity, and the local universities provided expertise in supporting additional health education programs. The mayor was also instrumental in raising the visibility of Nashville's health promotion efforts by including the community's health improvement plan in his annual New Year's resolution for the city. Even though the mayor strongly supported Nashville's MAPP process, the city's health promotion efforts were not prescriptive and implemented top down by the health department or the mayor's office; rather, the programs were designed by and for the citizens of Nashville with support from city leadership. Because the community was involved in every stage of the MAPP process, the resulting health promotion efforts to increase physical activity were tailored to the actual needs and concerns of the community. Overall, MAPP created a sense of community ownership of the process, increasing the sustainability of MAPP and the resulting health promotion activities in the city.

Although health promotion activities in MAPP communities like Nashville resemble successful health promotion efforts in other communities, MAPP ensures

- the need for health promotion programs are warranted, that is, the community wants and needs such programs;
- the health promotion activities are well informed by comprehensive data collection and collaborative data analysis and synthesis;
- the health promotion activities use assets and resources that already exist in the community;
- the community assesses the LPHS's capacity to implement health promotion programs;
- all the necessary LPHS entities and community members are involved in informing and implementing health promotion efforts;
- the health promotion efforts do not duplicate existing programs;

- the health promotion activities are continuously evaluated and improved upon; and
- the health promotion activities address the community's vision of a healthy community.

Figure 17-4 portrays how a traditional view of health promotion fits within the MAPP process. Although a traditional health promotion approach would respond to a public health problem by devising a strategy focused on changing behavior and then implementing the strategy, it would not require mobilizing the community and determining the importance and need for the health promotion intervention relative to other types of public health problems. Moreover, a traditional health promotion approach does not require an assessment of existing resources, identification of potential collaboration opportunities with nontraditional public health partners in the LPHS, or relevance to the overall vision of a healthier community. On the other hand, MAPP provides the framework for ensuring that health promotion activities are informed by the community and maximize the resources already existing in the community, thereby ensuring the relevance to the community's interests and perceived needs. MAPP also helps strengthen

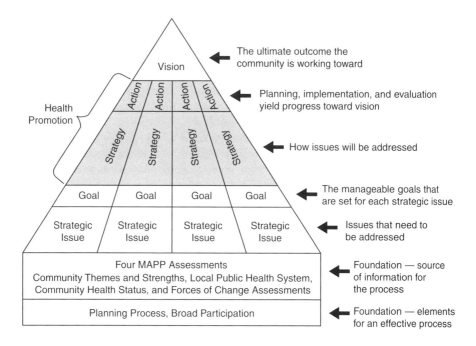

Figure 17-4 Traditional View of Health Promotion Within MAPP

Source: National Association of County and City Health Officials. (2001). *A strategic approach to community health improvement: Field guide.* Washington, DC: Author.

partnerships involved in health promotion and helps ensure that health promotion efforts work toward the community's vision of a healthy community.

MAPP and Other National Initiatives

In addition to aligning health promotion activities with the community's vision for public health, MAPP also connects health promotion efforts with larger national public health initiatives, such as the National Public Health Performance Standards Program (NPHPSP), the Operational Definition of a Local Health Department, and the voluntary accreditation of local and state health departments.

The NPHPSP comprises of three instruments that assist state, local, and governing bodies to measure the extent to which their public health systems provide the 10 essential public health services. As explained on the NPHPSP website, a partnership of 7 national organizations developed the state, local, and governance performance standard instruments, and the local NPHPSP instrument is used to complete the LPHSA within the MAPP process. Completion of the local NPHPSP instrument not only helps LPHSs evaluate how well they provide health promotion services, it also identifies the level of health promotion activities provided relative to the other essential public health services. Moreover, as noted on the NPHPSP website, the NPHPSP instruments serve as a "benchmark for public health practice improvements, by providing a 'gold standard' to which public health systems can aspire."

The Operational Definition of a Functional Local Health Department (2005) "describes what everyone, regardless of where they live, can reasonably expect from governmental local public health" (p. 2). Health promotion is one of the public health activities residents can expect from their local health departments. The local health department should either provide these essential services directly or assure they are being provided by another LPHS partner in the community. Going through the MAPP process, communities learn which LPHS entity, if any, provides services such as health promotion. Because the Operational Definition standards serve as a framework for the voluntary national accreditation of local health departments, determining how well health departments assure the provision of all the services outlined in the Operational Definition is important.[1]

The Benefits of the MAPP Process

The benefits gained by implementing the MAPP process translate into benefits for health promotion activities. Based on a 2005 evaluation of MAPP users, communities indicated the process strengthened and built partnerships and improved collaboration within the LPHS, which resulted in stronger public health infrastructure. Increased communication among the community and system partners resulted in more opportunities for decreasing gaps in

---

[1]For more information about the Operational Definition of Local Health Departments, see http://www.naccho.org/topics/infrastructure/operationaldefinition.cfm.

services, reducing duplication, and increasing LPHS efficiency. In many MAPP communities, stronger partnerships and new collaborations have led to increases in funding opportunities and sustainability of public health activities. The evaluation of MAPP communities also indicated that the process increased the visibility of public health. Many communities have commented that MAPP not only increases awareness of public health in the community, but it also creates advocates for public health. As a result, in some MAPP communities, elected officials and LPHS partners have worked to improve public health policies based on the data collected through their MAPP process and their strategic issues and actions plans resulting from their efforts. The data collected through the MAPP process, improvements in partnerships and LPHS infrastructure, and the process by which strategies are identified and selected have also allowed communities to better anticipate and manage trends and challenges that can affect how the LPHS performs. Finally, MAPP helps improve health and quality of life through an iterative strategic planning model, which is based in theory and demonstrated in practice. In turn, improvements in partnerships, public health infrastructure, public health visibility and advocacy, ability to anticipate and manage change, and the overall system for improving community health benefit health promotion activities by providing a solid foundation for their implementation and success.

Finally, MAPP provides a means for addressing the major challenge for health promotion identified by McGinnis and colleagues. As noted in chapter 1, they argue that a major factor affecting investment in health promotion initiatives has been gaining consensus on decisions regarding what should be done to change high-risk health behaviors and how to measure the effectiveness of these new initiatives. Through MAPP, communities own the process for community health improvement and use comprehensive sets of data and skills like dialogue to help reach consensus. The community's collective wisdom is used to identify effective strategies to change high-risk behaviors, which are based on assets and resources already in the community. Because the MAPP process requires data collection through an iterative process that also includes an evaluation component, MAPP also provides a means for measuring the effectiveness of health promotion initiatives over time. In short, MAPP provides a solid framework for advancing health promotion activities in local communities given current challenges in the field.

CONCLUDING REMARKS

Hundreds of communities have used the MAPP process to create and implement strategic plans. The six MAPP phases outline the steps involved in community-based strategic planning. The phases describe how communities can develop partnerships, convene LPHS partners, and create collective visions. MAPP helps communities collect assessment data that is used to identify the underlying strategic issues that need to be addressed in order for communities to achieve their visions. The process also provides guidance on formulating goals and strategies and identifying action steps needed to successfully implement strategic plans. After completing the six phases of the MAPP process, communities revisit earlier phases of the process. In subsequent iterations, communities strengthen and build new partnerships, revise visions, update assessment data, and rethink strategic issues, goals, strategies, and action steps. In this way, MAPP is an iterative process that institutes strategic planning into local public health practice.

The different elements that comprise MAPP are not novel to public health practice; however, MAPP is unique and effective because it consolidates these different elements into one process. MAPP recognizes the importance of viewing health as a physical, mental, spiritual, and social state of being. The protection of health is a shared responsibility that involves LPHS and community partners. In order to improve health, communities must strategically use partnerships, dialogue skills, and data to uncover the root causes of public health problems and the assets that can be used to address them. The principles underlying the MAPP process provide a strong foundation for improving public health.

Based on public health theory and practice, MAPP can help achieve health promotion goals even though MAPP is not a health promotion tool per se. The process ensures health promotion programs address community-identified needs and do not duplicate existing health promotion activities. MAPP also helps communities use assessment data, assets in the community, resources, and knowledge provided by local public health and community partners toward health promotion. In addition, the process assesses the capacity of the overall public health system to implement health promotion activities. Moreover, MAPP helps ensure health promotion activities are evaluated, improved upon, and ultimately address a community's collective vision.

MAPP is just one of many initiatives used to improve public health practice. Informed by public health experts, advancements in public health practice, and previous models for public health improvement, MAPP is an evidence-based process for improving community health. The process aligns with other public health improvement initiatives, such as the NPHPSP, the Operational Definition of a Local Health Department, and the voluntary national public health accreditation program. The benefits of the MAPP process have helped communities across the United States improve their capacity to address their public health issues and achieve their visions of healthy communities.

DISCUSSION QUESTIONS

1. How does MAPP provide a framework for creating a community, as opposed to a public health agency, strategic plan?

2. How does data from each of the four assessments collectively provide a comprehensive picture of a public health problem?

3. How would the MAPP process inform health promotion activities related to a particular public health problem? Reference all six phases of the MAPP process in your answer.

4. What are three potential challenges that might arise in using a MAPP approach to health promotion?

REFERENCES

Centers for Disease Control and Prevention. (n.d.) *National Public Health Performance Standards*. Available at http://www.cdc.gov/od/ocphp/nphpsp/overview.htm. Accessed April 1, 2009.

Judy Dias. (2007). MAPP Coordinator at the Metro Public Health Department of Nashville/Davidson County.

Harrell, J. A., & Baker, E. L. (1994). The essential services of public health. *Leadership Public Health*, 3, 27–30.

Institute of Medicine. (1997). *Improving health in the community: A role for performance monitoring*. Washington, DC: National Academy Press.

Institute of Medicine Committee on Assuring the Health of the Public in the 21st Century. (2001). *The future of the public's health in the 21st century*. Washington, DC: National Academy Press.

National Association of County and City Health Officials. (n.d.) *MAPP website*. Available at http://www.naccho.org/mapp. Accessed April 1, 2009.

National Association of County and City Health Officials. (2004). *Achieving healthier communities through MAPP: A user's handbook*. Washington, DC: Author.

National Association of County and City Health Officials. (2005). *Operational definition of a local health department*. Washington, DC: Author.

National Association of County and City Health Officials. (2001). *A strategic approach to community health improvement: Field guide*. Washington, DC: Author.

Lenihan, P. (2005). MAPP and the evolution of planning in public health practice. *Journal of Public Health Practice and Management, 11*, 381–388.

Liedtka, J. M. (1998). Linking strategic thinking with strategic planning. *Strategy & Leadership, 26*, 30–35.

World Health Organization. (1998). *Resolution EB101.R2*. Geneva, Switzerland: Author.

A

APPENDIX

Health Promotion and Health Education Resources for Health Educators and Health Promotion Specialists

Agency for Healthcare Research and Quality (AHRQ)

Consumers and Patients: information in English and Spanish on many health issues.

Fact Sheets: information on many health issues.

Patient Safety Network: a web-based resource featuring the latest news and essential resources on patient safety. The site offers weekly updates of patient safety literature, news, tools, and meetings ("What's New") and a vast set of carefully annotated links to important research and other information on patient safety ("The Collection").

Preventive Services: access to scientific evidence, recommendations on clinical preventive services, and information on how to implement recommended preventive services in clinical practice.

Treating Tobacco Use and Dependence: pathfinder page links to materials that help tobacco users quit.

American Cancer Society (ACS)

Asian Pacific Islander Cancer Education Materials Tool: searchable online database of Asian language cancer materials.

American College of Preventive Medicine (ACPM)

ACPM Practice Policy Statements: ACPM's Prevention Practice Committee coordinates the development of practice policy statements in areas of concern to college members. Practice policy statements provide guidance to clinicians.

American Public Health Association (APHA)

Get Ready Campaign: includes a blog, fact sheets, and podcasts to help the public prepare for a potential influenza pandemic and outbreaks of other emerging infectious diseases.

Health Disparities Database: sponsored by the APHA, this database contains projects and interventions provided by members of the public health community.

359

Healthy You: free public health materials from The Nation's Health newspaper. The materials are designed to be used with the public at health fairs, health departments, or community meetings.

American Self-Help Group Clearinghouse

Self-Help Group Sourcebook Online: a searchable database that includes information on over 1,100 national, international, and demonstrational model self-help support groups, ideas for starting groups, and opportunities to link with others to develop needed new national or international groups.

Association of Schools of Public Health (ASPH)

Pathways to Public Health: provides information and resources for talented young people interested in exploring careers in public health, and for the teachers, school counselors, and others who work with them.

What is Public Health?: describes the many areas of public health for prospective students or others who want to know more about the field.

Baylor College of Medicine

Salud en Accion: an initiative to address the burden of cancer disparities and stimulate behavior modification to improve public health in the Hispanic–Latino community.

California Distance Learning Health Network

California Distance Learning Health Network (CDLHN): promotes and provides access to continuing educational opportunities for health care workers at a time and a location convenient to where they live and work.

Cancer Control PLANET

Cancer Control PLANET: PLANET portal provides access to data and resources that can help planners, program staff, and researchers to design, implement, and evaluate evidence-based cancer control programs.

Center for International Rehabilitation Research Information and Exchange

Rehabilitation Provider's Guide to Cultures of the Foreign-Born: provides specific information on cultural perspectives of foreign-born persons in the United States.

Centers for Disease Control and Prevention (CDC)

BAM!: health topics from the CDC of interest to youth.

CDC en Español: CDC's gateway for health and safety information in Spanish.

CDCynergy: a multimedia CD-ROM used for planning, managing, and evaluating public health communication programs. This innovative tool is used to guide and assist users in designing health communication interventions within a public health framework.

Centers for Disease Control and Prevention Health Marketing: CDC's National Center for Health Marketing is responsible for creating, communicating, and delivering innovative health marketing programs, products, and services that are customer-centered, high impact, and science-based.

Excite: Excellence in Curriculum Integration through Teaching Health Promotion and Health Education.

Epidemiology: CDC teaching materials to introduce students to public health and epidemiology.

FASTATS A–Z: listing and quick links for basic public health statistical data.

Global Health Odyssey: CDC museum's home page with items of interest to children, teachers, and other CDC visitors.

Health Promotion Campaigns: health campaigns on a range of public health issues.

Health Topics A to Z: listing with quick links of health topics found on the CDC website.

Healthier Worksite Initiative: resource for workforce health promotion (WHP) program planners in state and federal government. Planners at non-government workplaces may also find this website useful in generating ideas for WHP in their organizations. The site provides information, resources, and step-by-step tool kits to help improve the health of employees.

National Immunization Program: childhood vaccination schedules and vaccine safety precautions.

Public Health Image Library (PHIL): contains a collection of public domain images.

Power to Prevent: curriculum to help educate African-American communities on how to prevent and control diabetes through healthy eating and physical activity.

TB Education & Training Resources: a searchable, comprehensive database of materials from national and international organizations. At this "one-stop" site of tuberculosis (TB) education and training resources, you can search for materials by language, target audience, and format.

Travelers' Health: health information on specific travel destinations.

VERB Youth Media Campaign: national, multicultural, social marketing campaign that encourages young people ages 9 to 13 years to be physically active every day.

Community Tool Box

Community Tool Box: provides over 6,000 pages of practical information to support your work in promoting community health and development. This website is created and maintained by the Work Group on Health Promotion and Community Development at the University of Kansas in Lawrence, Kansas. Developed in collaboration with AHEC/Community Partners in Amherst, Massachusetts, the site has been on line since 1995, and it continues to grow on a weekly basis.

Community-Campus Partnerships for Health (CCPH)

Community-Campus Partnerships for Health (CCPH): a nonprofit organization that promotes health through partnerships between communities and higher educational institutions. CCPH sponsors conferences, training institutes, and customized consultation to strengthen community-academic linkages in public health. The CCPH website contains a wealth of resources on practice-based learning, community-based participatory research, and community-engaged scholarship.

Department of Defense (DoD) U.S.	Health Promotion and Health Education.
	Deployment Health and Family Readiness Library: provides access to deployment health and family readiness information for service members, families, and health care providers. This online library includes fact sheets, guides, and other products on a wide variety of topics.
Department of Health and Human Services (DHHS) U.S.	**Healthfinder:** health education information, resources, and organizations from reliable sources (in English and Spanish).
	HealthierUS.gov: the HealthierUS initiative is a national effort to improve people's lives, to prevent and reduce the costs of disease and to promote community health and wellness. This website is part of a broad presidential agenda designed to help Americans, especially children, live longer, better, and healthier lives. The site provides credible, accurate information to help Americans choose healthier habits.
	PandemicFlu.gov
ECRI	**Patient Reference Guide:** comprehensive patient reference guides from ECRI, an international independent nonprofit agency and Collaborating Center of the World Health Organization. ECRI is designated as an Evidence-based Practice Center (EPC) by the U.S. Agency for Healthcare Research and Quality. ECRI's mission is to improve the safety, quality, and cost effectiveness of health care.
Education Development Center (EDC)	**Higher Education Center for Alcohol and Other Drug Abuse and Violence Protection:** the Higher Education Center's purpose is to help college and community leaders develop, implement, and evaluate programs and policies to reduce student problems related to alcohol and other drug use and interpersonal violence.
Food and Drug Administration (FDA) U.S.	**Consumer Health Information for You and Your Family:** features timely consumer health stories on pressing FDA topics, provides links to its most requested information, and includes interactive content.
	FDA & You. News for Health Educators and Students: an educational newsletter intended for use by health educators, secondary school students, and their parents. It contains news about medical products from each of FDA's five centers.
	FDA A–Z Index: an index of health topics available from the FDA.
	FDA Diabetes Information: helps people manage their diabetes and live a healthy life.
	FDA Heart Health Online: provides reliable information about the products used to prevent, diagnose, and treat cardiovascular disease. It includes full descriptions and patient instructions for many medications, medical devices, and diagnostic tests for cardiovascular disease.
	FDA Kids' Home Page: a website filled with fun activities for kids.
	FDA Radiological Health Program: provides information about FDA's Radiological Health Program, including its 2005–2010 plan to adapt to current public health needs.

FDA's Drug Safety Initiative: drug safety information for patients, consumers, and health care professionals.

Food Safety for Moms-To-Be: easy-to-understand information about foodborne illness for pregnant women. This site is in both English and Spanish.

Mammography: information for mammography facility personnel, inspectors, and consumers about the implementation of the Mammography Quality Standards Act of 1992 (MQSA).

Medical Device Safety: a resource to educate and inform health care professionals on patient safety issues relating to medical devices.

Medicines In My Home: an interactive and educational program about the safe and effective use of over-the-counter medicines.

MEDWATCH: The FDA Safety Information and Adverse Event Reporting Program: provides timely safety information on medical products and drugs regulated by the FDA. MedWatch also allows health care professionals and consumers to report serious problems with any FDA-regulated product and any serious adverse event.

Office of Women's Health: serves as a champion for women's health both within and outside the agency.

Personal Protective Equipment (PPE) and Patient Care: information about PPE that is regulated by the FDA for use in patient care activities, including surgical masks and surgical N-95 respirators, medical gloves, and surgical gowns.

Spanish Language Publications from the FDA: provides consumers with information on a variety of health-related topics. Also provides regulated industry information on drugs and veterinary medicine.

George Washington University, School of Public Health and Health Services

Center for Health and Health Care in Schools (CHHCS): links educators and health professionals to the information essential to building effective school health programs, tests new school-connected strategies to achieve better health outcomes for children, and promotes awareness of successful new directions in school-based programming.

Georgetown University, National Center for Education in Maternal and Child Health (NCEMCH)

Maternal and Child Health Library: provides the maternal and child health community with accurate and timely information on a broad range of topics.

Health Communication Partnership

Health Communication Partnership: five institutions working together to strengthen public health in the developing world through strategic communication programs.

Health Resources and Services Administration (HRSA)

Cultural Competence Resources for Health Care Providers: highlights HRSA-supported projects on cross-cultural health care in areas such as assessment, culture and language, specific diseases, health professions, research, special populations, technical assistance, training, and web-based learning.

Healthy Roads Media	**Healthy Roads Media:** this site contains free audio, written, and multimedia health education materials in a number of languages.
Kansas State University (KSU)	**RE-AIM.org (Reach, Efficacy–Effectiveness, Adoption, Implementation, and Maintenance):** provides a framework–model for planning, conducting, and evaluating health behavior interventions. Funded by the Robert Wood Johnson Foundation, the RE-AIM website provides calculators, checklists, citations to health behavior intervention studies that have used the RE-AIM framework, and other tools and resources for both researchers and community leaders.
Minnesota Department of Health (MDH)	**RN Barr Library:** provides resources of interest to the public health community, including links to hot topics, publications, and news resources.
National Eye Institute, National Institutes of Health (NIH)	**Healthy Vision Community Programs Database:** searchable collection of community-based eye health education programs from U.S. states and territories.
National Institute for Health and Clinical Excellence (NICE)	**Public Health Excellence at NICE:** provides guidance on the promotion of good health and the prevention and treatment of ill health.
National Institute on Aging (NIA)	**Helping Older Adults Search for Health Information Online—A Toolkit for Trainers:** training materials to help older adults find reliable, up-to-date online health information on their own. The training features two websites from the National Institutes of Health: NIH SeniorHealth.gov and MedlinePlus.gov.
National Institute on Alcohol Abuse and Alcoholism (NIAAA)	**Leadership to Keep Children Alcohol Free:** a coalition of governors' spouses, federal agencies, and public and private organizations, it is an initiative to prevent the use of alcohol by children ages 9 years and above.
National Institutes of Health (NIH)	**NIH Curriculum Supplement Series:** interactive teaching units that combine cutting-edge science research discoveries from the NIH with state-of-the-art instructional materials. Each supplement is a teacher's guide to 2 weeks of lessons on science and human health.
National Library of Medicine (NLM) U.S.	**American Indian Health:** an information portal to issues affecting the health and well-being of American Indians.
	Household Products Database: health and safety information on household products.
	MedlinePlus: provides extensive information from the NIH, DHHS, and other trusted sources on over 600 diseases and conditions.
	ToxTown: an interactive guide to commonly encountered toxic substances and environmental health risks.

National Library of Medicine, Specialized Information Services Division	**DIRLINE:** directory of health organizations and other resources in health and biomedicine.
Agency for Healthcare Research and Quality (AHRQ)	**Multilingual Consumer Health Information:** contains a list of links to consumer health information. Each link also contains a list of languages that are available for the resource.
Native American Connections	**Native American Connections:** provides culturally appropriate resources for Native Americans and special needs populations.
New York City Department of Health and Mental Hygiene	**Take Care New York:** contains Take Care New York action steps to improve your health, with specific things you can do, along with additional resources to help you follow through.
Agency for Healthcare Research and Quality (AHRQ)	**Health Communication Activities:** brings together work on the Healthy People 2010 Health Communication Focus Area, the Prevention Communication Research Database, and consumer and patient ehealth.
	Prevention Communication Research Database: searchable collection of audience research conducted or sponsored by DHHS agencies. The database was developed to highlight key prevention research findings that may not be widely known or published in peer-reviewed journals.
	Quick Guide to Health Literacy: provides an overview of health literacy concepts and techniques for improving health literacy. Designed for government employees, grantees and contractors, and community partners working in health care and public health fields. The tools can be applied to health care delivery, policy, administration, communication, and education activities aimed at the public.
Public Health Foundation (PHF)	**Public Health Foundation Learning Resource Center:** high quality training and health promotion materials that include information on preparedness, immunization, epidemiology, diabetes, infectious diseases, performance management, asthma and allergies, and health disparities. Materials are available in a variety of formats, including print, computer based, and video.
Public Health Indicators and National Data (PHIND)	**Public Health Indicators and National Data:** a web-based resource for community-level social indicators of health with links to community specific sites, indicators, and comparisons.
Rural Assistance Center (RAC)	**Rural Assistance Center:** a national resource on rural health and human services information. Information specialists are available to provide customized assistance for rural topics and funding resources, to link users to organizations, and to furnish relevant publications from the RAC resource library.

	USA–Mexico Border Health: resource for residents along the U.S.–Mexico border and others seeking information on health and human services for border communities.
Society for Public Health Education (SOPHE)	**Health Disparities and Social Inequities—Framing a Transdisciplinary Research Agenda in Health Education:** view panel presentations and the setting of a research agenda on the role of health education in eliminating racial and ethnic health disparities; webcast by the Henry J. Kaiser Foundation.
Substance Abuse & Mental Health Services Administration (SAMHSA)	**National Directory of Drug and Alcohol Treatment Programs, 2007:** a listing of federal, state, local, and private facilities that provide substance abuse treatment services.
Unite for Sight	**Unite for Sight:** works to build healthier communities through disease prevention, eye health promotion, and health education. This organization works nationally and internationally to develop sustainable solutions to reduce health disparities.
United Health Foundation	**United Health Foundation:** UnitedHealth Group established the United Health Foundation in 1999 as a nonprofit, private foundation with a mission to support the health and medical decisions made by physicians, health professionals, community leaders, and individuals that lead to better health outcomes and healthier communities.
University of Hawaii at Manoa	**Hawaii Public Health Information Virtual Emporium:** provides public health professionals hands-on training in the use of local and web-based health databases and with a website that can furnish them with timely, convenient access to information resources to help them improve the health of the public they serve.
University of Iowa, Hardin Library for the Health Sciences	**Iowa Public Health Information:** addresses the information needs of Iowa public health professionals by creating an easy-to-use website that emphasizes local and state resources and provides links to NLM and CDC resources.
University of Minnesota Libraries	**American Social Hygiene Posters, ca.1910–1970:** offers a searchable and browsable database of posters on a variety of social issues, such as dance, family, hygiene, mental health, reproduction, sexual abstinence, and more (from the Social Welfare History Archives at the University of Minnesota Libraries).
University of Minnesota	**Outbreak at Watersedge—A Public Health Discovery Game:** an interactive computer game developed by the University of Minnesota Midwest Center for Life-Long-Learning in Public Health that is designed to introduce high school students to the field of public health.

B

Case Studies of Successful Workplace Wellness Programs

Integrated Health, Safety, and Productivity Management Programs

Goetzel (2004) offers several examples of companies that have documented health improvements and cost savings from integrated health, safety, and productivity management programs.

DaimlerChrysler: UAW National Wellness Program

The program, targeted at DaimlerChrysler's 95,000 employees in the United States, aims to improve worker health and to help employees become wise health care consumers. In 1997, the health care costs of health risk appraisal (HRA) program participants were $114 to $146 lower than the costs of nonparticipants. Those who completed the HRA and then participated in at least one additional wellness program had costs that were $200 lower than for nonparticipants. Over time, differences in health care costs between participants and nonparticipants ranged from $5 to $16 per employee per month.

Fannie Mae Partnership for Healthy Living

The program, begun in 1994, is offered free of charge to all Fannie Mae employees and their spouses or domestic partners. The comprehensive program includes health screenings and targeted follow-up intervention programs. The program has achieved excellent overall participation and follow-up rates (60% to 80%). Multiple health risk assessments have shown that 53% of all high-risk employees drop at least one risk factor by their third annual HRA screening. The program has saved $1.5 million in medical costs and $1.0 million in employee absence. A return on investment (ROI) analysis based on 1,650 employees for the period of 1994 to 1996 concluded that the program returned $1.09 to $1.26 for every dollar invested.

Union Pacific Railroad (UPRR): Project Health Track

The Health Track Program is focused on 10 risk factors and chronic health conditions. Because Health Track has been successful in documenting health improvements and cost savings, it has been declared 1 of 8 Big Financial Deals (BDF) at UPRR for the years 2001 to 2006. An econometric analysis performed by outside evaluators for UPRR and published in a peer-reviewed journal found that the dollar difference between program elimination and successful program continuation, whereby a 1% reduction in 10 risk factors is achieved per year over a 10-year period, produced $99.4 million in savings for the railroad. A ROI of $4.07 for every dollar invested was projected for the company over 10 years, assuming the program continues at current performance levels.

Northeast Utilities (NU): WellAware Program

The WellAware Program targets all 15,000 NU employees and their spouses at 60 plus work sites throughout the northeast. Approximately 2,500 participants completed two HRAs between 1998 and 2000. Results were impressive—there was a 31% decrease in smoking, 29% decrease in sedentary lifestyle, 11% decrease in cholesterol risk, and 5% decrease in stress.

Citibank Health Management Program

In 1994, Citibank, a global financial services company with 130,000 employees worldwide and 51,000 employees in the United States, implemented a comprehensive health management program targeted at all U.S. employees and expatriate staff. The program, which attracted about half of the eligible population, included administration of an HRA, targeted high-risk interventions, and disease and demand management programming. An external economic evaluation, published in a peer-reviewed journal, documented a return on investment of $4.50 for every dollar invested in the program.

FedEx Corporation: Health Risk Reduction and Cost Reduction Programs

FedEx offers a variety of human capital management (HCM) programs to its over 200,000 employees. Its management philosophy and culture focuses on "people–service–profit," in that order. Its varied programs include FedEx Safety Above All; FedEx Employee Benefits (with programs directed at demand management, utilization management, catastrophic case management, and disease management); Cigna Well Aware; CareMark Care Patterns; Maternity Education Benefit Fairs; Smoking Cessation; LifeWorks; Health and Wellness Centers; and Employee Assistance Programs. Compared to expected values, FedEx's programs resulted in cumulative 5-year medical benefit cost savings of about $579 million. Additionally, 6-year cumulative cost savings related to decreases in medical-related lost time from work were estimated at approximately $497 million. FedEx Fitness Program participants reduced their overall benefit costs from $1,210 to $1,021 (16%) in the year following program enrollment, while nonparticipants' total benefits decreased from $2,104 to $1,947 (7%).

Motorola: Global Wellness Initiatives

Motorola offers wellness initiatives to its 56,000 U.S. employees. The company invests approximately $6.0 million annually in the development and operation of its wellness and work–life programs. Over a 3-year period, participants in the Wellness Centers and Wellness Reimbursement Benefit Programs increased their annual lifestyle-related health care costs by 2.5%, while nonparticipants' costs increased by 18%. This translated to an annual savings of $6.5 million in lifestyle-related medical expenses and $10.5 million in disability-related expenses. These savings yielded a $3.93 to $1.00 ROI. A flu vaccination program achieved a $1.20 to $1.00 ROI during the 2001 and 2002 flu season. Additionally, 46 individuals concluded an 8-week tobacco cessation program in which 15 became tobacco free.

Johnson & Johnson Health and Wellness

Johnson & Johnson Health and Wellness is an outgrowth of the company's "Live For Life" program, which originated in 1979. In developing its health and wellness initiatives, Johnson & Johnson brought together experts in health education, behavior change, risk reduction, and disease management to create programs to improve workers' health and productivity. Currently, the program integrates health promotion activities with disability management, occupational health, employee assistance, and work-life programs. In a study tracking health risks of workers over a 2-year period, researchers found significant reductions in health risks in the areas of cigarette smoking, sedentary lifestyle, high cholesterol, high blood pressure, nutrition, seat belt use, and drinking and driving. Certain risk factors worsened, however, including high body weight, high fat intake, risk for diabetes, and cigar smoking. A financial impact analysis performed by Medstat and spanning a 9-year study period found that the health and wellness program saved Johnson & Johnson about $225 per employee per year in medical care utilization costs. That savings, coupled with savings from administrative streamlining of the program, produced overall savings of about $8.6 million per year for the company, over a 4-year period examined by the researchers.

Fairview Health Services: Fairview Alive

The Fairview Alive Program, first introduced in 1996, now serves approximately 13,000 eligible employees. The program offers employees an employee health kit that includes a personalized health assessment and a self-care book. Employees are encouraged to obtain necessary preventive screenings. Incentives are offered to those who participate in health improvement programs. Fairview also provides on-site education classes, self-study materials, community health education programs, a high-risk personalized risk reduction and counseling program, and other programs designed to improve worker health and productivity. Of those eligible to participate, about 74% take advantage of some aspect of the program. A longitudinal assessment of risk factors in a subset of the population that participated in 2 HRA administrations found a reduction in average health risks from 4.4 to 3.6 risks per participant, a 19% reduction. An independent evaluation by Watson Wyatt Worldwide found that medical cost increases for participants in the program were about $100 lower than for nonparticipants, resulting in medical cost savings of about $400,000.

Practice Type	Best Practice	Relevant *Community Guide* Recommendation(s)[a]	Relevant USPSTF Recommendation(s) and Prevention Priorities[a] [CPB/CE/Total Scores[b]]
Insurance Benefits	**1.** Provide full coverage for tobacco cessation treatments, including prescription medications, over-the-counter nicotine replacement therapy, and counseling.	Reduce out-of-pocket costs for tobacco-cessation programs	Tobacco-use screening and cessation intervention [5/5/10]
	2. Provide full coverage for breast, cervical, and colon cancer screenings.	Reduce out-of-pocket costs for breast cancer screening	Breast: mammography [4/2/6] Cervical: Pap smear [4/3/7] Colorectal: any of 4 tests [4/4/8]
	3. Provide full coverage for influenza vaccination.	Reduce out-of-pocket costs for vaccinations	Annual vaccination for adults aged 50 years and older [4/4/8]
	4. Require health plans to send reminders to members and network providers about preventive health services.	Client and provider reminders for breast, cervical, and colon cancer screening and influenza vaccination	
	5. Require health plans to track delivery of preventive health services and send performance feedback to network providers.	Assess providers' delivery of recommended cancer screenings and influenza vaccination and give feedback	
Workplace Policies	**6.** Ban tobacco use at work sites.	Smoking bans and restrictions (to reduce environmental smoke)	
	7. Post "Use the Stairs" reminder signs near elevators.	Point-of-decision prompts to increase physical activity	
	8. Provide facilities for physical activity.	Enhance access to physical activity facilities in combination with informational outreach	

Table 1

Employers' Best Practices for Preventing Chronic Diseases, by Practice Type, 8 Pacific Northwest Employers, American Cancer Society Workplace Solutions Pilot Study, 2005–2006

Practice Type	Best Practice	Relevant *Community Guide* Recommendation(s)[a]	Relevant USPSTF Recommendation(s) and Prevention Priorities[a] [CPB/CE/Total Scores[b]]
Workplace Policies (continued)	**9.** Make healthy food choices available and affordable.	Multicomponent interventions aimed at diet, physical activity, and cognitive change	
	10. Require and provide sun protection for employees who work outdoors.	Insufficient evidence for occupational settings but recommended for adults in recreational settings	Currently under review by USPSTF
Workplace Programs	**11.** Sponsor a tobacco cessation quit line, including nicotine replacement therapy.	Multicomponent interventions that include client telephone support to increase tobacco cessation	Tobacco-use screening and cessation intervention [5/5/10]
	12. Provide annual influenza vaccination on-site.	Enhance access to vaccinations in combination with intervention to increase community demand	Annual vaccination for adults aged 50 years and older [4/4/8]
	13. Offer a workplace physical activity program.	Individually adapted health behavior change to increase physical activity	
Tracking	**14.** Survey employees' health behaviors to track effectiveness of health promotion efforts.	NA	
Communication	**15.** Conduct targeted health promotion campaigns, focusing on key health behaviors and use of preventive health care.	Multicomponent interventions to increase vaccination; small media to increase screening for breast, cervical, and colorectal cancers; and one-on-one education to increase breast and cervical cancer screening	

USPSTF, United States Preventive Services Task Force; CPB, clinically preventable burden; CE, cost effectiveness; NA.

[a] Summary of recommendations from the USPSTF (5) and the *Community Guide* (7), as well as health impact and cost-effectiveness scores from the Prevention Priorities (9).

[b] Possible scores for both CPB and CE range from 1 to 5, with 5 indicating greatest value. Scores in this column as cited in Maciosek et al (8). Empty cells in this column indicate practices that are not recommended by ACIP or USPSTF.

Table 1

Employers' Best Practices for Preventing Chronic Diseases, by Practice Type, 8 Pacific Northwest Employers, American Cancer Society Workplace Solutions Pilot Study, 2005–2006 (continued)

Reference

Goetzel, R. Z. (2004). *Health protection and promotion: policy and Practice. Steps to a healthier workforce symposium.* NIOSH. Washington, DC. October 26, 2004 Examining the Value of Integrating Occupational Health and Safety and health Promotion Programs in the Workplace.

APPENDIX

Partnership Steps Checklist

Task	Completed?	Owner	Time Frame	How Measured?
Determine public health problem, goals, and affected populations				
Conduct a preliminary analysis of the problem				
Assess the need for a partnership				
Assess if proposed partnership meets organizational policies and guidelines				
Identify potential partners–stakeholders				
Assess potential partners' appropriateness				
Convene a core group of potential partners				
Develop a draft mission statement and goals				
Identify other potential members				
Determine type of partnership and follow organizational policies and guidelines for approval				
Ensure variety and diversity among potential partners to enable a comprehensive understanding of issues being addressed				

CHECKLIST: Step 1 —Prepare–Groundwork

Task	Completed?	Owner	Time Frame	How Measured?
Plan of Action				
Convene an initial meeting of the partnership				
Systematically assess the problem				
Identify leverage points and shared investments				
Define a shared vision, mission, and goals that are supported by all members				
Develop an action plan				
Identify quick wins				
Organization				
Ensure the partnership has characteristics for success, not failure				
Ensure partner needs are met				
Delineate roles, responsibilities, and commitments				
Delineate financial needs and resources				
Prepare appropriate legal documents and obtain necessary approval–clearance				
Establish clear ground rules or by-laws				
Establish procedures that will minimize the barriers to successful partnerships				

CHECKLIST: Step 2—Create Action Plan–Organize Partnership

Task	Completed?	Owner	Time Frame	How Measured?
Implement the action plan and monitor progress				
Develop and maintain tracking system to record progress of partnership				
Adjust goals, objectives, and steps as necessary				
Provide oversight to partner commitments and ensure adherence to action plan				
Reward and recognize contributions of partners				
Maintain consistent communication				
Ensure regular opportunities for informal contact				
Publicize successes				
Share new materials and information that are relevant to their organization and partnership				

CHECKLIST: Step 3—Implement

Task	Completed?	Owner	Time Frame	How Measured?
Develop evaluation plan				
Evaluate progress of goals and objectives				
Record and track data according to established timeline				
Share results with the partners				
Compare results to project goals to determine level of achievement				
Use evaluation findings to inform the partnership, programs, and projects and to direct improvements in the programs and activities				
Write evaluation report				
Promote the partnership by sharing achievement with partners, the public, funders, the press, and stakeholders				

Checklist: Step 4—Evaluate

Task	Completed?	Owner	Time Frame	How Measured?
Focus on team building, decision making, and consensus development				
Adhere to established ground rules				
Monitor progress of activities				
Be able to document or demonstrate outcomes of the partnership				
Secure resources from internal and/or external sources				
Review the range of partners				
Create processes for recognizing and celebrating collective achievements				
Communicate clearly and frequently with members				
Communicate with the public, and the press when appropriate				
Record case study for documentation and use by others				

CHECKLIST: Step 5 — Sustain

D

MAPP Case Studies

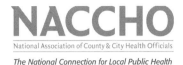

National Association of County & City Health Officials

The National Connection for Local Public Health

[STORY FROM THE FIELD]

November 2007

New Health Department MAPPs its way to a Successful Start: The East-Central Nebraska Story

In the spring of 2001, organizers of a fledgling health department in rural Nebraska huddled around a card table, where a borrowed home computer balanced precariously, to prepare a grant application involving a community assessment process. The department had come to life just three years earlier, with $30,000 and a commitment to figure out how to serve 41,000 people in two counties.

The grant-seekers' Web research turned up information about a community-driven system called MAPP—*Mobilizing for Action through Planning and Partnerships.* MAPP is the strategic planning and community assessment approach developed by the National Association of County and City Health Officials in collaboration with the U.S. Centers for Disease Control and Prevention. Unaware that MAPP itself was still in its infancy, the tiny outfit in the Cornhusker State was intrigued with the new concept and became, in effect, a MAPP pilot site.

> ...it has accomplished all this without access to a local tax base.

Six years later, the state's East Central District Health Department, now serving four counties with 51,000 people, boasts a staff of 56 and an annual budget of $3.75 million. The department is planning its next building expansion, has met ambitious goals in eight action areas, and is putting the final touches on a state-requested model strategic plan and manual for addressing the local health needs of special populations —and it has accomplished all this without access to a local tax base.

Doing MAPP and Not Knowing It

"MAPP really decided everything," relates Rebecca Rayman, a nurse who has served as the department's executive director since 1999. "It's a very focused assessment process."

Low childhood immunization rates led a handful of physicians and other health advocates, in the 1990s, to create a public health presence in the area. At the time, says Rayman, there was virtually no history or understanding about public health within the four counties (Platte, Colfax, Boone, and Nance) now covered by the department. Local health departments were rare in Nebraska, although they since have sprung up throughout the state, after the Legislature pumped in tobacco Master Settlement Agreement funds to establish multi-county-based departments.

Within 100 miles of Columbus, the area's municipal hub, one-fourth of all U.S. meat packing occurs, and area farmers raise cattle (four cows for every person) and grow corn, mostly to produce ethanol. Becky Rayman grew up there, left for 20 years that included a stint in public health around El Paso, and returned a few years before she was recruited to run the department. Ironically, she originally felt the job would be taken, due to the lack of local health funding or history, "only by an idiot."

As the new century dawned, the area was sorely in need of community health improvement. Despite generally stagnant overall population growth, the area has been experiencing a noticeable demographic shift. An influx of Latinos, many of whom labor in the packing plants, has led to a 50-percent rise in the Hispanic population in the five years following the 2000 Census in Platte County, the most populous of the area's four counties. Today, one in three residents of Colfax County, the second most populous, is Hispanic. (None of the counties is more than 0.5 percent black.) At the same time, as younger people have moved away, the population has grown older. Today, one in five residents of the two smaller counties, Boone and Nance, is elderly.

MAPP proved a perfect fit for the new department, because, Rayman says, "We were doing MAPP, and we didn't know it." Even before starting the MAPP process of recruiting partners, undertaking a four-pronged community assessment, and accomplishing an action cycle, the Nebraska group had reached out to local organizations with a stake in improving community health. The adoption of MAPP "strengthened and deepened the relationships," she says—and helped overcome turf defenses by focusing on community-wide interests.

MAPP

"The Best Thing for Our Community"

The prospect that MAPP would not consume excessive hours of pointless deliberation also helped the Nebraskans attract the top decision-makers in stakeholder organizations. In the end, the entire process took place during only nine months in 2002.

The MAPP process provided a volunteer force to carry out the work. For example, representatives of partner organizations chaired three of the four assessments, toiling tirelessly and effectively.

All in all, says Rayman, MAPP "was the best thing for our community, because it was community-driven."

As public health professionals are aware, the Ten Essential Public Health Services set a broad agenda, b ut to the people of east central Nebraska, the overriding need was for basic services. More than one in four residents is uninsured, a rate far above the national and state averages, partly because certain local employers cover workers but not their families. MAPP reinforced the emphasis on basic services. As Rayman explains, MAPP is "about the community and what it needs; it's not about the health department."

Thirty-eight agencies participated in the process. Meeting attendance fluctuated, as particularly important meetings attracted large numbers of professionals and consumers—energized in some cases by flyers distributed to every household in the area every two months during the action cycle. Rayman says that what mattered most was not the quantity of agencies involved but rather the quality of participation by key individuals, whose strengths ranged from political skills to a commitment to population-based mental health.

Still, setbacks were frequent, as each committee struggled to find the best way to contribute to the overall effort. Success, in other words, could not be plotted along a straight line.

Rayman has found interesting county-based patterns in participation. In Nance County, for instance, residents generally do not mobilize around planning but do come out in force for emergency preparedness drills. Emergency planning is indeed a serious matter in east central Nebraska. The area lies in a tornado belt, and the state pioneered the development of the 911 telephone response system.

A Governor Gets Involved

MAPP's four assessments—of community themes and strengths, the local health system, community health status, and forces of change—lead to the identification of

community-defined goals. With astonishing ambition, the Nebraska group generated eight service-related goals:

- Increasing access to culturally and linguistically appropriate primary care;
- Providing mental health services;
- Furnishing access to oral healthcare;
- Facilitating use of prescription drugs;
- Decreasing substance abuse;
- Reducing transportation barriers;
- Constructing a useful Web site; and
- Improving inter-agency communications.

Each goal has been served by a separate committee, which began its work by producing a vision of what it wanted the community to look like in five years. Rayman, who tends to refer to those responsible for the department's successes as "they" rather than "I" or "we," borrowed motivator Les Brown's motto, "Shoot for the moon. Even if you miss, you'll land among the stars."

> MAPP attracted the top decision-makers in stakeholder organizations.

The department and the primary care committee hit the moon early on, obtaining a "New Start" grant from the U.S. Health Resources and Services Administration to establish a community health center, staffed by bilingual clinicians.

Another committee took stock of a situation in which area mental health services were all but nonexistent. The committee included representation from hospitals, law enforcement agencies, boards of health, adult day centers, faith organizations, consumer groups, academic programs, and other sectors that could contribute to solutions. It drove creation of three outpatient psychiatric programs, more counseling by licensed alcohol and substance abuse counselors, and planning for the area's first inpatient psychiatric unit.

Governor Mike Johanns, later the U.S. secretary of agriculture, became sufficiently impressed with the mental health committee's efforts to meet with it to discuss reform of the state's mental health system. Eventually, the group became separately incorporated, as the Behavioral Health Consortium.

One of 150 in History

Successes in the prescription drug area have included conducting Medicare Part D educational programs at a hospital, hiring a social worker at the community health center to help residents navigate manufacturers' drug assistance programs, and backing legislation to distribute $80,000 worth of medications to low-income residents.

A remarkably user-friendly Web site also resulted from a committee effort. One particularly helpful feature of the site is demographic information that area agencies use in grant applications.

Although Rayman is modest in discussing her role in the department's achievements, others have acknowledged her accomplishments. The Columbus Chamber of Commerce selected her as its 2006 businesswoman of the year. The award recognizes both the importance of public health to business development and Rayman's personal commitment to place the local health department on a sound business footing. "When I leave," she says, "I want the department to be stronger without me than with me."

> The award recognizes the importance of public health to business development.

The town went further— in a rare accolade for a public health practitioner, Columbus named her one of the 150 most influential citizens in its 150-year history.

To Get Things Done

In the future, Rayman expects the now solidly established department to move beyond its focus on basic services to address environmental health. She also anticipates greater collaboration with schools and the business community. "Alliances," she predicts, "will grow."

Other east central Nebraskans share Becky Rayman's belief in MAPP. One participant said, "I [usually] hate meetings, but every one was useful—I felt good about them all." Another participant agreed that the MAPP meetings "led to results and accomplishments." MAPP, concluded another, "is the only way to get things done."

FOR MORE INFORMATION ON MAPP, PLEASE CONTACT:

Heidi Deutsch, MA, MSDM
Program Manager

P (202) 783-5550, Ext. 252
hdeutsch@naccho.org

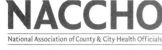
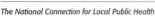

The National Connection for Local Public Health

www.naccho.org

Public Health
Prevent. Promote. Protect.

NACCHO is the national organization representing local health departments. NACCHO supports efforts that protect and improve the health of all people and all communities by promoting national policy, developing resources and programs, seeking health equity, and supporting effective local public health practice and systems.

1100 17th St, NW, 2nd Floor Washington, DC 20036
P (202) 783 5550 F (202) 783 1583

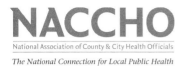

National Association of County & City Health Officials

The National Connection for Local Public Health

[STORY FROM THE FIELD]

November 2007

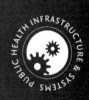

MAPP Helps 15-County Region Frame Comprehensive Public Health Policies: The East Tennessee Story

Starting with a "Homegrown Version"

The East Tennessee experience with community health planning predates MAPP, *Mobilizing for Action through Planning and Partnerships,* by several years. Influenced by the Institute of Medicine's landmark 1988 report, *The Future of Public Health*, the Tennessee Department of Health began to strengthen its public health capacity in the 1990s by focusing sharply on the assessment function. The state department promoted an assessment technique called Community Diagnosis, which the East Tennessee region instituted county-wide.

Similar to MAPP in several ways, Community Diagnosis is a community-based approach—touted as "community-owned"—for addressing where the community is now, where it wants to go, and how it can get there. The process is not as robust as MAPP, though, relying on less formal assessments and a less structured progression of stages. Paul Erwin calls Community Diagnosis a "homegrown version" of MAPP.

> Respect the Appalachian way of doing things, vigorously engage communities, and take into account local values.

Erwin is the physician who has served as East Tennessee regional director for the state department since the advent of the Community Diagnosis approach and on through the use of MAPP. He became such an extraordinary champion of MAPP that he served a term as chair of the national MAPP Workgroup, but his main focus has remained his 15-county region, one of 13 in the state.

Surrounding urban Knox County, a separate region that includes Knoxville, the rural East Tennessee region serves a population of 705,000 (according to 2005 Census figures). Only one in 40 of the region's residents is non-white. In most counties, poverty rates are high, while educational attainment tends to be relatively low, with as few as 56 percent of adults having graduated from high school. Generalizing can be hazardous, though; the region includes Oak Ridge National Laboratory, one of the nation's premier science and energy investigative facilities, where thousands of highly educated researchers work.

The Smoky Mountains' blue haze permeates the Appalachian region. Three of the 15 counties contain parts of the Great Smoky Mountains National Park, which logs more visitors than any other national park. Erwin, a native of Alabama, has found that winning East Tennesseans over to change requires respecting local values and the Appalachian way of doing things and vigorously engaging communities.

Convene, Facilitate, Provide Support, Ensure Quality

For the region as a whole, Erwin's view is that "poverty and lack of education and opportunity are at the root of all health and access-to-health problems." Chief among these problems, in his view, is obesity, followed closely by tobacco use.

Erwin introduced MAPP in 2001 as a way to evaluate the use of Community Diagnosis. In that same year, while County Health Councils throughout East Tennessee were gaining familiarity with MAPP for this initial purpose, Erwin organized a region-wide MAPP committee "to scope out how and where to proceed" over the longer term.

By 2002, the regional committee included representation from each county. The idea from the outset was that committee members, meeting quarterly, would gradually become more knowledgeable about MAPP and take this knowledge back to their counties.

Under this system of organization, the Regional Health Office convenes, facilitates, provides support, ensures quality, and acts, as Carlos Yunsan says, "with the engagement of the local leadership." Yunsan is the region's MAPP point person and also its director of health promotion. As this combination suggests, he's a bit of a force of nature in community health improvement in all 15 counties.

Opportunity for Workforce Development

The first of East Tennessee's unique MAPP aspects, an academic health partnership, is a feature of Yunsan's involvement. A Panamanian by birth, Yunsan came to the region in the 1990s as an undergraduate at the University of Tennessee, in Knoxville, and then stayed on to study public health. He recalls being "exposed to MAPP as a graduate MPH student in 2001."

> The Dialogue method fosters "thinking together."

Joining the regional office "fresh out of school," Yunsan says he became grounded in the belief that residents "know their community better than I do." MAPP, he says, became "my approach" to public health generally.

Yunsan's graduate student experience with MAPP came about because the regional committee used his "Theories and Techniques of Health Planning" class to evaluate the Community Diagnosis effort. The relationship between the class and the regional office endured. Each year the class spearheaded one of the four MAPP assessments, concentrating on a single county, until the cycle of all four types of assessment was completed in 2007. Yunsan has worked closely with the graduate students as they have zeroed in on a county and its community themes and strengths, local public health system, community health status, and forces of change—the four discrete MAPP assessments.

Paul Erwin describes the student contribution as "co-facilitating." He cites several advantages of the university partnership: the introduction of the MAPP philosophy of community engagement into the curriculum, the application of theory into practice for students' benefit, faculty involvement in community research, the expansion of staff resources to perform MAPP (which is important, because MAPP takes "deliberate, intentional inputs")—and the recruitment of new graduates, competent in community involvement, like Carlos Yunsan.

Model Regional Assessments

East Tennessee's second key MAPP characteristic, model regional assessments, came about as an exercise in efficiency. A student-assisted assessment in one county serves as a

template for the region's other counties. This is a rolling process—not, notes Erwin, a "neat and tidy" one.

Cocke County, a forested area with a population of 35,000, was the site of the initial, model assessment of community themes and strengths. Monroe County, gateway to the scenic Cherohala Skyway and home to 43,000 residents, was the site of both the initial community health status assessment and the initial forces-of-change assessment.

To the north and east, Jefferson County, a lakeshore area of 48,000 in the foothills of the Smokies—a county transitioning from an Appalachian-centered rural culture to greater prosperity and perhaps less distinctiveness as a Knoxville bedroom community—was the site of the first local public health system assessment.

The Jefferson County assessment was especially significant, because it used the National Public Health Performance Standards Program (NPHPSP) local instrument. This is considered the ideal way to conduct the MAPP local public health assessment. (Erwin and three colleagues have described the success of this Jefferson County endeavor in the *Journal of Public Health Management and Practice.*) Later, Monroe County also conducted a local public health system assessment, as a pilot site for an updated version of the NPHPSP tool, known as version 2.

Trio of Challenges

Stephanie Welch, then the regional office's strategic planning coordinator, facilitated MAPP efforts throughout the region. Welch encountered three main challenges. First, the region's 15 counties are demographically and structurally diverse. Second, many volunteers—in the Volunteer State—are stretched thin, are "doers" rather than "talkers," and felt a sort of assessment fatigue in the wake of the Community Diagnosis exercise. Third, some community leaders were reluctant to include their followers in decision-making, while some of the followers were reluctant to voice opinions on root issues.

To meet these challenges, says Welch, the MAPP process sparked greater community engagement, demonstrated the importance of identifying underlying causes of public health problems, generated renewed trust between leaders and followers, and promoted the rise of new ideas. Most of these gains were achieved during MAPP's Organizing for Success phase through the use of Dialogue, a facilitation method.

Every Voice Is Heard

An emphasis on facilitation, the third key characteristic of East Tennessee's use of MAPP, started at the outset. Invigorating the entire East Tennessee MAPP process from its earliest days has been the role of the Dialogue team, led by Leonadi Ward and Daniel Martin. After being introduced to the Centers for Disease Control and Prevention by New York state-based Cross River Connections, which Martin heads, Dialogue has become a feature of several MAPP projects across the country. Additionally, key Dialogue concepts are incorporated into MAPP's overall design.

As a facilitation method, Dialogue fosters "thinking together" in a group by clarifying each participant's assumptions and validating other participants' perspectives. It generates a shared understanding of problems in order to produce comprehensive and sustainable solutions. Leonadi Ward says Dialogue is a "deceptively simple" way to get better outcomes from difficult conversations.

Initially, Ward and Martin trained four regional office staff members, including Welch and Yunsan, as MAPP facilitators. Eventually, they trained about 60 MAPP participants in the region. Ward says the East Tennesseans are an interesting group to work with. They are "the salt of the earth" and "they care," he says, even if they do sometimes show a "reticence to adopt anything new."

Erwin credits Dialogue with making sure every voice is heard during MAPP discussions. "That's how we do things," he says. The result is a "spirit and philosophy" of active inter-personal involvement throughout the MAPP process.

MAPP, then, becomes a new way of practicing public health. Erwin, Yunsan, and their colleagues facilitate broad public-private, action-oriented conversations about community health improvement, rather than functioning as one layer in a government hierarchy.

Stephanie Welch, the region's former MAPP coordinator, says she has incorporated Dialogue techniques into her clinical work as a dietitian (and captain) serving an 18-month tour with the Army Reserves at Fort Campbell, Kentucky, where many of her clients are battle-tested members of the 101st Airborne Division. While in East Tennessee, she says, she relied on Dialogue "100 percent." She still actively promotes MAPP, having moved on to a more senior position with the health department in Knox County.

What MAPP Has Done for Tennessee

MAPP further provides a flexible framework for assessment. In a handout, the Regional Health Office urges participants and prospective participants to see MAPP as "not a project, but a tool to get your community organized to address health issues and their root causes." The simply formatted handout is capped with a visioning statement: "All stakeholders in East Tennessee will be engaged in creating conditions for improved health and quality of life."

What has MAPP done for public health in East Tennessee? "The best evidence of its effectiveness," Yunsan concludes, is "the comments from participants," including frequent expressions that MAPP made a participant feel "empowered instead of just a receiver of services." This feeling alone opens up the possibility of change, because it means the participants, in Yunsan's words, "are the most important part of solving their problems."

> he expects MAPP to improve people's real state of health.

As a concrete example, Yunsan says MAPP helped one county group become a statewide force of change in healthcare for the indigent. When 6,000 residents of the county faced the prospect of being dropped from the rolls of TennCare, the Volunteer State's controversial alternative to Medicaid, the group convened a series of meetings, leading eventually to creation of a committee that helped design new programs to serve people outside TennCare.

Such an activist response is exactly what Yunsan expects from groups experienced with MAPP, for MAPP focuses on "the roots of issues" and nurtures strategic thinking. This strategic aspect of MAPP makes it "a good fit" with the East Tennessee regional office, in his view.

A Simple Vision

Further, Yunsan sees benefits from MAPP in his other role, as director of health promotion. MAPP, he says, shapes the priorities of the regional office's health promotion staff, and he anticipates a positive long-term impact in health education and consumer behavior.

Erwin says that MAPP "revitalized" the region's County Health Councils. More people have become involved with the councils, he says, and several counties already have used MAPP data in grant applications and other materials. He considers MAPP a "unique" community planning approach, because it generates data that it then "filters" through community perspectives.

[STORY FROM THE FIELD]
November 2007

As a national leader, Erwin has traveled to several other states to conduct MAPP training, but he downplays this missionary role. "*I've* learned from *them*," he says, adding that he has been "overwhelmed and enlightened" by groups he has visited, such as leaders of Nebraska's East Central Health District, who used MAPP to construct a new local health department on a strategic foundation.

In the end, Paul Erwin has a simple vision for MAPP as a nationwide model: he expects MAPP to improve people's real state of health.

FOR MORE INFORMATION ON MAPP, PLEASE CONTACT:

Heidi Deutsch, MA, MSDM
Program Manager

P (202) 783-5550, Ext. 252
hdeutsch@naccho.org

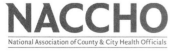

National Association of County & City Health Officials

The National Connection for Local Public Health

www.naccho.org

Public Health
Prevent. Promote. Protect.

NACCHO is the national organization representing local health departments. NACCHO supports efforts that protect and improve the health of all people and all communities by promoting national policy, developing resources and programs, seeking health equity, and supporting effective local public health practice and systems.

1100 17th St, NW, 2nd Floor Washington, DC 20036
P (202) 783 5550 F (202) 783 1583

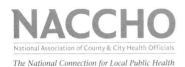

[STORY FROM THE FIELD]

November 2007

MAPP Helps County Show Public Health Success: The Cowlitz County Washington Story

Introduction

Picture yourself a public health champion in a semi-rural area reeling from a cascade of economic and natural blows. How can you respond effectively and take action to protect and improve community health? How can you demonstrate your effectiveness?

Washington State's western region is admired for its majestic conifer forests, rugged Pacific coastline, some of the nation's tallest peaks and most inspiring national parks, and a citizenry that values education, excels at technology, and takes environmental protection seriously. High unemployment, however, has rocked the Evergreen State's southwest corner, especially Cowlitz County, for more than a decade. The area has a resource-based economy, and the resources have been battered.

Cowlitz County has long prided itself as the "Gateway to Mount St. Helens," but in 1980, a 5.1-level earthquake famously tore

> The area has a resource-based economy, and the resources have been battered.

open the north face of the mountain, sparking the largest recorded landslide ever and greatest volcanic eruption in American history, with a release of energy equivalent to 27,000 Hiroshima atomic bombs. Ash was spewed everywhere, damage exceeded $one billion, and the death toll numbered 57 humans, 7,000 big-game animals, and 12 million fish.

In the 1990s, bitter controversy over the fate of the northern spotted owl contributed to a huge reduction in logging and cutbacks in the timber industry. In 2000–2001, the area was adversely affected by alleged manipulation of electric power prices by Enron Corp., and in 2001, the closing of a Reynolds aluminum plant cost the area at least 1,000 jobs.

From Heart Disease to Tobacco to WIC

Cowlitz County has a population of 97,000, over 94 percent White. Per capita income stands at $18,600, well below state and national averages. The county contains the cities of Longview, across the Columbia River from Oregon, and nearby Kelso; about half the population is rural.

For over four years, Sue Grinnell responded to the county's community health needs as the director of the Kelso-based Cowlitz County Health Department. In December 2006, Grinnell was named to head the Office of Community Wellness and Prevention in the Washington State Department of Health, in Olympia. Grinnell was a logical choice to oversee state chronic-disease activities because she led a successful effort to plan, coordinate, invigorate, and mobilize widespread local public health action based on the MAPP process.

MAPP—*Mobilizing for Action through Planning and Partnerships*—is the community health planning approach sponsored by the National Association of County and City Health Officials (NACCHO) in collaboration with the Centers for Disease Control and Prevention.

Grinnell learned about MAPP at a NACCHO pre-conference workshop and then researched the program further before committing to it. She explains the depth of her early exploration of MAPP by saying, "I'm kind of a hunter and a gatherer, constantly reading and researching."

Making Connections

In undertaking MAPP, Grinnell had two extraordinary human resource assets: her own capacity as a hard worker and self-described "very logical thinker" (she uses the term in a frank and not boastful way), and her MAPP co-leader, Paul Youmans.

Youmans heads a Cowlitz county-based community health mobilization program called "Pathways 2020," part of the county's Economic Development Council, located in Longview. The program's Web site prominently features MAPP, which it fittingly describes as "a community process to look at current public health services, missing or deficient services, community perceptions on the quality of life, and planning with action steps to address these public health issues."

MAPP

Reaching out to Youmans was exactly the sort of gathering of resources that Grinnell performed. Together, Grinnell and Youmans saw MAPP as a way to set priorities. What attracted her immediately to MAPP, says Grinnell, is that "it felt very comprehensive," rather than focusing on a single problem or aspect of a community.

Youmans, meanwhile, was drawn to MAPP's reliance on community partnerships, the vehicle that Pathways 2020 also uses in striving toward community health improvements. So, in 2001, after digesting mounds of MAPP material, Grinnell and Youmans initiated the process by "organizing for success" and securing partners.

Here is where the "logic" of the Cowlitz County approach to MAPP first becomes apparent. Key to Grinnell's approach was her insistence on using existing frameworks when possible, rather than designing new ones. Pathways 2020 already had a network of partners in place, and Grinnell saw the advantages of building on this existing network. With additional county health department support, the Pathways team morphed into the MAPP team.

The team's first project was a survey of the local public health waterfront. This survey produced a fascinating piece of information. Of the 167 agency respondents, about one-third already faced a requirement, usually as a condition of funding, to perform a community needs assessment. Presumably, other responding organizations also could benefit from assessment data. So, MAPP gained currency in the field as a route to develop a repository of MAPP data and other data that could be useful to participating organizations.

Finding Commonalities

Among the states, Washington is unusual in that it has implemented its own performance standards for local health departments. An outgrowth of the 1993 Washington Public Health Improvement Plan Act, the state program includes on-site reviews by a private contractor, which applies agency standards—not system-wide standards like those of the National Public Health Performance Standards Program (NPHPSP). The state standards address 12 functional areas, such as community health assessment, communications, prevention, and health education.

Again, to satisfy both state and MAPP requirements, Grinnell sought the most "logical" approach. She came up with a method to develop a survey tool for addressing each of the Ten Essential Public Health Services in a way that met the state standards and

> Through a unified assessment process, she could "kill two birds with one stone."

moved the MAPP process forward. The key, she learned, was to find commonalities between the two mechanisms. The advantage was that, through a unified assessment process, she could "kill two birds with one stone."

Actually, three. Grinnell also folded in the NPHPSP, which she portrays as a more comprehensive way to do MAPP. In her view, MAPP and NPHPSP together establish a "framework that follows a logical process that fits community needs."

Grinnell and her colleagues, including a department epidemiologist, using their own data template—rather than the more rigorous NPHPSP, as is generally recommended—distributed the local public health assessment survey instrument to 600 stakeholders. The survey revealed a county-wide trend toward significant workforce shortages that compromised public health.

Turning Data to Advantage

A second assessment, a quality-of-life survey, was conducted to assess community themes and strengths. It showed that county residents felt they were not sufficiently empowered to change the landscape. This finding led the MAPP team to engage in more coalition-building.

A third assessment, of community health status, revealed the need to address obesity, among other factors. Together, results of the quality-of-life survey and community health assessment pointed the way toward developing a coalition to combat obesity in the county.

Grinnell and Youmans also decided to undertake an asset-based community development exercise, modeled on the work of John McKnight at Northwestern University. This approach focuses on local strengths, rather than the needs and deficiencies that traditionally serve as the foundation for community change and organizational improvement. To lead the exercise, a disease prevention specialist in the county department first obtained training at Northwestern.

To assess forces of change, the Cowlitz MAPP team rode the shoulders of a Pathways 2020 project in scenario planning. This type of futures exercise leads participants to imagine alternative sets of problems and assets that might exist at a specified future date—such as 2020.

Results of this ambitious series of assessments and exercises pointed in the same general direction. The MAPP participants learned that Cowlitz County faces a formidable array of issues

MAPP

involving youth. They also learned they had the capacity to address daunting public health challenges.

To address obesity, which had experienced a troubling increase in the county in just two years, the team obtained a $50,000 state grant to launch their desired coalition, the Cowlitz County Healthy Lifestyle Coalition. This new entity succeeded in developing a five-year action plan called "Cowlitz on the Move," supplemented by a new Web-based physical activity information initiative funded by a $15,000 grant from the Kaiser Family Foundation.

From A to Z

"Everything comes from the data," Grinnell explains. The data served to justify hiring an epidemiologist. The data enabled additional improvements in the department's monitoring and surveillance infrastructure and the purchase of an integrated billing system. The data enhanced local grant development—in obesity and other areas—and helped the department register one of the highest scores in the state's performance standards survey (74 percent compliance, some four points below the state leader).

After all, thanks to the MAPP-related assessments and deliberations, each of the team's conclusions, problems, and initiatives was documented. MAPP became a data-rich platform for public health improvement and community action.

Besides congruence with the Washington standards and NPHPSP, several aspects of MAPP hold special appeal to Grinnell. With MAPP, she learned, "there's no right or wrong way," so participants can adapt the program to their own situations. She especially appreciated the support from NACCHO and the ability to address issues one at a time. "It's a phase-in process," Grinnell observes. "You don't get from A to Z overnight."

> "MAPP is a great process. You need the data, and it collects it. You build relationships. It's all a system."

Grinnell recalls that MAPP encountered virtually no resistance in Cowlitz County and that she herself "loved" working with it. She says that MAPP can be helpful to all local health departments, regardless of size or configuration, because "the cool thing about it is you can make it as big or little as you want—and there's no time frame, so it's very flexible." At the height of the MAPP project, the Cowlitz department had about 27 staff members and a budget of $2.5 million.

In Touch with the Real World

"Good public health," Sue Grinnell says, "is doing assessments, policy development, and assurance, and part of the assessment is about capacity-building." In facilitating these functions, MAPP, she adds, "is a great process. You need the data, and it collects it. You build relationships. It's all a system."

Although clearly excited about the prospects for improving chronic disease services on the state level, she regrets one aspect of her switch from Kelso to Olympia. "What I'm worried about working at the state level," she admits, "is forgetting the local level." She wants "to stay in touch with the real world"— by which she means communities— partly because "folks there are very committed" and she developed a wealth of close relationships in Cowlitz County.

Grinnell says the Cowlitz experience with MAPP began in 2001, but she does not put an end date on it. "It shouldn't ever end," she says.

FOR MORE INFORMATION ON MAPP, PLEASE CONTACT:

Heidi Deutsch, MA, MSDM
Program Manager

P (202) 783-5550, Ext. 252
hdeutsch@naccho.org

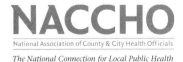

National Association of County & City Health Officials

The National Connection for Local Public Health

www.naccho.org

Public Health
Prevent. Promote. Protect.

NACCHO is the national organization representing local health departments. NACCHO supports efforts that protect and improve the health of all people and all communities by promoting national policy, developing resources and programs, seeking health equity, and supporting effective local public health practice and systems.

1100 17th St, NW, 2nd Floor Washington, DC 20036
P (202) 783 5550 F (202) 783 1583

Glossary

Americans with Disabilities Act: a civil rights law that prohibits discrimination based on a disability; defines a disability as a physical or mental impairment that substantially limits one or more major life activities

Analytical epidemiology: a type of epidemiological study aimed at testing a hypothesis

Assessment: involves data collection, synthesis, and analysis and can focus on different types of data such as health status, community priorities, local resources, and institutional capacity

BASICC approach: the approach developed by the CDC in 1995 for the evaluation of costs and consequences of preventive health programs

Behavioral theory: offers an explanation of the relationships among causal processes

Brand: a marketing device that links products with a set of ideas and values in the mind of the target consumer

Business partnerships: businesses who work collaboratively with other organizations to achieve a shared goal to protect and promote the safety and health of the public

Case management: an individualized approach to identifying needs and goals of the program participant, obtaining needed services, coordinating care, and monitoring improvement; tailors treatment and services to the needs of the individual participant, establishing linkages with appropriate agencies and service providers to address the participant's unique needs and goals

Chain of infection: a model used to explain the transmission of a communicable disease from an infected person to a new host

Charisma: a rare trait found in certain human personalities that usually includes extreme charm and a magnetic quality of personality

Chronic diseases: diseases of long duration and generally long incubation periods

Clinical preventive services: clinical services designed to prevent illness and disease and to improve the quality of life

Community conditions: the physical, economic, social, and cultural conditions of a community, all of which impact health outcomes and health equity

Community health: the state of wellness or well-being in a defined community; affected by forces in addition to health care services, including adequate housing, quality of schools, safe streets, economic stability, and the environment; a community health approach builds on strengths and assets within communities and advances community elements that have an impact on health, mental health, and safety

Community health problems: health problems found in a community usually discovered through a community health assessment

Countermarketing: a mass-media communication strategy that has been used by public health organizations in recent years to counter tobacco industry advertising and promotion and other protobacco media influences such as smoking imagery in movies

Continuous quality improvement: a management approach or process whereby processes are constantly evaluated and improved based on efficiency, effectiveness, and flexibility

Cost-benefit analysis: a method developed for the evaluation of public policy issues; it looks at the costs and benefits of programs and recommends continuation of programs only if there is a net positive impact from the program

Culture: collective mindset of a group that distinguishes itself from other groups

Developmental disability: disabilities that occur in the developmental period defined as birth to age 18 years

Deming cycle: an iterative four step (Plan, Do, Study, Act) problem-solving process typically used in quality control

Descriptive epidemiology: the part of epidemiology that involves describing health events in terms of time, place, and person

Determinants of health: include the social and economic environment, the physical environment, and the person's individual characteristics and behaviors

Dialogue: the development of shared understanding by simply holding differences together in a way that is open, empathetic, and equal; a methodology that (1) encourages the broadest possible participation by the various parties; (2) validates the legitimacy and equality of divergent perspectives; and (3) allows new ideas, solutions, and even wisdom to emerge that may well have been previously unseen or never before articulated

Disparity: difference or inequality; health disparities refers to specific populations and communities experiencing unequal (higher) rates of the same diseases affecting the country as a whole; disparities in health systematically put groups of people who are often already socially disadvantaged (by being poor, female, and/or members of a disenfranchised racial, ethnic, or religious group) at further disadvantage with respect to their health

Disabilities: restrictions or lack of ability to performance activity in a manner and range considered usual for a human being

Education partnerships: schools who work collaboratively with public health agencies to achieve a shared goal to protect and promote the safety and health of the public

Enablers: a characteristic that facilitates action required to attain a behavior

Environment–environmental approach: far more than air, water, and soil, the environment is anything external to individuals shared by members of the community, including community

Epidemiology: concerned with the distribution and determinants of health, disease, and injuries in the human population

Equity: equity in health is the absence of systematic disparities in health (or in the major social determinants of health) between groups with different levels of underlying social advantages–disadvantages, that is, wealth, power, or prestige; equity is an ethical principle; it also is consonant with and closely related to human rights principles

Evaluation design: the use of an evaluation strategy that has the best chance of being useful and accurate for the evaluators

Evaluation process: the method used to prove success or failure of a particular program

Evidence-based decisions: health care decisions based on the cost of the decision compared with the results of the decision

Evidence-based health promotion: allows funders to make reliable decisions on which health promotion efforts should be continued or expanded

Evidence-based intervention strategies: intervention strategies that have a history of achieving desired results at minimum cost

Faith-based organization partnerships: faith-based organizations who work collaboratively with other agencies to achieve a shared goal to protect and promote the safety and health of the public behavioral norms; according to the *American Heritage Dictionary*, it is the totality of circumstances surrounding an organism or group of organisms

Firearm-related injury: refers to all gunshot wounds regardless of whether intentional or accidental, self-inflicted or inflicted by another, or circumstance of the injury

Focus groups: personal interviews with a group of 8 to 10 participants that attempt to gain important data about the topic under consideration

Geodemographic segmentation: a common type of target segmentation, this is a multivariate statistical classification technique for discovering whether the individual or a population falls into different groups by making quantitative comparisons of multiple characteristics with the assumption that differences within any group should be less than differences between groups

Gross domestic product: the total amount of goods and services produced by a given country in a year

Healthy lifestyle: the practice of healthy behaviors and the avoidance of high-risk health behaviors

Health risk appraisal: a tool used by employees to increase employee's awareness of high-risk health behaviors that may predispose workers to the development of chronic diseases

Healthy People 2010: a third set of health goals and objectives for the United States that defines the nation's health agenda and acts as a guide to health policy

Health promotion: a planned combination of educational, political, and environmental activity designed to improve the health of the population

High-risk health behaviors: patterns, like tobacco use, associated with high-risk of developing disease

Incentives: mechanism used to increase employees willingness to participate in wellness initiatives

Influence: the power of winning devotion and acceptance by others for one's agenda

Injury surveillance: the collection of data on incidence, prevalence, and circumstance of injuries; the ability to track the incidence and characteristics of violence can serve as the basis to develop violence prevention strategies to reduce the impact and repercussions of violence on youth, families, and communities

Leadership: the art and science of influencing others to achieve a predetermined goal

Levels of prevention: generally organized in three levels: primary prevention in which activities are developed to control for risk factors in high-risk populations with the goal of stopping the occurrence of a disease before it starts; secondary prevention in which activities are targeted to already diagnosed populations with the goal of preventing progression or serious complications; tertiary prevention in which activities are directed to diagnosed members of the population in order the reduce the extent of disability or other negative complications of disease

Local public health system: all the public, private, and voluntary entities that work to ensure the public's health

Management information system (MIS): refers to a computer-based system that allows for client-level data input, organization, and storage as well as the generation of data reports

Marketing mix: the mix of controllable variables that are used in the business to pursue a desired level of profits; these variables are product, price, place, and promotion

Marketing research: the gathering of primary and secondary data to better define a problem

Mobilizing for Action through Planning and Partnerships (MAPP): a strategic approach to community health improvement; this process helps communities improve health and quality of life through community-wide strategic planning; using MAPP, communities seek to achieve optimal health by identifying and using their resources wisely, taking into account their unique circumstances and needs, and forming effective partnerships for strategic action

Morbidity Mortality Weekly Report: a weekly publication produced by the Centers for Disease Control and Prevention that includes reports of epidemiological investigation, surveillance activities, and morbidity and mortality data

Multisystem intervention: includes the participation and collaboration of a network of community and social service systems, such as schools, training programs, hospitals, behavioral health programs, and other specialized services in the intervention design and implementation

National Association of County and City Health Officials (NACCHO): the national organization representing local health departments; it supports efforts that protect and improve the health of all people and all communities by promoting national policy, developing resources and programs, seeking health equity, and supporting effective local public health practice and systems

Need: a condition in which there is a deficiency of something

Needs assessment: a method of identifying, analyzing, and prioritizing the needs of a population

Norms: behavior in a community or population that is socially accepted as normal; regularities in behavior with which people generally conform; often based in culture and tradition, they are attitudes, beliefs, and standards that are taken for granted; behavior shapers

Observation: a method of watching subjects and evaluating characteristics or patterns of behavior

Partnerships: comprehensive and widespread cross-sector collaboration to ensure sustainable development initiatives

Partners: individuals, organizations, or groups who work collaboratively to achieve a shared goal to protect and promote the safety and health of the public

Partnership evaluation: evaluation of the effectiveness of various partnerships that were designed to protect and promote the safety and health of the public

PATCH: the public health planning process called Planned Approach to Community Health

Positive locus of control: a positive coping behavior allowing a person to practice self-care when confronted with a chronic disease such as type 2 diabetes

Prescription for the American People: this prescription, offered by former Surgeon General Satcher, included all of the components required to remain healthy

Preventive medicine: measures taken to prevent illness or injury rather than to cure them

Primary prevention: a systematic process that promotes safe and healthy environments and behaviors, reducing the likelihood or frequency of an incident, injury, or condition occurring

PRIZM: developed by Claritas to provide a standard way of sorting the U.S. population in smaller groups based on demographics, lifestyle preferences, and consumer behavior

Probes: method used by the interviewer to gain additional information from focus group participants

Problem assessment: the first step in solving a problem; the perception of a difference between the desired state and the actual state

Process objectives: objectives that express the activities to be carried out by the planners of a program

Productivity: entails maximum output produced by minimum input

Program evaluation: determining the value or worth of a specific program

Program goals: the specific intent of a given action

Rate: the number of events that occur in a given period of time

Resilience: often refers to the ability of a person or community to positively adapt and develop in the face of new or different experiences and environments; fostering resiliency in people has been shown to improve academic, emotional, social, and cognitive outcomes; building community resilience factors or assets can counteract the negative effects of risk factors; research shows that, like risk, resiliency factors can accumulate such that those with more assets are less likely to engage in high-risk behaviors

Root factors: underlying issues and dynamics in society that contribute to inequality and ultimately lead to disparities in health, as well as other detrimental outcomes; examples include racism, discrimination, poverty, and other forms of oppression

Sensation seeking: a measurable personality trait that has been linked with high-risk behavior, including smoking, among youth

Stakeholders: individuals who have an interest in a health program

Social insurance: a program where risks are transferred to the insurance plan despite high-risk health behaviors

Social marketing: the application of marketing along with other concepts to achieve specific goals for a social good

Strategic planning: process for making decisions and taking action based on a defined vision and assessment data; in the MAPP process, strategic planning involves all community and local public health system partners and works to make sustainable, long-term systemic improvements in public health

SWOT: a situational assessment that deals with the strengths and weaknesses of the organization as well as the opportunities and threats relevant to the future of the business

Systems model: the use of the concept of input, throughput, and output to analyze and improve the operation of a particular system

Target segmentation: involves breaking a market into segments and then concentrating efforts on one or a few key segments

Theoretical constructs: the development of a concept for use with a particular theory

Tobacco industry: the major tobacco companies, collectively

Traits: distinctive characteristics that may account for the effectiveness of a leader. Examples would include: appearance, aggressiveness, self reliance or physical characteristics

Transformational leadership: this leadership style has the ability to move followers beyond their own self-interest

truth® Campaign: a branded antitobacco campaign designed to prevent youth smoking

Type 2 diabetes: over 90% of those with diabetes have type 2 diabetes, which is caused by lifestyle behaviors

Violence interventions: aim to help participants to recognize the conditions that may have contributed to their exposure to and increased risk of violence and to develop individual plans to help prevent further violence

Want: a wish or desire for something

Work site wellness: health programs offered at the work site that attempts to improve the health of employees while reducing the costs of health care

Years of potential life lost: the number of years lost when death occurs before the age of 65 or 75 years

Youth smoking: smoking among individuals under age 18 years

Index

Italicized page locators indicate a figure; tables are noted with a *t.*